W9-BGL-058

The Washington Manual™ Rheumatology Subspecialty Consult

The Washington Manual™ Rheumatology Subspecialty Consult

Faculty Advisor
Richard Brasington, M.D.
Associate Professor of Medicine
Director of Clinical Rheumatology
Department of Internal Medicine
Washington University School of
Medicine
St. Louis, Missouri

The Washington Manual™ Rheumatology Subspecialty Consult

Editors

Kevin M. Latinis, M.D., Ph.D.
Rheumatology Fellow
Department of Internal Medicine
Washington University School of Medicine
St. Louis, Missouri

Kathryn H. Dao, M.D.
Rheumatology Fellow
Department of Internal Medicine
The University of Texas Southwestern Medical Center at Dallas
Dallas, Texas

Ernesto Gutierrez, M.D.
Rheumatology Fellow
Department of Internal Medicine
Washington University School of Medicine
Barnes-Jewish Hospital
St. Louis, Missouri

Rebecca M. Shepherd, M.D.
Rheumatology Fellow
Department of Internal Medicine
Washington University School of Medicine
St. Louis, Missouri

Celso R. Velázquez, M.D.
Rheumatology Fellow
Department of Internal Medicine
Washington University School of Medicine
St. Louis, Missouri

Series Editor

Tammy L. Lin, M.D.
Series Editor
Adjunct Assistant Professor of Medicine
Washington University School of Medicine
St. Louis, Missouri

Series Advisor

Daniel M. Goodenberger, M.D.
Professor of Medicine
Chief, Division of Medical Education
Washington University School of Medicine
Director, Internal Medicine Residency Program
Barnes-Jewish Hospital
St. Louis, Missouri

LIPPINCOTT WILLIAMS & WILKINS
A **Wolters Kluwer** Company
Philadelphia · Baltimore · New York · London
Buenos Aires · Hong Kong · Sydney · Tokyo

Acquisitions Editors: Danette Somers and James Ryan
Developmental Editors: Scott Marinaro and Keith Donnellan
Supervising Editor: Steven P. Martin
Production Editor: Amanda Waltman Yanovitch, Silverchair Science + Communications
Manufacturing Manager: Colin Warnock
Cover Designer: QT Design
Compositor: Silverchair Science + Communications
Printer: RR Donnelley

© **2004 by Department of Medicine, Washington University School of Medicine**

All rights reserved. This book is protected by copyright. No part of this book may be reproduced in any form or by any means, including photocopying, or utilized by any information storage and retrieval system without written permission from the copyright owner, except for brief quotations embodied in critical articles and reviews. Materials appearing in this book prepared by individuals as part of their official duties as U.S. government employees are not covered by the above-mentioned copyright.

Printed in the USA

Library of Congress Cataloging-in-Publication Data

The Washington manual rheumatology subspecialty consult / editors, Kevin Latinis ... [et al.].
    p. ; cm. -- (Washington manual subspecialty consult series)
  Includes bibliographical references and index.
  ISBN 0-7817-4371-0
  1. Rheumatology--Handbooks, manuals, etc. 2. Rheumatism--Handbooks, manuals, etc. 3. Arthritis--Handbooks, manuals, etc. I. Latinis, Kevin. II. Series.
  [DNLM: 1. Rheumatic Diseases--diagnosis--Handbooks. 2. Rheumatic Diseases--therapy--Handbooks. WE 39 W319 2003]
  RC927.W375 2003
  616.7'23--dc21
                                                2003047699

The Washington Manual™ is an intent-to-use mark belonging to Washington University in St. Louis to which international legal protection applies. The mark is used in this publication by LWW under license from Washington University.

Care has been taken to confirm the accuracy of the information presented and to describe generally accepted practices. However, the authors, editors, and publisher are not responsible for errors or omissions or for any consequences from application of the information in this book and make no warranty, expressed or implied, with respect to the currency, completeness, or accuracy of the contents of the publication. Application of this information in a particular situation remains the professional responsibility of the practitioner.

The authors, editors, and publisher have exerted every effort to ensure that drug selection and dosage set forth in this text are in accordance with current recommendations and practice at the time of publication. However, in view of ongoing research, changes in government regulations, and the constant flow of information relating to drug therapy and drug reactions, the reader is urged to check the package insert for each drug for any change in indications and dosage and for added warnings and precautions. This is particularly important when the recommended agent is a new or infrequently employed drug.

Some drugs and medical devices presented in this publication have Food and Drug Administration (FDA) clearance for limited use in restricted research settings. It is the responsibility of health care providers to ascertain the FDA status of each drug or device planned for use in their clinical practice.

10 9 8 7 6 5 4 3 2

Contents

Contributing Authors

Milan J. Anadkat, M.D.
Dermatology Clinical Trials Research Fellow
Department of Dermatology
Washington University Medical Center
St. Louis, Missouri

Erin M. Christensen, Pharm.D., B.C.P.S.
Clinical Pharmacist
Department of Pharmacy
Barnes-Jewish Hospital
St. Louis, Missouri

Kathryn H. Dao, M.D.
Rheumatology Fellow
Department of Internal Medicine
The University of Texas Southwestern Medical Center at Dallas
Dallas, Texas

Ron J. Gerstle, M.D.
Resident
Department of Radiology
Washington University School of Medicine
St. Louis, Missouri

Ernesto Gutierrez, M.D.
Rheumatology Fellow
Department of Internal Medicine
Washington University School of Medicine
Barnes-Jewish Hospital
St. Louis, Missouri

Kevin M. Latinis, M.D., Ph.D.
Rheumatology Fellow
Department of Internal Medicine
Washington University School of Medicine
St. Louis, Missouri

Chakrapol Lattanand, M.D.
Anesthesiology Resident
Department of Anesthesiology
Barnes-Jewish Hospital
St. Louis, Missouri

Shannon C. Lynn, M.D.

Resident
Department of Internal Medicine
Washington University School of
Medicine
Barnes-Jewish Hospital
St. Louis, Missouri

Ami N. Mody, M.D.

Rheumatology Fellow
Department of Internal Medicine
Washington University School of
Medicine
St. Louis, Missouri

Giancarlo A. Pillot, M.D.

Resident
Department of Internal Medicine
Washington University School of
Medicine
St. Louis, Missouri

Rebecca M. Shepherd, M.D.

Rheumatology Fellow
Department of Internal Medicine
Washington University School of
Medicine
St. Louis, Missouri

Latha Sivaprasad, M.D.

Instructor of Medicine
Division of Cardiology
Washington University School of
Medicine
Barnes-Jewish Hospital
St. Louis, Missouri

Lawrence D. Tang, M.D.

Radiology Resident
Department of Radiology
Washington University School of
Medicine
Barnes-Jewish Hospital
St. Louis, Missouri

Ulker Tok, M.D.

Department of Rheumatology
Arizona Family Care Associates, Inc.
Sierra Vista, Arizona

Celso R. Velázquez, M.D.

Rheumatology Fellow
Department of Internal Medicine
Washington University School of
Medicine
St. Louis, Missouri

Jason D. Wright, M.D.

Gynecologic Oncology Fellow
Department of Obstetrics and
Gynecology
Washington University School of
Medicine
Barnes-Jewish Hospital
St. Louis, Missouri

Chairman's Note

Medical knowledge is increasing at an exponential rate, and physicians are being bombarded with new facts at a pace that many find overwhelming. The Washington Manual™ Subspecialty Consult Series was developed in this context for interns, residents, medical students, and other practitioners in need of readily accessible practical clinical information. They therefore meet an important unmet need in an era of information overload.

I would like to acknowledge the authors who have contributed to these books. In particular, Tammy L. Lin, M.D., Series Editor, provided energetic and inspired leadership, and Daniel M. Goodenberger, M.D., Series Advisor, Chief of the Division of Medical Education in the Department of Medicine at Washington University, is a continual source of sage advice. The efforts and outstanding skill of the lead authors are evident in the quality of the final product. I am confident that this series will meet its desired goal of providing practical knowledge that can be directly applied to improving patient care.

Kenneth S. Polonsky, M.D.
Adolphus Busch Professor
Chairman, Department of Medicine
Washington University
School of Medicine
St. Louis, Missouri

Series Preface

The Washington Manual™ Subspecialty Consult Series is designed to provide quick access to the essential information needed to evaluate a patient on a subspecialty consult service. Each manual includes the most updated and useful information on commonly encountered symptoms or diseases and highlights the practical information you need to gather before formulating a plan. Special efforts have been made to organize the information so that these guides will be valuable and trusted companions for medical students, residents, and fellows. They cover everything from questions to ask during the initial consult to issues in subsequent management.

One of the strengths of this series is that it is written by residents and fellows who know how busy a consult service can be, who know what information will be most helpful, and can detail a practical approach to patient care. Each volume is written to provide enough information for you to evaluate a patient until more in-depth reading can be done on a particular topic. Throughout the series, key references are noted, difficult management situations are addressed, and appropriate practice guidelines are included. Another strength of this series is that it was written in concert. All of the guides were designed to work together.

The most important strength of this series is the collection of authors, faculty advisors, and especially lead authors assembled to write this series. In addition, we received incredible commitment and support from our chairman, Kenneth S. Polonsky, M.D. As a result, the extraordinary depth of talent and genuine interest in teaching others at Washington University is showcased in this series. Although there has always been house staff involvement in editing The Washington Manual™ series, it came to our attention that many of them also wanted to be involved in writing and making decisions about what to convey to fellow colleagues. Remarkably, many of the lead authors became junior subspecialty fellows while writing their guides. Their desire to pass on what they were learning, while trying to balance multiple responsibilities, is a testament to their dedication and skills as clinicians, teachers, and leaders.

We hope this series fulfills the need for essential and practical knowledge for those learning the art of consultation in a particular subspecialty and for those just passing through it.

Tammy L. Lin, MD, Series Editor
Daniel M. Goodenberger, MD, Series Advisor

Preface

We have written this manual as a guide to inpatient and outpatient rheumatology consultations. The target audience includes medical students, residents, and other medical professionals who are caring for patients with rheumatologic problems. We believe that this manual could also serve as a pocket reference for medical professionals specializing in rheumatology. Of note, this manual is not intended to serve as a compendious overview of rheumatology. Rather, it focuses on how to approach rheumatologic problems, how to perform a musculoskeletal exam and arthrocentesis, which medications are appropriate (including dosages and recommended monitoring), and a brief overview of the major rheumatologic diseases.

The editors would like to thank the contributing authors for their participation in this project. A special thanks goes to Dr. Richard Brasington for playing an active role in content oversight and editing.

K.M.L.

Key to Abbreviations

APA	antiphospholipid antibody
ARF	acute rheumatic fever
AS	ankylosing spondylitis
AVN	avascular necrosis
BCP	basic calcium phosphate
beta$_2$GPI	beta$_2$-glycoprotein I
CAD	coronary artery disease
c-ANCA	cytoplasmic ANCA
CK	creatine phosphokinase
CMC	carpometacarpal
COX-2	cyclooxygenase-2
CSS	Churg-Strauss syndrome
CTD	connective tissue disease
CTS	carpal tunnel syndrome
CV	cryoglobulinemic vasculitis
CYC	cyclophosphamide
DIL	drug-induced lupus
DIP	distal interphalangeal
DM	dermatomyositis
DMARDs	disease-modifying antirheumatic drugs
EMG	electromyography
ENAs	extractable nuclear antigens
FMS	fibromyalgia syndrome
FSGN	focal and segmental glomerulonephritis
GC	gonococcal
GCA	giant cell arteritis
GU	genitourinary
HIV	human immunodeficiency virus
HSP	Henoch-Schönlein purpura
IBD	inflammatory bowel disease
IBM	inclusion-body myositis
Ig	immunoglobulin
IHS	idiopathic hypereosinophilic syndrome
IL	interleukin
LAC	lupus anticoagulant
LCV	leukocytoclastic vasculitis
MCP	metacarpophalangeal
MCTD	mixed connective tissue disease
MPA	microscopic polyangiitis
MPO	myeloperoxidase
MSA	myositis-specific antibodies
MTP	metatarsophalangeal
OA	osteoarthritis
PAN	polyarteritis nodosa
p-ANCA	perinuclear ANCA

PIP	proximal interphalangeal
PM	polymyositis
PMR	polymyalgia rheumatica
PR3	proteinase 3
PsA	psoriatic arthritis
RA	rheumatoid arthritis
ReA	reactive arthritis
RF	rheumatoid factor
RS3PE	relapsing seronegative symmetrical synovitis with pitting edema
SI	sacroiliac
Sm	Smith antigen
SS	Sjögren's syndrome
TA	Takayasu's arteritis
TAO	thromboangiitis obliterans
TNF	tumor necrosis factor
UCTD	undifferentiated connective tissue disease
WG	Wegener's granulomatosis

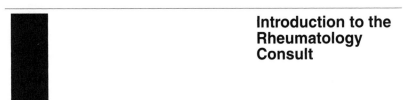

Introduction to the Rheumatology Consult

Approach to the Rheumatology Patient

Celso R. Velázquez

INTRODUCTION

Background

Rheumatologic diseases affect multiple systems and are therefore challenging to diagnose, complicated to treat, and often humbling to study. Rheumatic diseases mainly involve the musculoskeletal system and are often accompanied by systemic features (fever and weight loss) and other organ involvement (kidney, skin, lung, eye, blood). Musculoskeletal complaints account for a majority of outpatient visits in the community. Many of these patients have self-limited or localized problems that improve with symptomatic treatment. Other conditions (septic arthritis, crystal-induced arthritis, fractures) require urgent diagnosis and treatment.

Musculoskeletal problems may also be the initial presentation of diseases such as cancer and endocrinopathies. Inpatient consultations usually involve patients with known diagnoses (a patient with lupus admitted with a flare) or with multiple organ system involvement and the suspicion of a systemic rheumatic disease (a patient with respiratory and kidney failure with positive ANCA).

A comprehensive history and physical exam are often enough to make a diagnosis. A sometimes bewildering array of serologic tests is available to help support the diagnosis of many rheumatic diseases but should be used judiciously to avoid false-positive results and unnecessary testing.

The following is an approach to patients with musculoskeletal complaints and to common inpatient consults. Regional problems (i.e., nonsystemic musculoskeletal disorders) are discussed in Chap. 8, Regional Pain Syndromes.

Classification

Inflammatory vs Noninflammatory

See Table 1-1.

Inflammatory disorders are characterized by systemic symptoms (fever, stiffness, weight loss, fatigue), signs of joint inflammation on physical exam (erythema, warmth, swelling, pain), and lab evidence of inflammation (elevated ESR, elevated CRP, decreased albumin, increased platelets). **Joint stiffness** is common after prolonged rest (morning stiffness) and improves with activity. Duration of >1 hr suggests an inflammatory condition. Noninflammatory conditions may cause stiffness usually lasting <1 hr and the joint symptoms increase with use and weight bearing.

These distinctions are useful but not absolute. Inflammatory disorders may be immune-mediated [SLE, rheumatoid arthritis (RA)], reactive [reactive arthritis (ReA)], infectious [gonococcal (GC) arthritis], or crystal-induced (gout).

Noninflammatory disorders are characterized by the absence of systemic symptoms, pain without erythema or warmth, and normal lab tests. Osteoarthritis (OA), fibromyalgia, and traumatic conditions are common noninflammatory disorders.

Articular vs Nonarticular

Pain may originate from articular structures (synovial membrane, cartilage, intraarticular ligaments, capsule, or juxtaarticular bone surfaces) or periarticular structures

TABLE 1-1. NONINFLAMMATORY VS INFLAMMATORY DISORDERS

	Noninflammatory disorders (e.g., OA)	Inflammatory disorders (e.g., RA, lupus)
Symptoms		
Morning stiffness	Focal, brief	Significant, prolonged, >1 hr
Constitutional symptoms	Absent	Present
Peak period of discomfort	After prolonged use	After prolonged inactivity
Locking or instability	Implies loose body, internal derangement, or weakness	Uncommon
Symmetry (bilateral)	Occasional	Common
Signs		
Tenderness	Unusual	Over entire exposed joint area
Inflammation (fluid, tenderness, warmth, erythema, synovitis)	Unusual	Common
Multisystem disease	No	Often
Lab abnormalities	No	Often

Adapted from American College of Rheumatology ad hoc Committee on Clinical Guidelines. Guidelines for the initial evaluation of the adult patient with acute musculoskeletal symptoms. *Arthritis Rheum* 1996;39:1.

(bursae, tendons, muscle, bone, nerve, skin). **Articular disorders** cause deep or diffuse pain that worsens with active and passive movement. Physical exam shows deformity, warmth, swelling, effusion, or crepitus. Synovitis (inflammation of the synovial membrane that covers the joint) is a boggy, tender swelling around the joints and is easy to detect in finger and wrist joints.

Nonarticular disorders usually have point tenderness and increased pain with active, but not passive, movement. Physical exam does not usually show deformity or swelling. **Arthralgia** refers to joint pain, and **arthritis** implies the presence of signs of inflammation in the joint (warmth, swelling, erythema, tenderness).

CAUSES

Differential Diagnosis

Number and Pattern of Joints Involved
The number and pattern of joints involved are important in the diagnosis. **Acute monoarthritis** suggests infection but gout and trauma are possible. **Asymmetric, oligoarticular** (<5 joints) involvement, particularly of the lower extremities, is typical of OA and ReA. **Symmetric, polyarticular** (≥ 5 joints) involvement is typical of RA and SLE. Involvement of the spine, sacroiliac (SI) joints, and sternoclavicular joints is characteristic of ankylosing spondylitis (AS). In the hands, distal interphalangeal (DIP) joints are involved in OA (Heberden's nodes) and in psoriatic arthritis (PsA) but are spared by RA. Proximal interphalangeal (PIP) involvement is seen in OA (Bouchard's nodes) and RA. Metacarpophalangeal (MCP) joints are involved in RA but not in OA. Acute first metatarsophalangeal (MTP) joint arthritis is classic for gout (podagra) but is also seen in OA and ReA. Vasculitis and SLE may present with multiple organ system involvement without major joint complaints. Fibromyalgia presents with diffuse pain but without arthritis. Myositis presents with muscle weakness and rashes and occasionally peripheral arthritis.

The **review of systems** may identify other organ involvement and support the diagnosis. **Rashes** are seen in SLE, vasculitis, PsA, dermatomyositis (DM), adult-onset Still's disease, and Lyme disease. **Eye involvement** may be severe and occurs in Sjögren's syndrome (SS), RA, seronegative spondyloarthropathies, temporal arteritis, Behçet's disease, and Wegener's granulomatosis (WG). **Oral mucosal ulcers** are common in SLE, enteropathic arthritis, and Behçet's disease. **Raynaud's phenomenon** is a reversible, paroxysmal constriction of small arteries that occurs most commonly in fingers and toes and is precipitated by cold. The classic sequence is initial blanching followed by cyanosis and finally erythema due to vasodilation and is accompanied by numbness or tingling. It may be idiopathic or associated with scleroderma, SLE, RA, and mixed connective tissue disease (MCTD). **Pleuritis and pericarditis** may be seen in RA, SLE, MCTD, and adult-onset Still's disease. The **nervous system** may be involved in SLE, vasculitis, and Lyme disease. **GI involvement** is seen in enteropathic arthritis, polymyositis (PM), and scleroderma.

Certain diseases are more frequent in **specific age groups and genders.** SLE, juvenile RA, and gonococcal arthritis are more common in the young. Gout, OA, and RA are more common in middle-aged persons. Polymyalgia rheumatica (PMR) and temporal arteritis occur in the elderly. Gout and AS are more common in men. SLE, RA, and OA are more common in women. Gout is very rare in premenopausal women. Certain areas of the United States and Europe have an increased incidence of **Lyme disease.** A **family history** may be important in AS, gout, and OA. Rheumatology patients are often on medications with multiple side effects and immunosuppressive drugs that predispose to infections. Some medications may cause a lupuslike syndrome (e.g., hydralazine, procainamide), myopathies (e.g., statins, colchicine, zidovudine) or predispose to osteoporosis (e.g., corticosteroids, phenytoin). **Alcohol** commonly precipitates gout and may cause myopathies and avascular necrosis (AVN). Vasculitis, arthralgias, and rhabdomyolysis may be seen with substance abuse (e.g., cocaine, heroin).

PRESENTATION

Evaluation

The evaluation of musculoskeletal complaints should determine whether the disorder is inflammatory or noninflammatory, whether the joints or the periarticular structures are involved, and the number and pattern of joints involved. History, physical exam, and lab tests should identify other organ involvement.

Approach to Monoarthritis

Acute pain or swelling of a single joint requires immediate evaluation for septic arthritis that can rapidly destroy the joint if untreated (Fig. 1-1). It is also important to distinguish pain arising from periarticular structures (tendons, bursa), which usually requires only symptomatic treatment, and cases of referred pain (shoulder pain due to peritonitis or heart disease). Common causes of monoarthritis are infection, crystal-induced arthritis, and trauma (Table 1-2). The history should exclude trauma and can provide clues such as a history of tick bites (Lyme disease), sexual risk factors (GC arthritis), or colitis, uveitis, and urethritis (ReA). Physical exam usually distinguishes between articular and nonarticular disorders. Perform arthrocentesis in patients with acute monoarthritis (see Chap. 4, Synovial Fluid Analysis). Send synovial fluid for leukocyte count with differential, Gram's stain, culture, and crystal analysis. Leukocyte counts of >2000/mm suggest an inflammatory process. A wet mount of the fluid examined under polarizing microscopy may identify crystals, but the presence of crystals does not exclude infection. Culture other potential sources of infection (throat, cervix, rectum, wounds, blood). Synovial biopsy and arthroscopy are sometimes used to diagnose chronic monoarthritis. Radiographs are useful in cases of trauma and may show OA or chondrocalcinosis in calcium pyrophosphate deposition disease. Treatment (analgesics, colchicine, antibiotics) depends on etiology. **A patient with synovial fluid that is highly inflammatory requires empiric antibiotic therapy until the evaluation, including cultures, is completed.**

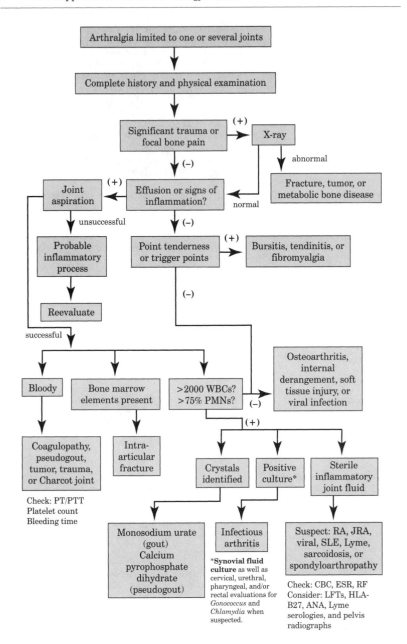

FIG. 1-1. Approach to monoarthritis. JRA, juvenile rheumatoid arthritis; PMNs, polymorphonuclear cells. (Adapted from American College of Rheumatology ad hoc Committee on Clinical Guidelines. Guidelines for the initial evaluation of the adult patient with acute musculoskeletal symptoms. *Arthritis Rheum* 1996;39:1.)

TABLE 1-2. FEATURES AND CAUSES OF MONOARTHRITIS

Type	Features	Causes
Infectious arthritis	Common; acute; may or may not have fever or leukocytosis; synovial fluid culture usually confirmatory in nongonococcal arthritis	Bacteria (gonococci and *Staphylococcus aureus*) most common. Also viruses (HIV, hepatitis B), fungi, mycobacteria, Lyme disease
Crystal-induced arthritis	Common; very acute onset; extremely painful; crystals on microscopic exam of synovial fluid	Monosodium urate crystals (gout), calcium pyrophosphate dihydrate crystals, and others
OA	Common; usually in lower extremities; synovial fluid is noninflammatory	May be primary or secondary to trauma, hemochromatosis
Trauma	Common; history is diagnostic; occurs rarely in inpatients	Fracture, hemarthrosis, internal derangement
AVN of bone	Uncommon; more common in hip, knee, shoulder	Risk factors include trauma, corticosteroid use, alcohol
Tumors	Uncommon	Benign or malignant, primary or metastatic
Systemic diseases with monoarticular onset	Uncommon (follow-up may be needed for diagnosis)	Psoriatic arthritis, SLE, ReA, RA

Approach to Polyarthritis

Polyarthritis is one of the most common problems in rheumatology (Fig. 1-2). The number and pattern of joint involvement suggest the diagnosis (Table 1-3). There are many nonarticular causes of generalized joint pain. Disorders of periarticular structures (tendons, bursae) cause joint pain but usually involve a single joint. Myopathies occasionally cause widespread pain, but muscle weakness is the primary symptom. PMR causes shoulder and pelvic girdle pain with morning stiffness, but there is usually no arthritis on exam. Neuropathies, primary bone diseases (Paget's disease), and fibromyalgia can also cause widespread pain but are distinguished by history and physical exam.

RA is the prototypical polyarticular arthritis, and, given its frequency (1%), it is important to recognize and distinguish RA from other types of arthritis. RA usually begins with symmetric peripheral arthritis of multiple small joints of hands, wrists, and feet that progresses over weeks to months. Morning stiffness is prominent. Other joints (knees, ankles, shoulders, elbows) are sequentially involved. Involvement of the cervical spine, temporomandibular joint, and sternoclavicular joint is also seen, but lumbar spine and sacroiliac involvement is very rare. **SLE** may present with polyarthritis similar to RA that may be intermittent. Fever, rashes, serositis, and other organ involvement may accompany arthritis in SLE. **Viral arthritis** (due to parvovirus B19, hepatitis B, rubella, HIV) may have an acute onset with fever and rashes and persist for months. **Palindromic rheumatism** causes recurrent attacks of symmetric arthritis that affect hands, wrists, and knees and are self-limited over several days. The **seronegative spondyloarthropathies** are characterized by spine and SI joint involvement, enthesopathy (pain at sites of tendon insertion to bone), and varying degrees of peripheral joint, eye, skin, and GI involvement. Peripheral joint involvement is usually asymmetric, oligoarticular, and of the lower extremities (knee, ankle). Dactylitis, a diffuse swelling of a digit ("sausage digit"), may be seen in fingers and toes and is characteristic of ReA and PsA. A symmetric, polyarticular form of PsA exists that is similar to RA. Oligoarticular disease may also be seen with Behçet's disease, sarcoidosis, and relapsing polychondri-

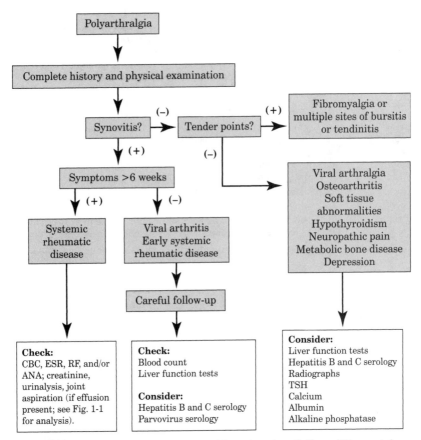

FIG. 1-2. Approach to polyarthritis. (Adapted from American College of Rheumatology ad hoc Committee on Clinical Guidelines. Guidelines for the initial evaluation of the adult patient with acute musculoskeletal symptoms. *Arthritis Rheum* 1996;39:1.)

tis. **Bacterial arthritis** may be polyarticular in patients with preexisting joint damage (RA). Gonococcal arthritis may be migratory and is accompanied by fever, pustular skin lesions, and tenosynovitis. Fever and migratory arthralgias or mild arthritis may be seen in early **Lyme disease,** and a persistent oligoarticular arthritis occurs months later. **Bacterial endocarditis** often presents with fever, low back pain, and arthralgias and may have a positive RF. **Gout** is usually monoarticular, but polyarthritis is sometimes seen. CPDD may present as "pseudo–RA" with bilateral hand and wrist involvement. **OA** is the most common form of noninflammatory polyarthritis. DIP, PIP, first carpometacarpal (CMC), knees, hips, and first MTP joints are involved in some patients. Hemochromatosis predisposes to OA in unusual joints (second and third MCP). **Rheumatic fever** occurs after streptococcal infection and is characterized by migratory arthritis of large joints, fever, and extraarticular involvement (carditis, chorea, rash).

The history and physical exam usually suffice for a diagnosis. Routine lab tests and imaging may be useful to identify other organ system involvement. Serologic tests (ANAs, RF, Lyme serologies) should not be ordered unless the suspicion for a particular diagnosis already exists. Many rheumatologic diseases have similar clinical pictures at onset and close follow-up is needed to make a diagnosis. A patient with

TABLE 1-3. CAUSES OF POLYARTHRITIS

Inflammatory
    Polyarticular peripheral (usually symmetric)
        RA (usually presents insidiously, additive)
        Viral arthritis (usually acute onset)
        SLE
        PsA (occasionally)
        Palindromic rheumatism (recurrent attacks)
    Oligoarticular with axial involvement (usually asymmetric, lower extremity joints)
        Seronegative spondyloarthropathies (AS, ReA, PsA, and enteropathic arthritis)
    Oligoarticular without axial involvement (usually asymmetric)
        PsA
        ReA
        Enteropathic arthritis
        Lyme disease
        Polyarticular gout (more commonly monoarticular)
        CPDD
        Bacterial endocarditis
        Septic arthritis (particularly in patients with RA)
        Sarcoidosis
        Behçet's disease and relapsing polychondritis (rare)
        Rheumatic fever (usually migratory)
Noninflammatory
    OA
        OA of the hands
        Generalized OA
        Posttraumatic OA
        OA secondary to metabolic diseases (hemochromatosis, ochronosis, acromegaly)
    Sickle cell disease
    Hypertrophic osteoarthropathy
    Other (rare)
        Leukemia
        Hemophilia
        Amyloidosis

symmetric, peripheral polyarthritis may have a self-limited viral arthritis, but persistence for >12 wks suggests that RA will be the final diagnosis. Urgent treatment is required in cases with active infection. Other patients may be treated with NSAIDs and should be referred to a rheumatologist if disease persists.

Approach to Patients with Positive Antinuclear Antibodies
ANAs are autoantibodies that target nucleic acids and nucleoproteins and are usually detected by indirect immunofluorescence (see Chap. 5, Lab Evaluation of Rheumatic Diseases) (Fig. 1-3). Tests for ANAs are frequently ordered in patients in order to rule out SLE. ANAs are very sensitive (their absence by current assays practically rules out SLE) but not too specific for SLE. ANAs are present in other rheumatic diseases (e.g.,

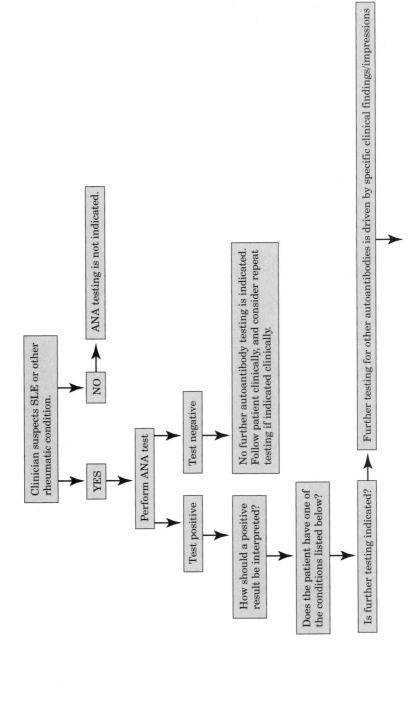

Clinician suspects SLE or other rheumatic condition.

NO → ANA testing is not indicated.

YES → Perform ANA test

Test negative → No further autoantibody testing is indicated. Follow patient clinically, and consider repeat testing if indicated clinically.

Test positive → How should a positive result be interpreted? → Does the patient have one of the conditions listed below? → Is further testing indicated? → Further testing for other autoantibodies is driven by specific clinical findings/impressions

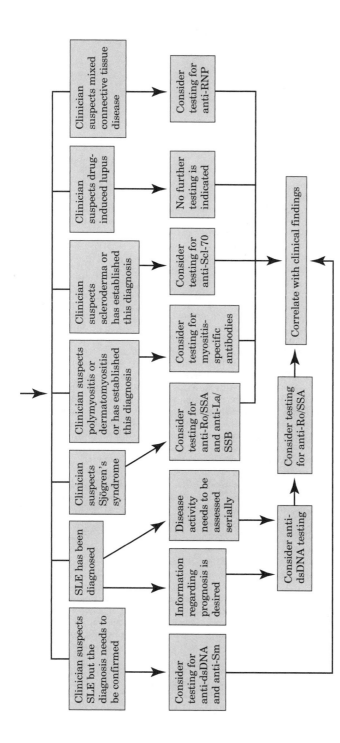

FIG. 1-3. Approach to a positive ANA. dsDNA, double-stranded DNA; Sm, Smith. (Adapted from Kavanaugh A, Tomar R, Reveille J, et al. Guidelines for clinical use of the antinuclear antibody test and test for specific autoantibodies to nuclear antigens. *Arch Pathol Lab Med* 2000;124:71–81.)

scleroderma, MCTD, PM, SS), in drug-induced lupus (DIL), in some infectious diseases (e.g., HIV), and in up to 5% of healthy individuals (in low titers). A positive ANA should be followed by a complete history and physical exam to identify those conditions. A history of hydralazine or procainamide use suggests DIL. Myositis, skin changes, and Raynaud's phenomenon suggest MCTD, myositis, or scleroderma. Sicca symptoms (dry eyes and dry mouth) suggest SS. SLE is a multisystem disease that is diagnosed clinically. Criteria developed for the classification of lupus (see Chap. 12, Systemic Lupus Erythematosus) can be used as a framework for assessing whether a patient has SLE. Certain other diseases (acute HIV infection, endocarditis, autoimmune hepatitis) may fulfill criteria for SLE. High titer ANAs (>1:160) should be followed by assays for antibodies to certain antigens (double-stranded DNA, SSA/Ro, SSB/La, RNP, Sm) that may be more specific for SLE and other rheumatic diseases. If no certain diagnosis is made, follow-up may be indicated: Up to 40% of patients referred to a rheumatologist for evaluation of positive ANAs who do not fulfill criteria on presentation do fulfill criteria for SLE after months to years of follow-up. Tests for ANAs should not be ordered unless the clinical suspicion of SLE exists.

Approach to Patients with Possible Systemic Vasculitis
The vasculitides are a heterogenous group of disorders characterized by inflammation of blood vessels. Vasculitis is often suspected in patients with multiple organ involvement. Perform a complete history and physical exam on these patients. Vessels in the respiratory tract, kidneys, GI tract, peripheral nerves, and skin may be involved in varying degrees depending on the category of vasculitis and the size of the blood vessel involved.

A frequent inpatient consultation is to evaluate possible pulmonary-renal syndromes. Pulmonary-renal syndromes are rare and are suspected in patients with lung involvement (ranging from asymptomatic radiographic findings to pulmonary hemorrhage and respiratory failure) and renal involvement (ranging from asymptomatic to nephritis and renal failure). Pulmonary-renal syndromes may be caused by vasculitis [WG, microscopic polyangiitis (MPA), Churg-Strauss syndrome (CSS)], other autoimmune diseases (SLE, Goodpasture's syndrome), certain infections, and sepsis.

Patients with suspected vasculitis should be questioned about fever, rashes, arthralgias or arthritis, abdominal pain and weight loss, and underlying rheumatic diseases (SLE, RA). The physical exam should identify other organ system involvement (purpura, peripheral neuropathy, joint abnormalities) that may not be obvious on initial presentation. ANCA are sensitive and specific for some vasculitides but may be seen in infections (such as HIV). Positive ANCA require confirmation with more specific assays for antibodies against myeloperoxidase (MPO) and proteinase-3 (PR3) (see Chap. 5, Lab Evaluation of Rheumatic Diseases). Other lab tests (ANA, complement levels, hepatitis panels, cryoglobulins, UA) may be useful to establish etiology. Chest and sinus radiographs may reveal occult respiratory tract involvement. Diagnosis may require pathologic exam of skin, nerve, kidney, or lung tissue. Infection should be ruled out before treatment with corticosteroids or immunosuppressives is considered.

MANAGEMENT

Perioperative

Patients with rheumatic diseases often undergo elective surgery to repair periarticular structures and repair or replace joints. Deformities that limit mobility, the medications the patient is taking, and existing end-organ damage need to be considered. Patients with RA, juvenile RA, and AS may have limited jaw opening, cervical spine fusion, and deformities that contribute to difficult intubation. The cervical spine is significantly affected in many patients with RA and preop radiographs (lateral in flexion) are done to detect severe instability. Fiberoptic or awake intubation may be needed. Patients with AS may also have thoracic expansion limitations that may complicate mechanical ventilation. Treat cystitis, skin infections, and possible sources of bacteremia such as caries before joint replacement to prevent seeding of the prosthesis.

Aspirin and other NSAIDs affect platelet aggregation and should be discontinued 5–7 days before surgery. Selective cyclooxygenase-2 (COX-2) inhibitors do not affect platelet aggregation and may be used until the day of surgery. Patients who are on or have received corticosteroids in the previous year may be at risk for adrenal insufficiency during the stress of surgery. Hydrocortisone (Cortef, Hydrocortone), 100 mg IV q8h, is the traditional "stress dose," but lower doses may be sufficient. Taper the corticosteroid dose to the daily dose (or to zero in patients not previously on corticosteroids) within a few days if the patient is stable. Methotrexate (Folex, Rheumatrex, Trexall) should be withheld 48 hrs before surgery and restarted within 1–2 wks to prevent a flare of arthritis. Nephrotoxic agents such as cyclophosphamide (CYC) (Cytoxan, Neosar) should also be withheld preop. Etanercept (Enbrel), infliximab (Remicade), adalimumab (Humira), and anakinra (Kineret) may be withheld for 1 wk before and after surgery.

Patients with Sjögren's syndrome are at risk for corneal abrasions in surgical settings and need to receive ocular lubricants before and after surgery. NPO orders may be made more tolerable with artificial saliva. Particular care is needed with intubation given the usual poor state of dentition in these patients.

Prophylaxis against deep vein thrombosis is mandatory in joint replacement patients. Aggressive physical therapy is essential for rehabilitation. Acute crystalline arthritis is common in the postop period, and management may be difficult in patients with renal dysfunction or who cannot have oral intake. In these patients, narcotic analgesics or intraarticular corticosteroids (after excluding infection) may be an option (see Chap. 13, Gout).

KEY POINTS TO REMEMBER

- Inflammatory conditions are characterized by at least 1 hr of morning stiffness, constitutional symptoms, and signs of inflammation.
- Mechanical arthritis is typically worse with activity and better with rest.
- Suspect infection in all cases of acute monoarthritis.
- A negative ANA has a high negative predictive value and essentially rules out SLE.

SUGGESTED READING

American College of Rheumatology ad hoc Committee on Clinical Guidelines. Guidelines for the initial evaluation of the adult patient with acute musculoskeletal symptoms. *Arthritis Rheum* 1996;39:1.

Baker DG, Schumacher HR. Acute monoarthritis. *N Engl J Med* 1993;329:1013.

Homburger HA. Cascade testing for autoantibodies in connective tissue diseases. *Mayo Clin Proc* 1995;70:183.

Klippel JH, ed. *Primer on the rheumatic diseases*, 11th ed. Atlanta: Arthritis Foundation, 1997.

Klippel JH, Dieppe PA, eds. *Rheumatology*, 2nd ed. London: Mosby, 1998.

Koopman WJ, ed. *Arthritis and allied conditions*, 14th ed. Philadelphia: Lippincott Williams & Wilkins, 2001.

Moder KG. Use and interpretation of rheumatologic tests: a guide for clinicians. *Mayo Clin Proc* 1996;71:391.

Phillips AC, Polisson RP. The rational clinical evaluation of the patient with musculoskeletal complaints. *Am J Med* 1997;103(6A):7S.

Pinals RS. Polyarthritis and fever. *N Engl J Med* 1994;330:769.

Ruddy S, Harris ED, Sledge CB, eds. *Kelley's textbook of rheumatology*, 6th ed. Philadelphia: WB Saunders, 2001.

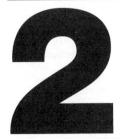

Rheumatologic Joint Exam

Shannon C. Lynn

INTRODUCTION

The full joint exam is often excluded from the general complete physical exam because it is considered too time-consuming for minimal diagnostic gain. The joints are addressed usually only if the patient has a specific complaint. Musculoskeletal disorders, however, are common in patients who present to physicians and are the most common reason for disability in the population. The joint exam, if done consistently, can be performed with increasing efficiency and brevity. A brief screening exam is presented in Table 2-1.

The history should focus not just on the abnormalities or complaints but also on how well the patient can perform activities of daily living (e.g., dressing, grooming, cooking) and how the musculoskeletal disorder interferes with occupation or hobbies. In general, one should begin with a visual inspection, noting asymmetry, swelling, deformities, and changes in color. One continues the exam by palpating for warmth, tenderness, and crepitus. Hard swelling around joints may be due to bony deformities, whereas tender, "boggy" swelling may be due to synovial inflammation (synovitis). Simultaneously notice the bulk, tone, and strength of the associated muscle groups. Finally, evaluate active and passive range of motion. Make note of a developing or lack of pattern of joint involvement.

Perform a general physical exam, paying close attention to the skin, eyes, and nervous system. Begin by noting the patient's gait as he or she walks in the room. Is the patient using any adaptations to protect a particular joint? How does the patient sit in the chair? Is the patient able to get up to the exam table unassisted? Note the use of canes or other assistive devices. Ask the patient if he or she has any limitations in activities of daily living as a result of the rheumatic condition.

INDIVIDUAL JOINTS

Hands

Instruct the patient to stretch out all fingers with the palms down. Then, palms up, have the patient make a fist and oppose the thumb to the base of the fifth finger. Note any finger lag. If abnormalities are noted, distinguish between a periarticular problem versus an articular disorder (see Chap. 1, Approach to the Rheumatology Patient). Palpate each joint for pain. Observe for any lumbrical or thenar atrophy. Note any deviation of the joints. Subluxation of the MCP joints with ulnar deviation of the digits is seen with RA, for example. Also note grip strength and ability to fine pinch. Normal patients should be able to make a completely closed fist.

Specific Findings

- Heberden's nodes: hard, painless nodules on the dorsolateral aspects of the DIP joints (characteristic in OA).
- Bouchard's nodes: similar to Heberden's nodes, except found on the PIP joints (also characteristic of OA).

TABLE 2-1. BRIEF JOINT SCREENING EXAM

Upper extremities

Squeeze across MCP joints collectively and ask patient if it is painful

"Make a fist"

"Touch your fingers to the tip of your thumb"

"Turn your hands over"

"Place your hands behind your head"

"Place your hands behind your back"

Neck and back

"Touch your chin to your chest"

"Look up at the ceiling"

"Turn your head to the left and to the right"

"Bend over and touch your toes"

Lower extremities

Squeeze across MTP joints collectively and ask patient if it is painful

Perform the FABER maneuver (of hip)

"Straighten your knee"

"Step on the gas" (plantar flexion)

"Pull your foot up" (dorsiflexion)

FABER, flexion, abduction, and external rotation.
Note: Exam may be performed in a few minutes. It may be easier to ask the patient to follow the examiner's lead and copy the movements. Any abnormality should be followed by a complete examination.
Adapted from Doherty M, Dacre J, Dieppe P, Snaith M. The "GALS" locomotor screen. *Ann Rheum Dis* 1992;51:1165–1169.

- "Swan neck" deformities: hyperextension of the PIP joint with fixed flexion of the DIP joint.
- "Boutonniere" deformity: fixed flexion of the PIP joint with hyperextension of the DIP joint.
- Other findings include tophi (hard or soft uric acid deposits seen in chronic gout), fingernail and cuticle abnormalities (seen in PsA, dermatomyositis) and sclerodactyly (thin, tapered fingers with tight overlying skin and loss of soft tissue seen in scleroderma).

Wrists

Passively flex, extend, and deviate the wrists medially (ulnarly) and laterally (radially). Note any swelling, effusion, or tenderness along the joint line. Normal range of motion is flexion and extension to 60–90 degrees.

Elbows

Passively flex, extend, pronate, and supinate the forearms. Normal range of motion is extension to 0 degrees (hyperextension occurs with >–10 degrees extension) and flexion to 145 degrees (the thumb should be able to touch the shoulder). With the elbow flexed at 90 degrees, the forearms should supinate and pronate to 90 degrees. Palpate along the extensor surface of the ulna for rheumatoid nodules. These nodules are usually firm, nontender, and mobile with respect to the overlying skin.

Shoulders

The shoulder is a highly mobile joint. The patient with normal shoulder joints should be able to raise the arms straight up (flexion). Normal external rotation and abduction are demonstrated by asking the patient to touch the scapula by reaching behind the neck; internal rotation and adduction are demonstrated by asking the patient to touch the scapula by reaching behind the back. The impingement test is positive in rotator cuff disorders and involves forward flexion of the arm while the examiner stabilizes the patient's scapula. A positive test produces pain with this maneuver.

Neck

Ask the patient to flex and extend the neck. Normal range of motion permits the chin to touch the chest. Ask the patient to turn his or her neck to the right then the left. 90 degrees of rotation in each direction is normal. To evaluate lateral flexion, ask the patient to bring his or her ear to each shoulder.

Back

Assess the curvature of the spine. The normal spine has three curves: lumbar lordosis, thoracic spine kyphosis, and cervical lordosis. Identify the presence of abnormal lordosis, kyphosis, scoliosis, or list (lateral tilt of the spine). Palpate for any tenderness along the spine. While the patient is standing, instruct him or her to bend forward, backward, right, and left.

If a spondyloarthropathy is suspected, perform the modified Schober test. With the patient standing, mark two midline points, one 10 cm above the lumbosacral junction (midline between the posterior iliac spines) and one 5 cm below the junction. The points will be 15 cm apart. Ask the patient to flex forward and measure the distance between the two points. In a normal individual, the span will increase by ≥ 4 cm.

Hips

While the patient is lying supine on the exam table, passively flex the hip and knee while the other leg is held straight. Normal flexion is 135 degrees (the patient should be able to touch the heel to the buttock). While the hip is flexed at a 90-degree angle, rotate the foot. Normal external rotation is 45 degrees, and normal internal rotation is 35 degrees. Internal rotation is often limited with arthritis of the hip. Note any limitation, crepitus, or pain. A quick screening maneuver is the FABER test: *F*lexion, *ab*duction, and *e*xternal *r*otation of the hip are tested by exerting light downward pressure on the knee while the hip is flexed with the heel touching the opposite knee. Pain suggests hip pathology.

Knees

Note alignment of the knees. Palpate along the joint margins for bony ridges (seen with OA). Passively flex and extend the knee while feeling for crepitus. The knee normally extends to 0 degrees and flexes to 135 degrees. Effusions are relatively easy to detect in the knee. Feel for joint effusion by palpating the medial and lateral aspects of the patella while using the other hand (placed proximal to the patella) to gently "milk" fluid toward the patella. One can also assess for fluid with the "bulge" sign: observe for a "bulge" medial or lateral to the patella as pressure is applied from the opposite side.

Ankles

Passively flex and extend ankles proper then medially (varus) and laterally (valgus) deviate the ankle to elicit abnormalities of the subtalar joint. To test the midtarsal joint, stabilize the heel with one hand, then use the other hand to invert and evert the forefoot. Normal dorsiflexion (from the ankle at a 90-degree angle to the leg) is 15 degrees, and normal plantar flexion is 55 degrees.

Metatarsophalangeal Joints

Ask the patient to plantar flex and dorsiflex the toes. Palpate each joint. Observe for hallux valgus, abduction of the great toe with respect to the first metatarsal. With hallux valgus, the head of the first metatarsal may enlarge on the medial side.

KEY POINTS TO REMEMBER

- A brief screening exam can be completed in just a few minutes and should be incorporated into most general physical exams.
- Exam of other organs such as the skin, nails, and eyes may provide valuable clues to rheumatologic diagnoses.

SUGGESTED READING

Bates B. *A guide to physical examination and history taking*, 6th ed. Philadelphia: JB Lippincott, 1995.

Canoso JJ. *Rheumatology in primary care*. Philadelphia: WB Saunders, 1997.

Doherty M, Dacre J, Dieppe P, Snaith M. The "GALS" locomotor screen. *Ann Rheum Dis* 1992;51:1165–1169.

Hoppenfeld S. *Physical examination of the spine and extremities*. New York: Appleton Communication, 1976.

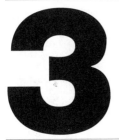

Arthrocentesis: Aspirating and Injecting Joints

Kathryn H. Dao

INTRODUCTION

Arthrocentesis is an essential tool for evaluating and treating many rheumatic diseases.

Indications

- Suspected crystalline disease or infection
- Posttraumatic effusion (to rule out hemarthrosis)
- New effusions with uncertain diagnosis
- Intraarticular injections (with steroids or contrast for arthography)

Contraindications

- Overlying cellulitis.
- Clotting disorder (platelets <50,000, coagulopathy, anticoagulant therapy). This is a relative contraindication.
- Contraindications to *injecting a joint with steroids* include septic arthritis/bursitis, unstable joints, fractures, Charcot joint, bacteremia, prior failure to respond to injections.

Possible Complications

- Bleeding (local hematoma or hemarthrosis)
- Iatrogenic infection (this is rare and is estimated to occur in only 1:50,000 procedures)
- Rupture of tendon or periarticular structure
- Nerve damage (e.g., median nerve atrophy following a steroid injection)
- Allergic reaction to the equipment used or to the injected medications
- Postinjection flare
- SC atrophy with steroid injection (more common with fluoridated steroids: dexamethasone, betamethasone, and triamcinolone) (Table 3-1)

EQUIPMENT

- Iodine/surgical scrub
- 3-, 5-, 10-cc syringes
- 18- , 20-, 25-gauge needles
- 1% lidocaine
- Hemostat/Kelly clamp
- Gloves
- Gauze, bandages
- Alcohol pads
- Glass slides with coverslips
- Test tubes (EDTA and heparinized)
- Blood culture bottles, culture swab
- Ballpoint pen

TABLE 3-1. STEROID PREPARATIONS FOR JOINT INJECTIONS

Steroid	Concentration (mg/mL)	Dose (mg)
Hydrocortisone acetate	24	200
Dexamethasone acetate[a]	8	4
Methylprednisolone acetate	20, 40, 80	40
Triamcinolone hexacetonide[a]	20	40
Triamcinolone acetonide[a]	10, 40	40
Betamethasone acetate[a]	6	6
Prednisolone tebutate	20	40

Note: Doses listed are for large joints (knee, shoulder, hip). For medium joints (wrist, ankle, elbow) use half the dose and for small joints (finger and toe) use one-tenth to one-fifth the dose.
[a]Fluorinated steroids.

GENERAL APPROACH

To access the joint space, palpate the desired area and mark it with a retracted ball-point pen (which will leave a circular impression when pressure is applied to the skin). Clean the skin thoroughly and perform the procedure with aseptic technique. Infiltrate lidocaine into the skin and SC tissues for local anesthesia. Attach the needle to a syringe, introduce it into the desired joint space, and aspirate fluid. If injecting a steroid preparation (see Table 3-1), there should be no resistance during the injection. The Kelly clamp/hemostat may be used to change out syringes during the procedure. If joint aspiration is unsuccessful or assistance is needed for anatomically complex joints, ultrasound guidance may be useful. Recommendations are made to limit steroid injections to 3–4 injections/site/yr. After any aspiration procedure, record the amount of synovial fluid drawn and grossly examine the fluid for viscosity, clarity, and color. Place a small drop onto a slide with a coverslip for microscopic viewing. Send the synovial fluid to the lab for cell count (in an EDTA lavender tube), routine Gram's stain and culture, and crystal analysis. Glucose, protein, autoantibodies, pH, and complement levels from the fluid are rarely helpful. Acid-fast bacilli, fungal cultures (in a culture bottle/swab), and cytology can be ordered if clinically indicated.

Knee

Fully extend or slightly flex the knee with complete relaxation of the quadriceps muscles and identify margins of the patella. The needle may be introduced from the medial or the superolateral aspect of the knee; it should enter underneath the patella (Fig. 3-1).

Ankle

The leg should be rested with the foot at a 90-degree angle. The tibialis anterior tendon and the medial malleolus should be identified. The needle should enter the skin medial to the tendon and lateral to the mid-superior portion of the malleolus. It is directed posteriorly to enter the joint space (Fig. 3-2).

Shoulder

Posterior Approach to Glenohumeral Joint

With the patient sitting, palpate the posterior margin of the acromion. The needle is inserted anteriorly 1 cm below and 1 cm medial to the posterior corner of the acro-

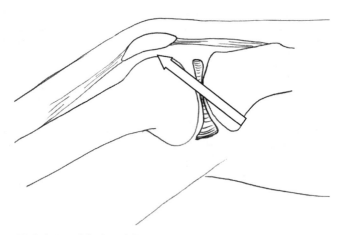

FIG. 3-1. Medial view of the knee joint.

mion. Direct the needle toward the coracoid process until bone is touched at the articular surface (Fig. 3-3).

Anterior Approach to Glenohumeral Joint

The patient should be sitting with the affected shoulder externally rotated. The point medial to the head of the humerus and slightly inferior and lateral to the coracoid process is located. Introduce and direct the needle posteriorly. Redirect superiorly and laterally if bone is hit. Some recommend rotating the arm internally and externally to find the joint space (Fig. 3-4).

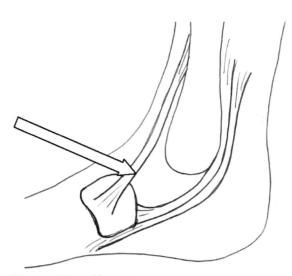

FIG. 3-2. Medial view of the ankle joint.

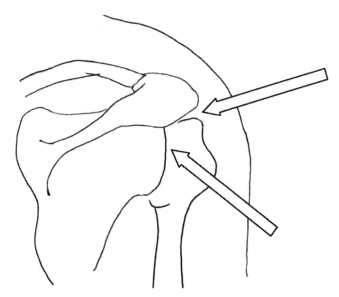

FIG. 3-3. Posterior view of the shoulder.

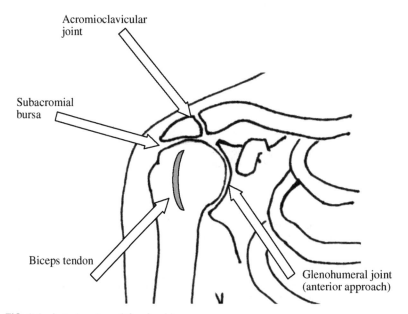

FIG. 3-4. Anterior view of the shoulder.

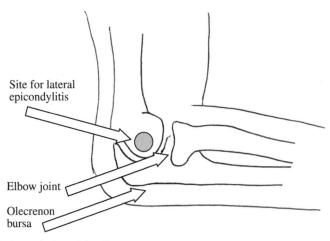

Site for lateral
epicondylitis

Elbow joint

Olecrenon
bursa

FIG. 3-5. Lateral view of the elbow.

Acromioclavicular Joint

The acromioclavicular joint may be injected at the groove by the lateral end of the clavicle, medial to the acromion.

Subacromial Bursa

Using the posterolateral approach, enter the subacromial bursa with the needle directed anteromedially under the acromion.

Biceps Tendon Sheath

Palpate the biceps tendon; aim the needle superiorly to the tendon at a tangential angle. Take care with injecting near the biceps tendon because tendon rupture is relatively common. Avoid injecting the tendon itself.

Elbow

The elbow should be flexed at 90 degrees. To approach the elbow joint, a mark may be made below the lateral epicondyle but above the head of the radius. Insert the needle perpendicular to the skin into the elbow joint. For lateral epicondylitis ("tennis elbow") injections, the needle should enter at the most tender point and be inserted until periosteum is contacted (Fig. 3-5).

Wrist

The joint is most easily accessible distal to the radius and ulnar to the extensor pollicus longus tendon in the radiocarpal groove (Fig. 3-6).

Hand

Finger and MCP joints. Flex fingers slightly and inject with a small needle dorsally and under the extensor tendons (going either medial or lateral to the tendon).

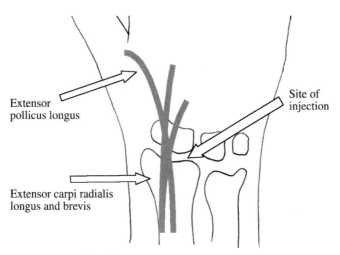

FIG. 3-6. Dorsal view of the right wrist.

Hip

The trochanteric bursa may be injected with the patient lying on the unaffected side. Insert the needle vertically into the site of maximal tenderness (usually located at the posterior corner of the greater trochanter) until the periosteum is contacted.

Aspiration of the hip joint is not described because it is generally reserved for orthopedists and interventional radiologists; the neurovascular bundle can easily be damaged if the procedure is done incorrectly (Fig. 3-7).

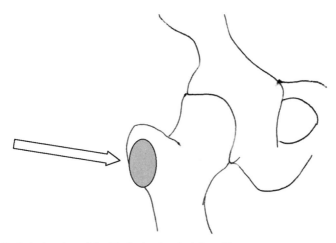

FIG. 3-7. Anterior view of the hip for trochanteric bursitis.

KEY POINTS TO REMEMBER

- Acute monoarthritis necessitates immediate aspiration to rule out septic joint.
- For superficial injections (trigger points, anserine bursitis, and lateral epicondylitis), avoid fluorinated steroid compounds to prevent SC atrophy.

SUGGESTED READING

Canoso JJ. Aspiration and injection of joints and periarticular tissues. In: Klippel JH, Dieppe PA, eds. *Rheumatology*, 2nd ed. London: Mosby, 1998; 2.12.1–12.

Chen H, Sola JE, Lillemoe KD, eds. *Manual of common bedside surgical procedures*. Baltimore: Williams & Wilkins, 1996.

Sack H. Joint aspiration and injection: a how-to guide. *J Musculoskeletal Med* 1999;16:419–427.

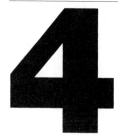

Synovial Fluid Analysis

Kathryn H. Dao

GROSS APPEARANCE

Normal synovial fluid is an "ultrafiltrate of plasma" that contains small amounts of high molecular weight proteins (fibrinogen, complement, globulin) complexed with hyaluronan. The fluid should be evaluated to distinguish between noninflammatory, inflammatory, septic, or hemorrhagic states (Table 4-1).

MICROSCOPIC EXAM

After aspirating a joint, place 1–2 drops of synovial fluid onto a slide with a coverslip. If the syringe appears empty after attempted aspirations, try to draw some saline into the syringe (0.50–1 cc), then use this fluid for your microscopic exam (Table 4-2). With a polarized microscope, crystals can be seen easily (Fig. 4-1).

KEY POINTS TO REMEMBER

- Gout crystals are yellow and calcium pyrophosphate deposition disease crystals are blue when the long axis of the first order red compensator is parallel to the long axis of the crystals.
- Calcium pyrophosphate deposition disease crystals are often difficult to visualize.
- Corticosteroid crystals (used for intraarticular injections) may be confused with pathologic crystals.

TABLE 4-1. GENERAL EVALUATION OF SYNOVIAL FLUID

Exam	Normal	Noninflammatory	Inflammatory	Septic	Hemorrhagic
Viscosity	High (dripping synovial fluid yields a strand of 2.5–5 cm)	High	Low	Variable	Variable
Color	Colorless to straw	Straw to yellow	Yellow	Variable	Bloody
Clarity[a]	Transparent (can read a newspaper or the numbers on the syringe through this)	Transparent	Cloudy; may have rice bodies[a]	Opaque	Opaque
WBCs	<200	50–1000	1000–75,000	>60,000	RBCs>>WBCs
Differential diagnosis		OA, SLE, amyloidosis, osteonecrosis, Charcot's joint, trauma, tumors, ochronosis, Wilson's disease	RA, PsA, ReA, crystalline arthropathies, SLE, scleroderma, infections (tuberculosis, viral, fungal, bacterial)	Bacteria, mycobacterium, fungal infections, crystalline disease, RA	Trauma, hemophilia, Charcot arthritis, pigmented villonodular synovitis, torn ligament

[a]Occasionally in chronically inflamed joints, rice bodies may be seen; these are cellular debris, fibrin, and collagen precipitate. Black speckled fluid ("ground pepper sign") may result from fragmentation of a prosthetic arthroplasty.

TABLE 4-2. MICROSCOPIC CRYSTAL ANALYSIS OF SYNOVIAL FLUID

Crystal	Morphology	Birefringence	Color[a]	Disease
Monosodium urate	Needles	Negative	Yellow	Gout
CPPD	Rhomboid, rods	Positive	Blue	Pseudogout, chondrocalcinosis
Cholesterol	Rectangles	Variable	Yellow/blue	Chronic RA or OA
Calcium oxalate	Bipyramidal	Positive	Blue	Renal disease
Immunoglobulin	Polymorphic	Variable	Yellow/blue	Multiple myeloma, cryoglobulinemia, amyloid
Hydroxyapatite	Round, irregular	None	None	Acute/chronic arthritis
Charcot-Leyden	Spindle	Variable	Yellow/blue	Eosinophilic synovitis

[a]Color when slow vibration of light is parallel to crystal. In a polarized microscope, there are 2 polarizing lenses that are arranged 90 degrees to each other. Light can pass through the first lens in a single plane but is blocked by the second lens, causing a dark field. If crystal is between the lenses, it can deflect the rays of light, resulting in new angles and visibility against a darkened field. A first-order red compensator is a tool to distinguish the difference in birefringence. For urate, if the slow rays are parallel to the crystals (fast rays parallel to the compensator), a yellow color (negative birefringence) will appear. When the stage is rotated 90 degrees, the crystal will appear blue. CPPD, calcium pyrophosphate deposition.

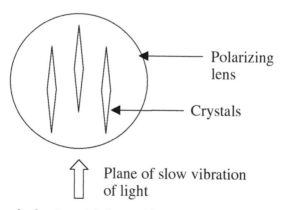

Polarizing lens

Crystals

Plane of slow vibration of light

FIG. 4-1. Example of urate crystals that would appear yellow when parallel to the slow rays of light.

SUGGESTED READING

Cush JJ, Kavanaugh AF. *Rheumatology: diagnosis and therapeutics*. Baltimore: Williams & Wilkins, 1999:61–73.

Owen DS. Aspiration and injection of joints and soft tissues. In: Ruddy S, ed. *Kelley's textbook of rheumatology*, 6th ed. Philadelphia: WB Saunders, 2001:583–619.

Schmerling RH, Delbanco TL, Tosteson AN, Trentham DE. Synovial fluid test: what should be ordered? *JAMA* 1990;264:1009–1014.

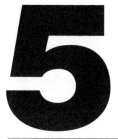

Lab Evaluation of Rheumatic Diseases

Ernesto Gutierrez

AUTOANTIBODIES

Antinuclear Antibodies

ANAs are directed against nuclear antigens. Testing for the presence of ANAs is widely available and is a useful tool for the diagnosis of many autoimmune diseases including SLE and other CTDs. Unfortunately, it is also misunderstood and inappropriately used by many physicians. As the specificities and sensitivities of ANA titers vary not only for each disease but also with the type of lab assay used, overreliance on the ANA may lead to inappropriate diagnosis and treatment. Furthermore, titers of ANA do not necessarily correlate with disease activity. Hence, the presence or absence of ANA titers must be interpreted within a clinical context. As most CTDs are defined as systemic diseases with clinical and lab findings, *ANA titers should be ordered after appropriate clinical and lab data are obtained and a differential diagnosis has been formulated.* With the exception of SLE, ANA testing should not be used as a screening tool for CTDs. The best screening tool for CTDs is a thorough history and physical exam with basic lab data of organ function. Although the absence of ANAs virtually excludes a diagnosis of SLE, the presence of ANAs does not establish the diagnosis.

ANAs are detected using indirect immunofluorescence or immunoenzyme assays. The substrates, substrate fixatives, and buffering solutions may vary from one lab to the next, hence the sensitivity and specificities may vary. Most labs perform a standard assay using a human epithelial cell line as the substrate. Several staining patterns of ANAs have been described. With the exception of the association between a discretely speckled anticentromere pattern and the CREST variant of scleroderma, the significant overlap between the patterns of ANA staining and specific CTD makes staining patterns diagnostically unhelpful.

Extractable nuclear antigens (ENAs) are specific antigenic targets for ANA that can be extracted from the nucleus with physiologic saline and include the ribonucleoprotein and Smith (Sm) antigens. Both ENAs are peptides complexed with small nuclear RNA. Antibodies to ribonucleoprotein are associated with MCTD, and antibodies to Sm are specific for SLE. Before standardization of ANA assays, many patients with reported "ANA-negative SLE" had positive antibodies to ENA. Standardization of ANA assays ensures that negative ANA titers result in the absence of antibodies to ENA, although positive ANA titers do not necessarily result in detectable antibodies to ENA.

Other specific ANAs include anti–double-stranded DNA (anti-dsDNA), anti–Scl-70, anti-histone, anti-Ro (or anti–SS-A), and anti-La (or anti–SS-B) antibodies. The roles that ANAs play in the pathogenesis of diseases are not well understood. Particular ANA may be associated with certain CTDs and may carry prognostic information as described in Table 5-1.

Rheumatoid Factor

RF is a polyclonal autoantibody directed against the Fc portion of immunoglobulin (Ig), most commonly IgM directed against IgG. RF is associated with chronic inflammatory diseases including RA (see Table 5-1). It is believed that a change in glycosyla-

TABLE 5-1. AUTOANTIBODIES AND THEIR ASSOCIATED DISEASES

Antibody	Disease association	Comments
ANA	SLE, MCTD, SjS, PM, DM, scleroderma	Nonspecific (present in 5% of population and prevalence increases with age); sensitivities: SLE >95%, MCTD >95%, SjS 75%, PM/DM >75%, scleroderma >60–90%, RA 15–35%; also present in other autoimmune disorders, cancer, and infections.
Anti-centromere (pattern of ANA)	CREST	Sensitivities: CREST >90%, idiopathic Raynaud's 25%, associated with progression to CREST in patients with idiopathic Raynaud's; staining pattern is easily identifiable on ANA stain.
RF	RA	Nonspecific, prevalence increases with age (false-positive in up to 25% of subjects aged >70); sensitivities: RA 80%, scleroderma 50%; also present in WG, bacterial endocarditis, chronic hepatitis, chronic infection, sarcoidosis, malignancy, and cryoglobulinemia; in RA, may have loose correlation with clinical activity and predicts poorer prognosis and extraarticular disease.
Anti-dsDNA	SLE	Very specific for SLE, only 20–30% sensitive; associated with lupus nephritis and may correlate with disease activity in SLE; also present in chronic active hepatitis.
Anti-Sm	SLE	Very specific for SLE, only 30% sensitive; associated with lupus nephritis and anti-ribonucleoprotein.
Anti-Ro (SS-A)	SS	Sensitivities: SS 75%, SLE 25%; associated with sicca symptoms in other CTDs, extraglandular disease in SS, heart block in neonates with anti-Ro positive mothers; correlates with SCLE rash, photosensitivity, or thrombocytopenia in SLE.
Anti-La (SS-B)	SS	Sensitivities: SS 40%, SLE 10%; association with anti-Ro; correlates with benign course in SLE if no other autoantibody present except ANA.
Anti-histone	DIL	Sensitivities: DIL >90%, SLE >50%; associated with RA and Felty's syndrome.
Anti–Scl-70	Scleroderma	Very specific but only 20–30% sensitive for scleroderma.
c-ANCA	WG	Confirm positive values with anti-PR3; very sensitive (>80%) and specific for active disease in fulminant WG but less sensitive in limited WG; levels tend to correlate with disease activity but titers vary from patient to patient; less sensitive for MPA 45%, CSS 10%, and PAN 5%.
p-ANCA	CSS, MPA	Nonspecific; confirm positive finding with anti-MPO; sensitivities for anti-MPO: CSS 65%, idiopathic crescentic glomerulonephritis 65%, MPA 45%, PAN 15%, WG 10%; non anti-MPO p-ANCA present in RA, SLE, PM/DM, relapsing polychondritis, APS, and other autoimmune diseases.

(continued)

TABLE 5-1. CONTINUED

Antibody	Disease association	Comments
Anti–Jo-1	PM	30% sensitive in PM; predicts deforming arthritis, "mechanic's hands," Raynaud's, and pulmonary fibrosis in DM and PM.
Anti–Mi-2	DM	5% sensitive in DM; associated with V-sign, shawl sign, cuticular overgrowth, good response to therapy and good prognosis.
Anti-SRP	PM/DM	<5% sensitive in PM/DM; associated with acute onset, severe weakness, palpitations, and poor prognosis.
Lupus antico-agulant	Hypercoagu-lable states, APS	APA; Screened for by detecting prolonged PTT, KCT, or dRVVT that fails to correct with mixing studies and confirmed with phospholipid neutralization studies that confirm a phospholipid-dependent in vitro anticoagulant.
Anti-cardio-lipin anti-body	Hypercoagu-lable states, APS	APA; Association with thrombosis: IgG>>IgM>IgA; titers tend to correspond with disease activity.
$beta_2GPI$–dependent aCL	Hypercoagu-lable states, APS	A type of aCL that binds to complex of $beta_2GPI$ and cardiolipin; positive values associated with higher risk of hypercoagulable states than non–$beta_2GPI$-dependent aCL.
Cryoglobulins	HCV, LPD, CTD	Type I: monoclonal Ig (usually IgM or IgG) that self-aggregate; may have RF activity, associated with LPD; Type II: monoclonal Ig (usually IgM) with activity against polyclonal IgG (i.e., RF activity), most commonly idiopathic, may be associated with HCV or CTD; Type III: polyclonal Ig (usually IgM) with activity against polyclonal IgG (i.e., RF activity), most commonly idiopathic, may be associated with HCV or CTD.

APS, antiphospholipid syndrome; CREST, CREST variant scleroderma; dRVVT, dilute Russel viper venom time; HCV, hepatitis C virus; KCT, kaolin clotting time; LPD, lymphoproliferative diseases; SCLE, subacute cutaneous lupus erythematosus.

tion patterns of the Fc portion of IgG in patients with RA leads to development of neoantigens and to the production of RF.

RF is classically detected using a latex immunofixation test and reported as a titer. Newer methods, including nephelometric assays, report results in international units. The inverse ratio of the nephelometric result correlates roughly with the titer result; for example, 120 IU correlates roughly with a titer of 1:120. The role of RF in the pathogenesis of disease is unclear.

Antineutrophil Cytoplasmic Antibodies

ANCAs are directed against cytoplasmic antigens in human neutrophils and are identified with immunofluorescent staining assays using ethanol-fixed neutrophils. Two distinct staining patterns have been described: cytoplasmic-ANCA (c-ANCA) and perinuclear-ANCA (p-ANCA). ANCAs are not ANAs, although proximity of p-ANCA staining to the nucleus may be mistaken for an ANA. Hence, a positive ANA or p-ANCA may result in false-positive results for p-ANCA or ANA, respectively. c-ANCA is associated with WG and p-ANCA is associated with CSS, MPA, and PAN. The specific antigen for most c-ANCA is PR3 and for most p-ANCA is MPO; testing for anti-PR3 and anti-MPO antibodies is performed by enzyme-linked immunosorbent assays at a reference lab. PR3 is a protein present in azurophil granules in neutrophils and is involved in the function and activation of neutrophils. Antibodies to PR3 have high sensitivities and specificities for active fulminant WG. It is believed that neutrophil modification by anti-PR3 antibodies in WG may account for some of the disease manifestations. MPO is a protein involved in the generation of reactive oxygen species and in the modulation of macrophage function. Because p-ANCA and anti-MPO antibodies are present in a large number of diseases, their roles in pathogenesis are poorly understood.

Myositis-Specific Antibodies

The three best described myositis-specific antibodies (MSA) are anti–Jo-1 (directed to t-RNA histydyl synthetase), anti–signal recognition protein (anti-SRP), and anti–Mi-2. Their sensitivities for inflammatory myopathies are low. Specific MSA may be associated with certain clinical features and prognosis (see Table 5-1).

Antiphospholipid Antibodies

Antiphospholipid antibodies (APAs) are directed against phospholipids and are associated with hypercoagulable and thrombotic states. APA is detected by assays for the lupus anticoagulant (LAC), anticardiolipin antibodies (aCL), and false-positive serologies for syphilis.

Of the three APAs, LAC has the strongest association with hypercoagulation. The name *LAC* is derived from the fact that the antibody was first described in patients with SLE and from its tendency to cause prolonged aPTT. We now know that LAC can be found in other CTDs or in isolation.

LAC is identified in a stepwise manner using functional phospholipid-dependent clotting assays that reveal a coagulation inhibitor that is neutralized by phospholipids. First, phospholipid-dependent clotting assays such as a dilute prothrombin time, aPTT, kaolin clotting time, and a dRVVT are drawn; prolonged times are considered positive results. Each test has different sensitivities in detecting LAC, and the use of more than one test is recommended. Patients with LAC are more likely to have prolonged dRVVT, kaolin clotting time, or PTT and less likely to have a prolonged PT. Mixing studies are then performed on samples with prolonged times to exclude factor deficiencies. If a prolonged time corrects in mixing studies, the sample is further incubated in different temperatures to exclude a temperature-sensitive inhibitor of coagulation. A sample that does not correct with mixing studies or with variable-temperature incubation is identified as having an inhibitor of coagulation. This sample is then incubated with excessive phospholipids to characterize the inhibitor as either a phospholipid-dependent or a phospholipid-independent inhibitor. Excessive phospholipids neutralize the LAC and the prolonged times correct. Although LAC is a phospholipid-dependent inhibitor of coagulation in lab assays, in vivo the LAC's interactions with phospholipid-rich endothelial and platelet surfaces are thought to activate both platelets and the coagulation cascade and result in hypercoagulation and thrombosis.

The association between aCL and hypercoagulable states is related to antibody titers and immunoglobulin isotype. As a general rule, increasing titers of aCL are associated with increasing risk of hypercoagulation and thrombosis. IgG aCL carry more risk than IgM aCL, and the risk of IgA aCL is questionable. Some aCL bind to complexes composed of phospholipids and beta$_2$-glycoprotein I (beta$_2$GPI), a natural serum anti-coagulant. Beta$_2$GPI-dependent aCL are associated with increased risk of hypercoagulable states, but the role of testing for specific beta$_2$GPI-dependent aCL has yet to be defined.

Serologic assays for syphilis such as the VDRL and RPR use cardiolipin phospholipids. When VDRL or RPR are positive, perform a confirmatory test such as the FTA-

ABS (looking for antibodies against treponemes). A false-positive test for syphilis identifies an APA. A false-positive VDRL for syphilis in a patient with APA has a characteristic beaded pattern. These APA have a weak association with hypercoagulation and thrombosis.

Cryoglobulins

Igs that are soluble at body temperature but reversibly precipitate at lower temperatures are known as *cryoglobulins*. Cryoglobulins are classified into three types depending on the characteristics of the Igs, and each type is associated with different diseases. A cryocrit is obtained using a minimum of 10–20 cc of fresh venous blood that is drawn into prewarmed test tubes and transported to the lab in sand or water warmed to 37°C. The specimen is allowed to clot at 37°C for 30–60 mins before centrifugation. The supernatant is then left at 4°C for as long as 7 days; types I and II usually precipitate within 24 hrs, whereas type III may take days. Newer methods such as electrophoresis can detect and quantify cryoglobulins, but preheated tubes and warm transportation are still required.

ERYTHROCYTE SEDIMENTATION RATE

ESR is the measurement of the rate of erythrocyte settling in anticoagulated blood and is a nonspecific marker of tissue inflammation. The presence of asymmetric macromolecules produced during inflammation promotes erythrocyte aggregation and increases the ESR. The ESR is affected by many conditions, some of which may be present in patients with rheumatologic diseases. Noninflammatory conditions that tend to raise the ESR include anemia (except sickle cell anemia), renal disease (including nephrotic syndrome and glomerulonephritis), hypercholesterolemia, female sex, pregnancy, oral contraceptives, malignancy, thyroid disease, and increasing age. Patients with elevations >100 mm/hr usually have metastatic malignancy (including multiple myeloma), infection (classically TB or osteomyelitis), or CTD. Conditions that can lower the ESR include high-dose steroid use, sickle cell anemia, polycythemia, anisocytosis, spherocytosis, microcytosis, hepatic failure, and cachexia.

An ESR >50 mm/hr is part of the American College of Rheumatology classification criteria for giant cell arteritis. The ESR is sometimes used to monitor the activity of inflammatory conditions such as SLE and RA, although other markers of disease activity such as clinical signs and symptoms and lab indicators of organ function are more useful.

C-REACTIVE PROTEIN

CRP is a beta globulin normally present in the serum in trace amounts. Serum concentrations rapidly increase during inflammation. CRP is a component of the innate immune response whose major function is to recognize foreign pathogens and damaged cells by binding to phosphocholine surfaces. Activation of complement proteins or phagocytic cells follows. Similar to ESR, CRP levels are elevated in acute or chronic inflammatory states. Obesity, smoking, coronary artery disease, malignancy, and diabetes mellitus may also elevate CRP levels.

The use of CRP levels in addition to the ESR in the rheumatic diseases is limited. Evidence suggests CRP levels may provide prognostic information in patients with RA in whom elevated and sustained CRP levels are associated with radiographic progression of joint disease and with long-term disability. CRP levels may also be useful in patients with SLE. CRP levels are usually normal in active SLE except in chronic synovitis or acute serositis. In SLE patients with fever in whom synovitis or serositis can be excluded, elevated CRP levels suggest a bacterial source of inflammation and fever.

COMPLEMENT

The complement cascade involves >30 proteins and accounts for 15% of the globulin portion of plasma protein. Three pathways have been identified. The classical pathway involves the opsonization and/or lysis of cells covered with antibodies to cell surface antigens; the alternative pathway involves the nonspecific opsonization and/or lysis of foreign cells that lack cell membrane complement regulators; the mannose-binding lectin pathway involves the opsonization and/or lysis of foreign cells with mannose groups on the cell membrane.

The rheumatic diseases that involve immune complex formation and subsequent activation of the classic pathway include SLE, cryoglobulinemic vasculitis (CV), and Henoch-Schönlein purpura (HSP). The total hemolytic complement activity is a functional assay that tests the integrity of the classical pathway. Low total hemolytic complement activity suggests a deficiency of ≥ 1 factors. C3 and C4 are individual components of the complement cascade. In SLE, low C3 and C4 complement levels may correlate with disease activity, especially in lupus nephritis. Not all patients have complement levels that correlate with disease activity, and the pattern of correlation may vary with each patient. Nevertheless, once a pattern is established in a particular patient, levels may be used to monitor disease activity. Low C4 levels are present in patients with cryoglobulinemic vasculitis, reflective of the complement activation by immune complex deposition.

KEY POINTS TO REMEMBER

- A negative ANA virtually excludes the diagnosis of SLE.
- Specific rheumatologic lab tests are used primarily to support a specific diagnosis and are rarely independently diagnostic.
- Few tests aside from the ESR with temporal arteritis/polymyalgia rheumatica, C3, C4, and anti-DNA titers in lupus nephritis correlate with disease activity.

SUGGESTED READING

Arnout J. Antiphospholipid syndrome: diagnostic aspects of lupus anticoagulants. *Thromb Haemost* 2001;86:83–91.

Brandt JT, et al. Criteria for the diagnosis of lupus anticoagulant: an update. On behalf of the Subcommittee on Lupus Anticoagulant/Antiphospholipid Antibody of the Scientific and Standardisation Committee of the ISTH. *Thromb Haemost* 1995;74:1185–1190.

Dispenzieri A, Gorevic PD. Cryoglobulinemia. *Hematol Oncol Clin North Am* 1999;13:1315–1349.

Egner W. The use of laboratory tests in the diagnosis of SLE. *J Clin Pathol* 2000;53:424–432.

Hahn BH. Antibodies to DNA. *N Engl J Med* 1998;338:1359–1368.

Hoffman GS, Specks U. Antineutrophil cytoplasmic antibodies. *Arthritis Rheum* 1998;41:1521–1537.

Levine JS, et al. Medical progress: the antiphospholipid syndrome. *N Engl J Med* 2002;346:752–763.

Mayet WJ, et al. The pathophysiology of anti-neutrophil cytoplasmic antibodies (ANCA) and their clinical relevance. *Crit Rev Oncol Hematol* 1996;23:151–165.

Moder KG. Use and interpretation of rheumatologic tests: a guide for clinicians. *Mayo Clin Proc* 1996;71:391–396.

Mongey A, Hess EV. *Adv Intern Med* 1991;36:151–169.

Shmerling RH, Liang MH. Evaluation of the patient: laboratory assessment. In: *Primer on the rheumatic diseases*, 11th ed. Atlanta: Arthritis Foundation, 1997:94–97.

Sox HC, Liang MH. The erythrocyte sedimentation rate. *Ann Intern Med* 1986;104:515–523.

Walport MJ. Complement (parts 1 and 2). *N Engl J Med* 2001;344:1058–1066, 1140–1144.

Radiographic Evaluation of Rheumatic Diseases

Ron J. Gerstle and
Lawrence D. Tang

APPROACH TO BONE AND JOINT RADIOGRAPHS

A simplified systemic approach using the mnemonic ABCDS can be used to interpret bone and joint plain films. *A* refers to joint alignment, *B* refers to bone, *C* refers to cartilage and joint space, *D* refers to distribution, and *S* refers to soft tissue findings. Not all features described for each disease below are present at any one time, and no individual abnormality is pathognomonic.

See Table 6-1 for commonly ordered x-rays for evaluation of arthritic joints and Table 6-2 for radiographic findings of common types of arthritis.

OSTEOARTHRITIS

Primary OA is the most common arthropathy encountered by bone and joint radiologists. The most characteristic findings are nonuniform joint space narrowing and osteophyte formation, also known as bone spurs. Joint involvement can be unilateral or bilateral. Joint erosions commonly seen in inflammatory arthropathies are not present in OA. Subchondral bone cysts or subchondral bone formation is secondary to joint disease. OA most commonly affects the hands, feet, hips, knees, and the lumbar and cervical spine. Involvement of the shoulders, elbows, and ankles is uncommon.

Primary OA in the hand involves the DIP and PIP joints with relative sparing of the MCP joints. Bouchard's and Heberden's nodes refer to osteophyte formation and soft tissue swelling at the DIP and PIP joints, respectively.

The most commonly affected joint in the feet is the first MTP joint. It is commonly associated with hallux valgus (lateral deviation of the tip of the first toe) or hallux rigidus (stiffness in the first MTP joint) deformities of the great toe. Subchondral bone cyst formation is more common in the feet than in the hands.

The hips and knees are also commonly involved with OA. In the knees, bone growth may form and extend into the joint space when cartilage has been lost. Joint space narrowing is usually asymmetric and worse on the medial side.

OA of the spine is commonly referred to as *degenerative disk disease* and involves osteoarthritic changes of the apophyseal joints between the vertebral bodies. Disk space narrowing or apophyseal joint space narrowing and bone sclerosis are commonly seen. An important complication of severe degenerative disk disease in the spine is spondylolisthesis, which is movement of a vertebral body on the vertebral body below it or on the sacrum. Movement occurs either forward (anterolisthesis) or backward (posterolisthesis).

RHEUMATOID ARTHRITIS

RA is the most common systemic rheumatologic disease encountered in bone and joint plain radiographs. RA affects the appendicular skeleton and the cervical spine. The distribution of arthritis is usually bilateral and symmetric in the small joints but unilateral in large joints. Joint changes are most frequently seen in hands, feet, knees, and hips, and less commonly in the shoulder and elbow joints. Radiographs show peri-

TABLE 6-1. COMMONLY ORDERED X-RAYS FOR EVALUATION OF ARTHRITIC JOINTS

Hand	Hip
Posteroanterior	Anteroposterior
Norgaard (supinated oblique)	Frog-leg of affected hip
Foot	SI joint
Anteroposterior	Straight anteroposterior view
Lateral	Anteroposterior: modified Ferguson view
Knee	Cervical spine
Standing anteroposterior	Lateral view in a flexed position
Non-standing flexed lateral	

articular soft tissue swelling and joint malalignment such as subluxations and dislocations. Bony structures commonly have initial marginal erosions that subsequently develop severe subchondral bone erosions. Osteoporosis due to hyperremia from chronic joint inflammation starts in the juxtaarticular region and progresses to generalized osteoporosis. New bone formation is not a feature of RA. Joint space loss is uniform with synovial cyst formation.

The earliest changes seen radiographically in RA are soft tissue swelling around the involved joints in the hands and feet. The distribution of soft tissue swelling is usually symmetric and is accompanied by juxtaarticular osteoporosis. Early marginal erosions

TABLE 6-2. RADIOGRAPHIC FINDINGS OF COMMON TYPES OF ARTHRITIS

	RA	OA	PsA	Gout
Alignment	Affected early	Affected late	Affected late	Not affected
Erosions	Symmetric, marginal	None	Occur with bony proliferation	Asymmetric, with overhanging edges
Periarticular osteoporosis	Present	Absent	Absent	Absent
Joint space	Uniformly narrowed	Non-uniformly narrowed	Narrowed in severe cases	Preserved
Distribution	Symmetric, peripheral joints: hands, wrists, feet, knees, and others, but spares lower spine	May be asymmetric, hands, hips, knees, lumbar and cervical spine	May be asymmetric, hands, wrists, feet, knees	Asymmetric, hands, feet
Soft tissue swelling	Present	Mild swelling	May be very swollen "sausage digit"	Asymmetric when tophi are present (tophi are not radiopaque)

are subtle. In the hand, the MCP and PIP joints are involved. In the wrist, early erosions often occur at the waist of the capitate, the articulation of the hamate with the base of the fifth metacarpal, and at the ulnar styloid. Later into the disease course, the MCPs and PIPs are uniformly involved and all the carpal bones are affected as a unit in the wrist. Subluxations occur at MCP joints. Soft tissue atrophy and SC rheumatoid nodules develop in late stages of the disease.

The feet are also very commonly involved in RA. In general, the feet are evaluated with posteroanterior and lateral views. As in hands, early involvement of the feet results in juxtaarticular osteoporosis and erosion of the bare areas at the metatarsal heads. The lateral aspect of the head of the fifth metatarsal is usually involved first with erosive changes and later with loss of the white cortical line. The heads of other metatarsals are generally eroded first medially and later laterally. At later stages of the disease, there are progressive erosive changes, uniform loss of the MTP joint cartilage space, and lateral subluxations of the proximal phalanges. Similar to the carpal bones, the tarsal bones are involved as a unit with uniform joint space loss.

The hip joint is affected in approximately 50% of RA patients. The involvement is characterized by uniform loss of the cartilage space with secondary migration of femoral head in the femoral head–acetabulum axis, resulting in acetabuli protrusion (protrusion of the femoral head into the acetabulum).

ANKYLOSING SPONDYLITIS

AS primarily affects the axial skeleton and less commonly the appendicular skeleton. It is more ossifying than erosive when compared to other inflammatory arthropathies. The axial distribution of disease and the classic "bamboo spine" changes are the two features that make the radiographic diagnosis relatively easy. Bone density is usually normal before ankylosis and becomes osteoporotic after ankylosis. The distribution is the spine and the SI joints, with the SI joints and lumbar spine being the most frequently involved. The hips, shoulders, knees, hands, and feet are less commonly involved. Subluxations as seen in RA and PsA are not seen in AS.

The first abnormalities usually seen are in the SI joints. The SI joints are commonly involved bilaterally and symmetrically and commonly fuse completely. Erosions and sclerosis are mild and sometimes subtle. The modified Ferguson view provides a better assessment of the SI joints than standard anteroposterior views of the pelvis.

Lumbar spine changes are the first changes noted in the spine. They progress in a caudocranial direction to involve thoracic and cervical spines. An early sign of spine involvement is erosion of the vertebral body corner with secondary sclerosis. The changes give the vertebral body a "squared" appearance. The anterior longitudinal ligaments are the first visible sites of ossification (syndesmophyte). Erosions of the odontoid process may occur in cases of cervical spine AS and result in atlantoaxial subluxation.

PSORIATIC ARTHRITIS

PsA differs from RA radiographically in many important ways, particularly with regard to bone proliferation. PsA usually has periosteal bone proliferation, whereas RA does not. PsA usually has a bilateral asymmetric distribution, normal bone mineralization, and can have fusiform soft tissue swelling. In decreasing order of frequency, PsA involves the hands, feet, SI joints, and spine.

The periarticular soft tissue swelling can be striking in hands. The swelling often extends beyond the joint into the soft tissue in the digit, forming a "sausage digit." The arthritis may be erosive. In severe cases, erosions can destroy large portions of the underlying bone and give a widened joint space appearance. The ends of the bones involved in severe erosive cases become pointy and produce "pencil-in-cup" deformities. Bony proliferation is relatively unique to PsA. It occurs adjacent to areas of erosions, along the shafts of the bones, across joints, and at tendinous and ligamentous insertion sites. Initial bone proliferation appears fluffy and spiculated.

Different patterns of distribution can be encountered in hands. Other features of PsA, such as bone proliferation and DIP involvement, differentiate it from RA.

The radiographic changes in the feet are similar to those in the hands. Erosive changes, soft tissue swelling, bony proliferation characterized by periostitis, and interphalangeal joint ankylosis are present. In particular, involvement is seen at the posterior and inferior aspects of the calcaneus. The shoulders, elbows, knees, and ankles may be involved in similar fashions.

SI joint involvement is usually bilateral and asymmetric. Erosions and bone proliferation are the usual findings. Bony ankylosis may occur in the SI joints but is much less frequent than in AS. Spondylitis usually occurs along with SI joint involvement. Large, bulky, and unilateral or asymmetric paravertebral ossification is a characteristic finding in PsA. The cervical spine may be involved with atlantoaxial subluxation similar to that in RA and AS.

REACTIVE ARTHRITIS

Many of the radiographic findings in ReA are indistinguishable from those in PsA. As in PsA, bone erosions, bone proliferation, uniform joint space narrowing, ligamentous and tendinous ossification, bilateral asymmetric distribution, and fusiform soft tissue swelling are common in ReA. However, ReA has a different distribution, affecting the feet, ankles, knees, and SI joints and less frequently the hands, hips, and spine. Clinical correlations are particularly important in differentiating ReA from PsA.

SYSTEMIC LUPUS ERYTHEMATOSUS

Characteristic radiographic findings of SLE include SC calcifications, deforming non-erosive arthritis, and osteonecrosis. Unlike inflammatory arthropathies, there are no erosions or joint space loss in SLE. However, subluxations and dislocations are often seen in SLE. The arthropathy is most commonly seen in the hands, wrists, hips, knees, and shoulders.

Bone infarcts or osteonecrosis can occur as a result of vasculitis or chronic steroid use. The femoral heads, femoral condyles, tibial plateaus, humeral heads, and tali are the most frequently involved in osteonecrosis.

CALCIUM PYROPHOSPHATE DIHYDRATE DEPOSITION DISEASE

Calcium pyrophosphate dihydrate (CPPD) deposition disease is the most common crystalline arthropathy and affects about 5% of the elderly population. The radiographic spectrum of disease ranges from subtle to striking, but certain features are constant.

The hallmark of CPPD deposition disease is chondrocalcinosis, the deposition of calcium salts in cartilage. This finding is quite specific for CPPD deposition disease, and it is most commonly seen in the knee menisci and in the triangular fibrocartilage of the wrist. Other sites that are affected are the hips, elbows, and pubic symphysis.

Other findings in the disease are uniform joint space loss and involvement of the radiocarpal joint, which helps to distinguish it from OA. Like OA, there are subchondral cysts, but they are typically more prominent in CPPD deposition disease. As with other nonrheumatoid arthritides, bone mineralization is normal.

GOUT

Although tophi are not radiopaque unless they calcify, their effects on the surrounding tissues allow for radiographic detection. Periarticular tophi produce "punched-out" lesions in the adjacent bone. The bone proliferation adjacent to these lesions produce "overhanging edges." This combination of findings is characteristic of gout. Because tophaceous gout does not involve the cartilage directly, joint space is preserved. This allows differentiation from the primary arthropathies. The most commonly affected joints are those of the feet, knees, and hands. Multiple joints are typically affected, and the distribution is asymmetric. Bone mineralization is unaffected by tophaceous gout.

SEPTIC ARTHRITIS

No single radiographic feature distinguishes septic arthritis from the other arthropathies, and typically the history and physical exam lead one to suspect the diagnosis. Further complicating the picture is the possibility of superinfection of an already abnormal joint.

The arthritis is typically monoarticular, with a rapidly progressive radiologic course. Loss of the cortical line from the articular surfaces also suggests the diagnosis. Diffuse osteoporosis is followed by symmetric joint space narrowing. The most commonly involved joints are the hip and knee.

KEY POINTS TO REMEMBER

- RA appears bilateral and symmetric with periarticular osteopenia and early erosions occuring in bare areas of bone adjacent to cartilage.
- OA is characterized by nonuniform joint space narrowing and formation of bone spurs.
- Spinal involvement in AS occurs in a caudal-to-cephalad direction.
- PsA can lead to inflammatory changes in DIP joints.

SUGGESTED READING

Brower AC. *Imaging of rheumatic disorders*. Summit, NJ: CIBA-GEIGY Corp., 1992.

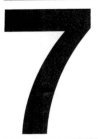

Rheumatologic Emergencies

Kevin M. Latinis

INTRODUCTION

Rheumatologic emergencies are relatively uncommon; however, some consultations require quick action to prevent serious clinical sequelae. The following are considered rheumatologic emergencies and should be addressed immediately on the patient's arrival in the office or receipt of inpatient consultation.

INFECTIOUS ARTHRITIS

The differential diagnosis of acute-onset arthritis always includes infectious arthritis, especially if accompanied by a fever and constitutional symptoms. Always evaluate onset of monoarticular or oligoarticular arthritis using early synovial fluid analysis. Empirically start IV antibiotic treatment if fluid is inflammatory. Bedside arthrocentesis can be performed for accessible joints such as the knee, wrist, elbow, and ankle. Otherwise, order radiologically assisted arthrocentesis. Joints with orthopedic hardware warrant urgent consultation to the orthopedic surgery service. The consequences of improperly treated infectious arthritis include rapid joint destruction and permanent disability. For further details about diagnostic workup and treatment see Chap. 32, Infectious Arthritis.

GIANT CELL (TEMPORAL) ARTERITIS

Given the risk of sudden and permanent vision loss, manage GCA emergently. The diagnosis is based on presumptive clinical evidence of jaw claudication, headache, scalp tenderness, and sometimes acute, usually unilateral vision loss. The diagnosis often accompanies polymyalgia rheumatica, which includes symptoms of fever, morning stiffness, and arthralgias in shoulder, hip, neck, and torso. Lab studies usually show a high ESR (>50) and anemia. Definitive diagnosis involves temporal artery biopsy of an affected segment.

When the diagnosis of GCA is suspected, especially when associated with symptoms of transient vision loss, initiate immediate treatment with oral prednisone, 60 mg/day. Obtain lab tests followed by arrangement for a temporal artery biopsy within 1 wk of initiating steroids. Symptoms often rapidly resolve with steroid initiation. Once symptoms have resolved and ESR returns to normal, taper steroids. For further details see Chap. 22, Giant Cell Arteritis and Polymyalgia Rheumatica.

SCLERODERMA RENAL CRISIS

Renal crisis is a severe, sometimes life-threatening complication that occurs in approximately 10–15% of patients with scleroderma. A scleroderma renal crisis is characterized by rapidly progressive azotemia, malignant HTN (although approximately 10% of patients are normotensive), microangiopathic hemolytic anemia, and thrombocytopenia. Risk factors include diffuse, rapidly progressive skin disease, cool ambient temperatures, races with higher prevalence of essential HTN (i.e., African Americans), and use of corticosteroids or cyclosporin. The pathogenesis reflects a severe vasculopathy leading to ischemic activation of the renin-angiotensin system. Treatment involves BP control with the use of short-acting ACE inhibitors, in particular captopril (initiate at 25 mg bid and titrate to maximum of 50 mg PO tid). For patients intolerant to ACE inhibitors, angiotensin receptor blockers may be effective. Avoid IV antihypertensives, such as nitroprusside and labetalol, and all nephrotoxins. Calcium channel blockers can be added to the regimen of ACE inhibitor if necessary for BP control. Dialysis may be necessary for those patients with end-stage renal failure. For more details on diagnosis and management of scleroderma see Chap. 38, Scleroderma.

CERVICAL SPINE ABNORMALITIES

Cervical spine involvement is a common manifestation of RA or severe, long-standing OA. Neurologic deficits can occur, even in the absence of pain, and, when present, should be addressed urgently. C1-C2 instability may result from tenosynovitis of the transverse ligament of C1, erosion of the odontoid process, ligament laxity, ligament rupture, or apophyseal joint erosion. The lesions most likely to lead to myelopathy (disease of the spinal cord) are nonfixed atlantoaxial anterior subluxation or downward/upward subluxation of the C1-C2 facet joints. Cranial settling (also known as *basilar invagination*) in which the odontoid process pushes up into the foramen magnum may also occur. Radiographic changes of the C1-C2 joints are common but do not always correlate with neurologic deficits. Symptoms of myelopathy are usually slowly progressive but may have rapid onset if associated with cord compression. Although neurologic symptoms are infrequent, they should be addressed with a neurosurgical evaluation for possible stabilization procedures. Additionally, patients with cervical spine arthritis are at increased risk of traumatic injury during intubation and should be appropriately managed perioperatively.

TRANSVERSE MYELITIS

Transverse myelitis develops as an acute or subacute inflammatory disorder of the spinal cord. The majority of cases occur following an infection or immunization. Additionally, transverse myelitis can be associated with MS, SLE and other collagen vascular diseases, SS, Behçet's disease, antiphospholipid syndrome, and sarcoidosis.

Symptoms of transverse myelitis may include focal neck and back pain, paresthesias, weakness, sensory loss, urinary retention or incontinence, fecal incontinence, and fever. Symptoms typically start in the lower extremities and ascend. The disease usually progresses over hours to days and varies in severity from mild neurologic involvement to functional transection of the spinal cord.

Diagnostic workup includes urgent spinal MRI, brain MRI (to evaluate for MS), and CSF analysis. MRI of the spinal cord reveals variable spinal edema and signal enhancement. Obtaining normal CSF is useful to rule out acute infections. Alternatively, pleocytosis, elevated protein, and decreased glucose may be present.

Treatment of transverse myelitis has not been well researched. However, high-dose IV corticosteroids are usually initiated within 24 hrs of diagnosis.

CAUDA EQUINA SYNDROME

Cauda equina syndrome is a rare complication of the seronegative spondyloarthropathies (related to arachnoiditis), in particular AS, as well as lumbar disk rupture, spinal or epidural anesthesia, or mass lesions from malignancies or infections. In patients with AS, symptoms may be slowly progressive. Cauda equina syndrome from any cause, however, has the potential for rapid onset and progression. Symptoms include severe low back pain, rectal pain, and pain in both legs. Additionally, with progressive disease patients can develop saddle anesthesia with loss of bladder and bowel control, poor anal sphincter tone, and impotence. Patients may also develop variable lower extremity areflexia and asymmetric leg weakness or loss of sensation. Cauda equina syndrome should be distinguished from sciatica or plexopathy, which do not involve symptoms of incontinence or impotence. MRI can help confirm the diagnosis, and urgent neurosurgical consultation is required to prevent irreversible neurologic changes. Steroids and localized radiation treatment may be beneficial with lesions caused by malignancies.

PULMONARY HEMORRHAGE

Pulmonary hemorrhage can be a complication of several rheumatologic and nonrheumatologic diseases. Common presenting signs and symptoms include progressive dyspnea with hypoxemia, hemoptysis, radiographic appearance of alveolar or interstitial infiltrates, anemia or a drop in hemoglobin level of 1.5–4 g/dl. Correction of hypoxemia and appropriate control of airway (possibly requiring intubation and mechanical ventilation) and correction of coagulopathies should be addressed immediately. Obtain early consult with a pulmonologist to assess the need for urgent bronchoscopy to help refine the diagnosis. Demonstration of active bleeding or hemosiderin-laden macrophages in bronchoalveolar lavage or sputum helps confirm the diagnosis of pulmonary hemorrhage.

The differential diagnosis of pulmonary hemorrhage includes pulmonary-renal syndromes, including Goodpasture's syndrome or WG, SLE, extraarticular manifestations of RA, Behçet's disease, and other systemic vasculitides such as HSP, CSS, MPA, and cryoglobulinemia. Other possible etiologies include uremia, congestive heart failure, infection, pulmonary infarction, pulmonary HTN, and coagulopathy.

Lab evaluation should include routine chemistries, liver function tests, CBC, and coagulation studies as well as antinuclear antibodies, antiglomerular basement membrane antibody, ANCA, and complement levels (C3, C4, and CH50). Lung (or other involved tissue) biopsy may be required for a definitive diagnosis.

In addition to supportive treatment, target specific therapies at the underlying disorder. Pharmacologic therapy may involve a combination of corticosteroids (usually in high IV doses), cytotoxic agents, and sometimes plasmapheresis.

INTESTINAL INFARCTION

Intestinal infarction is a rare complication associated with SLE and polyarteritis nodosa. The disease is manifested by diffuse vasculitis of the mesenteric blood vessels. Patients typically present with symptoms of an acute abdomen, which may be masked, however, by corticosteroids or may occur late in the clinical presentation. Emergent surgical exploration and resection is important, but overall prognosis is poor.

KEY POINTS TO REMEMBER

- Acute onset of mono- or oligoarthritis requires immediate workup for septic arthritis, including urgent diagnostic arthrocentesis.
- Clinical suspicion of GCA should prompt immediate treatment with high-dose corticosteroids and arrangement for temporal artery biopsy within 7 days.
- Toxic patients should be sent immediately to the nearest ER.

SUGGESTED READING

Braunwald E, Fauci A, Isselbacher KJ, et al., eds. *Harrison's principles of internal medicine,* 15th ed. New York: McGraw-Hill, 2001.

Halla J. Rheumatologic emergencies. *Bull Rheum Dis* 1997;46:4–6.

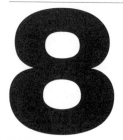

Regional Pain Syndromes

Celso R. Velázquez

INTRODUCTION

Regional pain syndrome refers to pain localized to one area of the body and not caused by systemic disease. Regional pain syndromes (also called *soft tissue rheumatic pain syndromes*) are very common. They include disorders of bone, cartilage, ligaments, muscle, tendons, entheses (sites where tendons attach to bone), bursa, fascia, and nerve. Regional pain syndromes may be caused by trauma, injury from overuse, or degeneration with aging. Consider infections, fractures, or other serious problems (e.g., deep venous thrombosis in a patient with leg pain) in patients who develop regional pain while in the hospital.

History and Physical Exam

History and physical exam are usually enough to make a diagnosis and exclude systemic diseases such as cancer, infection, and arthritis (inflammatory and noninflammatory) that may present as regional pain. Certain features suggest systemic disease (Table 8-1) and should lead to further investigation.

Question patients about the location and characteristics of their pain, radiation of the pain, presence of numbness or tingling, their ability to function, precipitating events, aggravating and ameliorating factors, underlying diseases and systemic complaints (fever, weight loss). It is helpful to ask the patient to locate the pain with one finger. The physical exam should include inspection (looking for atrophy, asymmetry, swelling, erythema), palpation (warmth, crepitus, point tenderness), evaluation of active and passive range of motion, and a neurologic exam. Specific maneuvers exist to help identify involvement of specific structures. An exam that is too focused may miss abnormalities in other parts of the body or sources of referred pain.

Diagnostic Workup

Order lab tests only if there is suspicion of systemic disease. In particular, tests such as ESR, RF, and ANAs have a low predictive value in the general population. Abnormal results may be seen in patients with diseases other than inflammatory arthritis or in healthy persons.

Imaging is rarely indicated at the initial evaluation. Problems of tendons, bursae, or nerves are not detected by plain radiographs. OA is a very common finding on plain radiographs but may be misleading as in the case of patients with OA of the knee on radiographs but knee pain due to anserine bursitis. Consider imaging in patients with a history of trauma. Specific tests (e.g., nerve conduction studies, MRI) may be needed to confirm a diagnosis or before considering surgery. Order these tests sparingly.

Treatment and Follow-Up

Most regional pain syndromes improve with conservative treatment. Table 8-2 presents a general guideline for managing regional pain syndromes. Some patients benefit from assistive devices such as splints or referrals to physical or occupational

TABLE 8-1. FEATURES THAT SUGGEST SYSTEMIC DISEASE

Fever, chills	Pulse abnormalities
Weight loss	Lymphadenopathy
Skin color changes	Neurologic deficits
Bilateral involvement	Muscle wasting or atrophy
Joint warmth, swelling, or tenderness (synovitis)	Lab abnormalities

therapy to increase flexibility, strength, and endurance. Stretching and heat or cold application may be beneficial. When needed, treat pain with medications; exercises, physical modalities, and splinting are often more helpful, however. Some conditions improve with intralesional injections of lidocaine or corticosteroids. Reassure patients that with time, most regional pain syndromes improve.

NECK PAIN

Neck pain is less common than lower back pain but still affects one-third of the population at some time. Pain may be due to involvement of the spine or surrounding soft tissues, spinal cord, or nerve roots, or referred from other structures or organs (Table 8-3). The history and physical exam are usually enough to make a diagnosis.

The neck is frequently involved in arthritis, both inflammatory (RA, AS) and non-inflammatory (OA). Suspect a serious cause of neck pain (meningitis, septic diskitis, metastatic lesions) in patients with a history of cancer or IV drug use, weight loss, progressive neurologic findings, or fever. The physical exam of the patient with neck pain should include cervical range of motion (which normally decreases with age) and a neurologic exam. Radiographic abnormalities are extremely common in the elderly and correlate poorly with symptoms. Consider imaging in patients with neck pain after trauma or with neurologic findings and in cases of suspected fractures, metastatic lesions, or infections. CT and MRI are more accurate in cases of suspected tumor or infection.

Most cases of neck pain are nonspecific and due to **muscle spasm or sprain** and occur in young patients after unusual or repetitive neck movement. The sternocleidomastoid and trapezius muscles are frequently involved. These cases may improve with heat application or rest and usually resolve with time. Neck pain after trauma may be due to soft tissue injury (**"whiplash" injury** due to acceleration-deceleration injury in a rear-end collision motor vehicle accident) or fractures.

OA is a common cause of chronic neck pain in adults and the elderly. OA of the cervical spine that progressively causes extensive osteophyte formation, instability, and subluxation (a process known as **cervical spondylosis**) may cause **radiculopathy.** Encroachment on neural foramina may compress the nerve roots and cause neck pain that radiates to the shoulder or arm. Severe degenerative changes may cause sensory or motor disturbances that vary according to the root involved (Table 8-4). Neck pain with radiculopathy may also be caused by **degenerative disk disease** and disk herniation. Radiographs may identify osteophytes and intervertebral space narrowing that

TABLE 8-2. GUIDELINES FOR MANAGEMENT OF REGIONAL PAIN SYNDROMES

1. Exclude systemic disease with history and physical exam
2. Recognize aggravating and ameliorating factors
3. Provide an explanation of the problem and the likely outcome to the patient
4. Provide relief from pain
5. In patients who do not improve, consider other diagnoses and referral

TABLE 8-3. CAUSES OF NECK PAIN

Soft tissue disorders
Nonspecific neck pain (muscle sprain, spasm)
Whiplash injury
Arthritis[a]
OA and cervical spondylosis
Degenerative disk disease with disk herniation
RA
AS
Juvenile RA
Bone disease[a]
Fracture (due to trauma or osteoporosis) or dislocation
Metastatic lesions
Osteomyelitis
Other
Meningitis
Septic diskitis
Thyroiditis
Referred from intrathoracic or intraabdominal disease

[a]May be associated with signs and symptoms due to radiculopathy or myelopathy.

suggests disk degeneration. Nerve conduction studies may be used to document the nerve root involved but are seldom necessary unless surgery is contemplated. MRI is the best technique to identify the cause and location of root impingement. Treatment of neck OA is conservative. Some activity restriction is beneficial. Soft cervical collars may provide symptomatic relief. Use rigid cervical collars only in cases with instability and under close supervision. NSAIDs are helpful, and local injections and cervical traction are sometimes used. Severe, intractable pain may require surgery.

Myelopathy is less common but more serious than radiculopathy. It is caused by osteophytes, protruding disks, thickening of the ligamentum flavum, or other processes that narrow the cervical spinal canal and exert direct pressure on the cord or compress the spinal arteries. Clinical manifestations include weakness and incoordination of the hands, lower extremity weakness with hyperreflexia, Babinski's sign, and gait disturbances. Incontinence is a late finding. Neck pain is frequently absent. Progressive myelopathy requires surgical decompression.

RA frequently affects the cervical spine. Synovitis and bony changes may encroach on the nerve roots. Ligament involvement leads to laxity, instability, and C1-C2 sub-

TABLE 8-4. NEUROLOGIC FINDINGS IN CERVICAL RADICULOPATHY

Nerve root	Sensory loss	Motor loss	Reflex loss
C5	Neck to lateral shoulder, upper arm	Deltoid	Biceps
C6	Lateral arm to thumb, index finger	Biceps	Brachioradialis
C7	Dorsal and palmar forearm, middle finger	Triceps	Triceps
C8	Medial forearm, ring, middle fingers	Finger flexion	—

TABLE 8-5. DIFFERENTIAL DIAGNOSIS OF LOW BACK PAIN

Mechanical low back pain (97%)

    Idiopathic low back pain (lumbago, lumbar strain)

    Degenerative disk disease

    Herniated disk

    Spinal stenosis

    Spondylolisthesis

    Trauma

Neoplasia (<1%)

    Metastatic lesions

    Multiple myeloma

    Lymphoma and leukemia

    Primary vertebral tumors

    Spinal cord tumors

Infection (<1%)

    Osteomyelitis

    Paraspinous abscess

    Epidural abscess

    Septic diskitis

    Bacterial endocarditis

Rheumatic diseases (<1%)

    AS

    PsA

    ReA

    Inflammatory bowel disease–related arthritis

Visceral disease and referred pain (<1%)

    Aortic aneurysm

      GI disease (pancreatitis, cholecystitis)

      Genitourinary (nephrolithiasis, pyelonephritis, pelvic inflammatory disease)

    Hip disease

luxation. Acute subluxation causes severe pain and may compress the cord and become life-threatening. Subluxation may be spontaneous or follow mild trauma, so maintain a high index of suspicion with RA patients who develop neck pain. **AS** also affects the cervical spine, usually following progressive involvement of the lumbar and thoracic spine. The cervical spine becomes stiff and fractures may occur even with mild trauma.

LOW BACK PAIN

Introduction

Low back pain is one of the most common problems people face. It is the second most common reason to seek medical care (after upper respiratory problems) and is the most common cause of disability in young workers. Many different conditions cause low back pain (Table 8-5).

Mechanical disorders (muscle sprain, herniated nucleus pulposus, OA) are by far the most common causes of back pain. Most patients improve with conservative treatment over time, so education and reassurance are important to prevent unnecessary testing and anxiety. About 1% of patients who present with new-onset back pain have systemic diseases (cancer, infection, inflammatory disease). **A careful history and physical exam are often enough to identify systemic disease** (Table 8-6).

History and Physical Exam

Clues to **cancer** in the history are age >50 yrs, history of cancer, unexplained weight loss, lack of relief with bed rest, duration of pain and failure to improve over 1 mo, and nighttime pain [1]. In a study of >2000 patients with low back pain, no cancer was found in any patient aged <50 yrs without a history of cancer, unexplained weight loss, or failure of conservative therapy [2]. Fever and a history of IV drug use suggest **infection** (spinal osteomyelitis, diskitis.) Also suspect infection in patients who develop low back pain while hospitalized. Morning stiffness of >1 hr with improvement with exercise and onset before age 40 suggests **AS**. Localized tenderness over the midline is seen in **vertebral fractures** due to multiple myeloma, cancer, or osteoporosis. **Disk herniation** may cause sciatica: pain, numbness, and paresthesias radiating to the lower extremity below the knee. Bowel or bladder dysfunction, saddle anesthesia, and bilateral lower extremity weakness are signs of **spinal cord compression** (cauda equina syndrome). Patients with these symptoms should undergo immediate imaging and surgical referral (see Chap. 7, Rheumatologic Emergencies).

The **general physical exam** may provide clues to underlying systemic disease. Murmurs (endocarditis), breast masses (metastases), pulsatile abdominal masses, and pulse abnormalities (aortic aneurysm) are important findings. Range of motion may be decreased in many causes of back pain. The **neurologic exam** should identify spinal nerve root involvement (Table 8-7). A positive **straight-leg raising test** suggests nerve root compression. The test is performed with the patient supine, and the leg is raised straight at the knee. A positive test reproduces pain radiating below the knee when the leg is raised >60 degrees. Low back pain without radiation below the knee does not constitute a positive test.

Diagnostic Workup

Lab tests (ESR, UA, CBC, cultures) may occasionally help exclude systemic disease. Plain radiographs are overutilized. They are recommended only for patients with **fever, unexplained weight loss, history of cancer, neurologic deficits, alcohol or injection-drug abuse, and trauma.** CT scans and MRI are more sensitive than x-rays. However, they often reveal abnormalities even in asymptomatic adults. On MRI, up to 40% of young, asymptomatic volunteers have herniated disks and >90% of subjects >60 yrs have degenerative disks [3,4]. CT and MRI should be reserved for cases with a strong suspicion of cancer or infection or for patients with persistent neurologic deficits.

Treatment

Acetaminophen, NSAIDs, and muscle relaxants are effective for idiopathic acute low back pain. Physical therapy may be useful for patients with persistent pain. Encourage patients to return rapidly to their normal activities, but avoidance of heavy lifting may be prudent until the pain improves. Patients with herniated disks may require short-term opioids for pain control. Bed rest does not accelerate recovery in idiopathic low back pain or sciatica. Patients should be reassured that pain resolves in most cases within 12 wks. Spinal stenosis may also benefit from NSAIDs, but the prognosis for relief of symptoms is not as good. **Surgical evaluation** should be immediate in patients with cord compression or progressive neurologic deficits. Patients with spinal stenosis and persistent and disabling pain and patients with herniated disks and persistent sciatica with neurologic findings may benefit from surgical referral. Chronic

TABLE 8-6. EVALUATION OF SELECTED CAUSES OF LOW BACK PAIN

	Idiopathic low back pain	Herniated disk	Spinal stenosis	AS	Metastases	Spinal infection
Character-istics of pain	Dull, lower back; may radiate to buttocks; improves with rest.	Sudden, sharp, intense; radiates below the knee (sciatica); usually unilateral.	Pseudoclaudication: bilateral pain (buttocks, thighs, legs) brought on by standing or walking and relieved by sitting or flexing spine.	Insidious, chronic, worse in the morning, improves with exercise.	Chronic, severe, not improved with bed rest.	Severe, sharp; may radiate to thighs.
History	History of lifting or straining.	History of lifting or straining.	Occurs in patients >60 yrs with degenerative disease of the spine.	Occurs in patients <40 yrs; may have family history, or history of uveitis or axial arthritis.	Age >50 yrs, history of cancer, weight loss, failure of conservative management.	Immunocompromised patients; history of IV drug abuse, alcohol abuse, infections; fever not always present.
Physical exam	May have pain with movement or in certain positions; neurologic exam is normal.	Pain with straight-leg raise; may have altered dermatomal sensation, weakness or decreased reflexes; 95% S1 root.	May have sensory, motor, and reflex abnormalities.	Decreased range of motion, arthritis.	May show evidence of primary tumor; rule out spinal cord compression in patients with neurologic findings.	Neurologic findings present and depend on the level of involvement.
Lab studies	None needed.	None needed.	None needed.	ESR often elevated; HLA-B27 may be present but is not a good screening test.	ESR may be elevated.	ESR often elevated; positive blood cultures, leukocytosis not always present.
Imaging	None needed.	MRI recommended in patients with neurologic deficits.	MRI may be needed for diagnosis.	X-rays may show sacroiliitis; "bamboo spine" is a late finding.	CT or MRI; emergent imaging needed in suspected cord compression.	MRI indicated.

TABLE 8-7. NEUROLOGIC FINDINGS IN LUMBAR SPINAL NERVE ROOT INVOLVEMENT

Nerve root	Sensory loss	Motor loss	Reflex loss
L4	Lateral thigh, medial leg to medial malleolus	Knee extension, thigh adduction, foot dorsiflexion	Knee
L5	Posterolateral thigh, lateral leg to dorsal foot	Great toe extension and foot dorsiflexion	—
S1	Posterior leg, lateral and plantar foot	Plantar flexion of great toe and foot	Ankle

lower back pain is difficult to manage and sometimes requires a multidisciplinary approach to address rehabilitation, depression, or substance abuse.

SHOULDER PAIN

Shoulder pain is the second most common musculoskeletal complaint after low back pain. There are many causes of shoulder pain (Table 8-8). The shoulder is exceedingly mobile at the expense of some stability. It is made up of four joints that are typically affected in different types of arthritis: glenohumeral joint (affected in RA, calcium pyrophosphate deposition disease), acromioclavicular (OA), sternoclavicular (AS, septic arthritis), and scapulothoracic. The rotator cuff is composed of the tendons of the supraspinatus, infraspinatus, teres minor, and subscapularis muscles and attaches to the humeral tuberosities. Its location between the acromion and the humeral head explains why pain from rotator cuff disease worsens with elevation of the arm.

Rotator cuff tendinitis is the most common cause of shoulder pain. It may be acute or chronic and be associated with calcium deposits in the tendon (calcific tendinitis). Pain is usually over the lateral deltoid and worsens with overhead activity. Night pain due to difficulty positioning the painful shoulder is common. The **impingement sign** is almost always positive (but may also be seen in other shoulder diseases). The sign is elicited by passively forward flexing the patient's arm with the examiner holding down the scapula with the other hand. This produces pain in cases of impingement. Rotator cuff tendinitis may be due to overuse, trauma, age-related degeneration, and osteophytes on the inferior portion of the acromion. **Subacromial bursitis** may be associated with rotator cuff tendinitis and causes point tenderness under the acromium. Treatment includes rest and specific exercises to strengthen the rotator cuff and improve range of motion. Prolonged immobilization of the shoulder in any shoulder disease should be avoided as it may cause adhesive capsulitis. NSAIDs and local anesthetic with corticosteroid injections are also used. **Rotator cuff tears** may be partial or complete and may be due to trauma or the result of gradual degeneration. Complete tears cause inability to abduct the shoulder. MRI (or ultrasound) may distinguish between partial and complete tears. Surgery is necessary to repair complete tears.

Bicipital tendinitis usually causes anterior shoulder pain. The bicipital groove along the anterior humeral head may be tender on palpation. Pain with supination of the forearm against resistance or forward flexion against resistance is seen. Treatment is similar to rotator cuff tendinitis.

Adhesive capsulitis ("frozen shoulder") causes generalized pain with severe loss of active and passive range of motion. It may be due to diabetes, inflammatory arthritis, or prolonged shoulder immobilization. Treatment is with physical therapy, injections, and occasionally surgery.

ELBOW PAIN

Elbow pain is usually caused by periarticular disorders. The elbow is frequently involved in RA but rarely in OA.

TABLE 8-8. CAUSES OF SHOULDER PAIN

Periarticular disorders
    Rotator cuff tendinitis
    Calcific tendinitis
    Rotator cuff tear
    Subacromial bursitis
    Bicipital tendinitis
    Adhesive capsulitis
Articular disorders
    Inflammatory arthritis (RA)
    Glenohumeral arthritis
    Acromioclavicular arthritis
    Sternoclavicular arthritis
    Septic arthritis
    Osteonecrosis (of humeral head)
    Fractures, dislocations
Neurovascular diseases (usually have neurovascular symptoms)
    Brachial plexopathy
    Suprascapular nerve entrapment
    Thoracic outlet syndrome
Referred pain (should be suspected in cases with normal range of motion)
    Cervical spine disease
    Intrathoracic or intrabdominal disease
Other
    PMR (usually bilateral)
    Fibromyalgia
    Reflex sympathetic dystrophy

Olecranon bursitis may be septic or idiopathic or due to inflammatory conditions (RA, gout) or trauma. The bursa is located just proximal to the olecranon. The surrounding area may be swollen, warm, and erythematous in septic bursitis. Septic bursitis usually does not compromise elbow mobility as a septic elbow joint does. Olecranon bursitis may be aspirated and injected with corticosteroids but may recur. Septic bursitis should be aspirated (taking care to avoid penetrating into the elbow joint), and patients should receive antibiotics.

Lateral and medial epicondylitis are known as tennis and golfer's elbow, respectively, but may be due to any type of activity. Lateral epicondylitis is more common. Tenderness is localized to the lateral epicondyle at the insertion of the common extensor tendon. Pain is exacerbated by resisted wrist extension and forearm supination in lateral epicondylitis and by resisted wrist flexion and forearm pronation in medial epicondylitis. Rest, avoidance of exacerbating activities, or NSAIDs may be helpful for both conditions. Corticosteroid injections may be needed.

HAND AND WRIST PAIN

The hand and wrist are frequently affected by arthritis, both inflammatory (RA, lupus, PsA) and noninflammatory (OA). The presence or absence of synovitis, joint deformities, and the specific joints involved may lead to a diagnosis. Hand and wrist pain may also be due to periarticular disorders and to infections. Unilateral pain is often due to trauma, overuse or infection; consider arthritis or systemic diseases in patients with bilateral pain. Order radiographs in patients with hand pain and trauma.

Carpal tunnel syndrome (CTS) is a very common cause of hand pain. The median nerve and the flexor tendons pass through a tunnel at the wrist limited by the carpal bones and the transverse carpal ligament. CTS may be idiopathic but is also seen in pregnancy, RA, diabetes, obesity, and myxedema and with disorders that encroach on the nerve (osteophytes, tophi, amyloid deposits). Pain and tingling of the hand is characteristic but may extend to the wrist, forearm, arm, and sometimes, shoulder. Numbness and paresthesias are felt in the distribution of the median nerve (thumb, index, and middle fingers; radial aspect of ring finger). The hand may be weak and clumsy and feel swollen. Bilateral disease is common. Women are affected more frequently. The history is usually diagnostic, but the exam should identify median nerve involvement and exclude cervical or brachial plexus abnormalities. Weakness and atrophy of the thenar muscles are usually late findings. Tinel and Phalen's signs may be present but are neither sensitive nor specific [5]. **Tinel sign** is distal paresthesias with sharp tapping over the median nerve at the wrist. **Phalen's sign** is reproduction of symptoms when the wrists are held flexed against each other. The **"flick" sign** [6] may be more accurate: When asked "What do you actually do with your hand(s) when the symptoms are at their worst?" patients with CTS do a flicking movement with their hand(s) similar to how someone would shake a mercury thermometer. Nerve conduction studies are usually diagnostic in unclear cases. Nighttime splinting in a neutral position, NSAIDs, and careful injection with corticosteroids are helpful. Surgical release of the transverse carpal ligament is beneficial if conservative measures fail. The **ulnar nerve** may become entrapped at the elbow, causing hand pain and numbness or paresthesias of the ulnar side of the ring and little fingers. Compression of the ulnar nerve at the wrist causes similar symptoms and may be due to trauma or fracture of the carpal or fifth metacarpal bones.

De Quervain's tenosynovitis is the inflammation of the extensor pollicis brevis and abductor pollicis longus tendons at the level of the radial styloid that causes pain, tenderness, and occasionally swelling of that area. It may be due to repetitive thumb pinching while moving the wrist. **Finkelstein's test** is positive when passive ulnar deviation of the wrist while the fingers are flexed over the thumb reproduces pain. Rest, splinting, and NSAIDs are helpful. Surgery may be indicated in refractory cases. **Tenosynovitis** may also occur in other flexor and extensor tendons besides those involved in De Quervain's. Localized pain and tenderness on palpation and with resisted movement are seen. Tenosynovitis may be due to overuse, trauma, or RA, or may be idiopathic.

Infectious tenosynovitis may be seen in gonococcal arthritis and as a result of puncture wounds. Drainage and antibiotics are indicated.

Ganglions are the most common soft tissue tumors of the hand and wrist. They are mucin-filled cysts that arise from adjacent tendon sheaths or joint capsules. They usually appear on the dorsal aspect and are painless but may limit movement if large. Aspiration and surgical excision are indicated in those cases.

Trigger finger is a common cause of hand pain and discomfort. Painful clicking on the palmar aspect and locking of the finger in flexion occurs and may be intermittent. Trigger finger is due to thickening of the retinacular pulley in the palm or a fibrous nodule on the tendon that interferes with flexion. The thumb, ring, and long fingers are most commonly affected. Corticosteroid injections or surgery are helpful.

Dupuytren's contracture is a thickening and shortening of the palmar fascia that result in visible thickening and cording of the palm that is usually painless. The ring finger is affected more frequently. It is seen in diabetics or in patients with chronic alcohol abuse. Stretching and corticosteroid injections are useful in the initial stages, but surgery may be needed to release chronic contractures.

HIP PAIN

Hip pain is a very common complaint and may be due to articular and periarticular disorders or may be referred from other structures (Table 8-9). Different disorders cause pain in different areas around the hip joint, which may be useful for diagnosis. Ask the

TABLE 8-9. CAUSES OF HIP PAIN

Articular disorders
  Noninflammatory
    OA
    Osteonecrosis (AVN) of the femoral head
    Fracture
  Inflammatory
    Seronegative spondyloarthropathies
    Septic arthritis
    Juvenile RA
    RA (usually late in the disease)
Periarticular disorders
  Trochanteric bursitis
  Ischiogluteal bursitis
  Iliopsoas bursitis
  Septic bursitis
Referred pain
  Lumbar spine OA and sciatica
  Spinal stenosis
  Sacroilitis
  Knee disorders
  Vascular insufficiency
  Meralgia paresthetica

patient to point to the location of maximal pain. Imaging is reserved for cases of trauma and suspected fracture, for patients with hip pain and risk factors for AVN (corticosteroid use, alcohol abuse), and for patients with chronic hip pain.

Hip OA is a very common cause of hip pain and increases with age. True hip joint arthritis usually causes pain in the anterior groin that worsens with weight bearing (see Chap. 11, Osteoarthritis). Lumbosacral spine and SI joint disease cause buttock pain, as do spinal stenosis and vascular insufficiency. Trochanteric bursitis causes proximal lateral thigh pain. The hip joint is affected in RA (usually late in the disease) and in juvenile RA and the seronegative spondyloarthropathies. **Fractures** of the femoral neck are common in elderly women with osteoporosis and may occur after a fall. **AVN** commonly affects the hip joint. Refer patients with fractures and osteonecrosis for orthopedic consultation.

Trochanteric bursitis is very common and causes lateral hip pain that may radiate down the thigh and can be severe. It is more common in the elderly and is often associated with OA of the lumbar spine or hip. Pain is worse with walking and lying on the affected side. Localized tenderness on palpation of the trochanteric area (the uppermost area with the patient on his or her side) and pain with resisted abduction are seen. Stretching exercises, weight loss, and NSAIDs are beneficial. Injection of the trochanteric bursa area with lidocaine and corticosteroids is a relatively simple procedure and may bring relief.

Ischiogluteal bursitis is caused by trauma or prolonged sitting on hard surfaces. The pain is over the buttocks, may radiate down the thigh, and is worse with sitting. **Iliopsoas bursitis** is caused by inflammation of the bursa located between the hip joint and the overlying psoas muscle. Anterior thigh and groin pain are present. Pain on palpation or with hyperextension or resisted flexion is seen. Both ischiogluteal and iliopsoas bursitis respond to conservative measures or corticosteroid injections.

Meralgia paresthetica is caused by compression of the lateral femoral cutaneous nerve at the waist. Anterior or lateral thigh pain may be accompanied by numbness or paresthesias. This condition is seen in pregnant or obese patients and in people who wear tight garments or heavy belts. Eliminating the source of compression and, occasionally, corticosteroid injections are useful.

KNEE PAIN

Knee pain is a very common complaint and can be due to articular or periarticular disorders (Table 8-10). Common arthritides such as OA, RA, and gout frequently affect the knee. **Knee OA** is a very common cause of knee pain. Brief morning stiffness and pain with activity are common. On physical exam, tenderness along the joint line, small effusions, and crepitus may be found (see Chap. 11, Osteoarthritis). There are multiple intraarticular structures (articular cartilage, meniscal cartilage, cruciate ligaments) that may degenerate with age, overuse, or trauma and lead to **internal derangement.** Suspect internal derangement in patients, often young adults, who complain of "locking" or "catching" sensations after trauma (particularly sports injuries). Acute, painful swelling (due to hemarthrosis) often follows. Specific maneuvers on physical exam may detect damage to the internal structures [7]. Multiple bursae are around the knee and may become inflamed causing point tenderness on palpation, pain with active motion, but no obvious swelling. Knee pain may be referred from hip disorders (as knee problems can cause hip pain). In general, reserve imaging for posttraumatic pain and for patients with chronic pain. Arthrocenthesis is relatively simple to perform on the knee and should be done in cases of monoarthritis to exclude infection, crystal-induced arthritis, or hemarthrosis.

Anserine bursitis derives its name from the pes anserinus, composed of the conjoined tendons of the sartorius, gracilis, and semitendinosus muscles that insert in the medial proximal tibia. The associated bursa often becomes inflamed, causing medial knee pain and point tenderness on palpation just below the joint line. Anserine bursi-

TABLE 8-10. CAUSES OF KNEE PAIN

Articular disorders
   Noninflammatory
      OA
      Internal derangement (due to meniscal cartilage or cruciate ligament injuries)
      Osteonecrosis (AVN)
      Fracture
   Inflammatory
      RA
      Gout and calcium pyrophosphate deposition disease (CPPD)
      Seronegative spondyloarthropathies
      Viral arthritis
      Septic arthritis
Periarticular disorders
      Bursitis (anserine, prepatellar, infrapatellar)
      Tendinitis (patellar, quadriceps)
      Patellofemoral pain syndrome
      Popliteal cysts

tis often coexists with knee OA. Rest, stretching, and corticosteroid injections are helpful.

Prepatellar bursitis causes pain (and occasionally erythema, warmth, and swelling) anterior to the patella and is common in people who spend a lot of time on their knees. Avoiding kneeling may help resolve the bursitis, but aspiration may be needed in cases with abundant fluid. This bursitis is occasionally septic, so send fluid for cultures. Surgical excision may be necessary for frequent recurrences. **Infrapatellar bursitis** presents similarly to prepatellar bursitis.

Tendinitis: Inflammation of the tendons around the knee may occur with overuse and in inflammatory arthritis and may be confused with bursitis. **Patellar tendinitis** is seen in young athletes who engage in repetitive jumping or kicking (jumper's knee). Pain is over the patellar tendon. Treatment is rest, ice application, and stretching exercises. Corticosteroid injections are contraindicated due to the risk of tendon rupture. **Popliteal tendinitis** causes posterolateral knee pain. The quadriceps and patellar tendons may rupture due to trauma and repetitive injuries and in patients with RA and SLE and those who are receiving corticosteroids. Sudden pain and inability to extend the knee result. **Iliotibial band syndrome** is due to inflammation of the thickened part of the fascia lata that inserts over the lateral tibial condyle. It causes lateral knee pain and is common in runners.

Patellofemoral pain syndrome is characterized by pain in the patellar region that is worse with stair climbing or knee flexion. Stiffness after prolonged sitting is common. The pain is reproduced when the patella is held immobile while the patient contracts the quadriceps muscle. Bilateral symptoms in young patients may be due to **chondromalacia patellae.** Rest, ice, and taping of the knee may alleviate the pain.

Popliteal cysts (Baker's cysts) may be asymptomatic or cause swelling in the popliteal fossa area. Cysts may be seen in patients with OA or RA and often communicate with the knee joint cavity. Large popliteal cysts may rupture and cause pain, swelling, and erythema of the calf, mimicking venous thrombosis. Ultrasound is diagnostic in these cases. Aspiration and injection with corticosteroids are indicated for symptomatic cysts.

Osgood-Schlatter disease is seen in adolescents and presents with pain at the site of the insertion of the patellar tendon to the tibial tuberosity. It usually resolves as the patient grows older.

ANKLE AND FOOT PAIN

Ankle and foot pain are common problems and may be due to periarticular disorders, arthritis, or trauma and are often worsened by inappropriate footwear. The history and physical exam usually lead to a diagnosis. A history of diabetes, peripheral neuropathy, or peripheral vascular disease is particularly important. The physical exam should include inspection (looking for deformities, abnormal calluses), palpation (of tender areas), testing of sensation, and evaluation of distal pulses. Examine the patient's footwear: signs of abnormal (or unilateral) wear or frequent use of high heels or narrow pointed shoes are important clues. Radiographs are rarely useful except in cases of trauma. Treatment of foot and ankle pain is conservative. Rest, stretching exercises, and NSAIDs are frequently used. Orthoses and appropriate footwear are an essential part of care in many cases. Assistance from podiatrists and orthotists is invaluable.

Arthritis frequently affects the ankle and foot. **OA** spares the ankle but often involves the first MTP joint causing inward deviation (**hallux valgus** or **bunion**). Patients are more commonly women and complain of pain and deformity of the great toe. A shoe with a wide toe box provides symptomatic relief but surgery is often performed for cosmetic reasons. **RA** affects the ankle and forefoot in the majority of patients. Bilateral ankle pain and synovitis and forefoot pain usually accompanies other joint involvement. The first MTP is the most commonly affected joint in acute **gout.** Tophi and deformities may be seen in chronic gout. Motor, sensory, and autonomic neuropathy (seen in diabetic and other peripheral neuropathies) may lead to ankle and foot pain and severe deformity in **neuropathic arthropathy.**

Ankle sprains are very common in outpatients and usually follow ankle inversion after a misstep or fall. According to the Ottawa guidelines, **obtain radiographs** to rule out fracture in patients with medial or lateral malleolar tenderness or with inability to bear weight after the event or in the ER [8]. **Stress fractures** are common causes of foot pain and occur as a result of overuse. They are often seen in dancers, runners, or military recruits and affect the second or third metatarsals most frequently. Radiographs sometimes do not detect stress fractures. Bone scan or MRI may be used for diagnosis. Treatment is usually conservative.

Plantar fasciitis is the most common cause of plantar foot pain and is due to inflammation of the plantar fascia at its insertion into the calcaneus. Pain is worse in the morning and after prolonged standing or walking and may be severe. It may be idiopathic or due to overuse and is sometimes seen in patients with seronegative spondyloarthropathies. Stretching exercises, heel inserts, NSAIDs, and occasionally corticosteroid injections are used.

Achilles tendinitis occurs when the Achilles tendon may become inflamed due to trauma or overuse (dancers, runners). Heel pain due to Achilles tendon enthesopathy is characteristic of the seronegative spondyloarthropathies. The tendon may rupture due to trauma or spontaneously in patients taking corticosteroids. Injection of the Achilles tendon with corticosteroids may also lead to rupture. Patients with tendon rupture have difficulty walking and foot dorsiflexing. Treatment of Achilles tendinitis is conservative, but rupture requires surgical evaluation. Inflammation of the **retrocalcaneal bursa** may be difficult to distinguish from Achilles tendinitis. **Posterior tibial tendinitis** causes pain behind the medial malleolus and **peroneal tendinitis** causes pain anterior to the lateral malleolus.

Tarsal tunnel syndrome is characterized by pain, numbness, and paresthesias of the sole. The posterior tibial nerve is compressed at the flexor retinaculum, posterior to the medial malleolus. Tapping over the nerve may reproduce symptoms. Corticosteroid injections are helpful but should be done carefully. Surgical decompression may be needed.

Morton's neuroma is due to compression of the interdigital nerve between the third and fourth toes. It causes forefoot pain and numbness and tingling of these toes. It occurs more frequently in middle-aged women and is exacerbated by walking and by wearing tight shoes or high heels. Properly fitting footwear or a metatarsal pad is helpful. Corticosteroid injections are sometimes used for relief. Some patients require surgery. **Metatarsalgia** (pain arising from the metatarsal heads) may be due to high heels, everted foot, arthritis, trauma, or deformities and is quite common. Proper footwear and a metatarsal pad are helpful.

SUGGESTED READING

Deyo RA, Diehl AK. Cancer as a cause of back pain: frequency, clinical presentation and diagnostic strategies. *J Gen Intern Med* 1988;3:230–238.

Hadler NM. *Occupational musculoskeletal disorders*, 2nd ed. Philadelphia: Lippincott Williams & Wilkins, 1999.

Pryse-Phillips W. Validation of a diagnostic sign in carpal tunnel syndrome. *J Neurol Neurosurg Psychiatry* 1984;47:870–872.

REFERENCES

1. Deyo RA, Rainville J, Kent DL. What can the history and physical examination tell us about low back pain? *JAMA* 1992;268:760–765.
2. Deyo RA, Weinstein JN. Low back pain. *N Engl J Med* 2001;344:363–370.
3. Boden SD, Davis DO, Dina TS, et al. Abnormal magnetic resonance scans of the lumbar spine in asymptomatic subjects: a prospective investigation. *J Bone Joint Surg Am* 1990;72:403–408.
4. Weishaupt D, Zanetti M, Hodler J, et al. MR imaging of the lumbar spine: prevalence of intervertebral disk extrusion, and sequestration, nerve root compression, end plate abnormalities, and osteoarthritis of the facet joints in asymptomatic volunteers. *Radiology* 1998;209:661–666.

5. D'Arcy CA, McGee S. Does this patient have carpal tunnel syndrome? *JAMA* 2000;283:3110–3117.
6. Shoen RP, Moskowitz RW, Goldberg VM. *Soft tissue rheumatic pain: recognition, management, prevention*, 3rd ed. Philadelphia: Lea & Febiger, 1996.
7. Solomon DH, Simel DL, Bates DW, et al. Does this patient have a torn meniscus or ligament of the knee? *JAMA* 2001;286:1610–1620.
8. Stiell IG, McKnight RD, Greenberg GH, et al. Implementation of the Ottawa ankle rules. *JAMA* 1994;271:827–832.

Drugs Used in the Treatment of Rheumatic Diseases

Erin M. Christensen

INTRODUCTION

Despite the many rheumatic diseases and syndromes, there are only a few classes of drugs available for their treatment. Multiple agents directed at various pathophysiologic targets are often used to achieve different therapeutic effects. The information that follows provides a brief review of the therapeutic classes of agents as well as more specific information about individual agents.

MANAGEMENT

Analgesics

Inflammation is common among rheumatic diseases. Simple analgesics (Table 9-1) do not have an effect on inflammation; therefore, their role in the treatment of these diseases is small. However, the treatment of OA is an exception. Inflammation does not have a large role in the pathophysiology of OA, and because analgesics are generally well tolerated, they are often considered first-line therapy. The goal of therapy with these agents is simply the relief of pain.

NSAIDs/Selective Cyclooxygenase-2 Inhibitors

As mentioned previously, inflammation is common among rheumatic diseases. It is for this reason that NSAIDs and the related selective COX-2 inhibitors (Table 9-2) have such a prominent role in therapy. These agents have both analgesic and antiinflammatory properties, making them ideal agents for use in many of the rheumatic diseases. *Antiinflammatory agents alone are not effective in altering disease progression.* Therefore, they are often used in combination with other agents. The primary mechanism of action of the NSAIDs is the reduction of prostaglandin synthesis by inhibition of the cyclooxygenase enzymes COX-1 and COX-2. These agents are indicated for reduction of pain and inflammation.

The related selective COX-2 inhibitors preferentially inhibit COX-2, an inducible isoenzyme that is involved in inflammation. In contrast, the COX-1 enzyme is present in most tissues and is expressed constitutively rather than inducibly. The inhibition of COX-1 is thought to be responsible for the GI, platelet, and renal toxicity associated with traditional NSAIDs. Therefore, under ideal conditions, selective COX-2 inhibitors would reduce inflammation and pain with a lower risk of adverse events commonly associated with NSAIDs. Indeed, there is a lower incidence of GI adverse events with the selective COX-2 inhibitors. Like the NSAIDs, the selective COX-2 inhibitors are indicated for the reduction of pain and inflammation.

It is important to note that patient response to both NSAIDs and COX-2 inhibitors is variable. Base the selection of a specific agent on individual patient history and preference, compliance, and cost. It is not uncommon for a patient to respond to one agent but not another; therefore, treatment failure with one or even two agents does not preclude a trial of an alternative NSAID or COX-2 inhibitor.

TABLE 9-1. ANALGESICS

Drug	Brand name(s)	Dosage (PO)	Mechanism	Side effects	Contraindications and precautions
Acetaminophen	Aspirin-free Anacin, Excedrin, Panadol, Tylenol	325–650 mg q4–6h or 1000 mg q6–8 h; max: 4 g/day	Inhibition of prostaglandin synthesis in CNS	Generally well tolerated. Liver or kidney damage can occur with chronic use, especially high dose or in combination with alcohol. INR elevation can occur when large doses are given with warfarin.	Chronic alcohol use, liver disease, glucose-6-phosphate dehydrogenase deficiency, concomitant warfarin
Tramadol	Ultram	50–100 mg q4-6h	Binds to opiate receptors in CNS in addition to inhibiting reuptake of norepinephrine and serotonin	Dizziness, headache, fatigue, nausea, vomiting.	History of alcohol or drug abuse, chronic respiratory disease, liver disease, concomitant administration of TCAs, MAOIs, SSRIs, history of seizure disorder

TABLE 9-2. NSAIDS AND SELECTIVE COX-2 INHIBITORS

Classification	Drug	Brand name(s)	Dosage (PO, adult dose unless indicated)	Mechanism	Side effects	Contraindications and precautions
Carboxylic acid: acetylated[a]	Aspirin	Anacin, Ascriptin, Bayer, Bufferin, Ecotrin, Empirin, Excedrin	2400–5400 mg/day in 4 divided doses	Inhibition of prostaglandin synthesis through inhibition of COX-2	Abdominal pain, nausea, GI ulceration, increased risk of bleeding, liver or kidney toxicity (increased risk in combination with alcohol), sodium and water retention, HTN, hypersensitivity, tinnitus	History of hypersensitivity to related agents, bleeding disorder, asthma, peptic ulcer disease, hepatic or renal insufficiency, chronic alcohol use, HTN, congestive heart failure
Carboxylic acid: non-acetylated salicylates[a]	Salsalate	Amigesic, Artha-G, Disalcid, Mono-Gesic, Salflex, Salsitab	3 g/day in 2–3 divided doses			
	Diflunisal	Dolobid	500–1500 mg/day in 2 divided doses			
	Choline salicylate	Arthropan	870–1740 mg/dose given qid			
	Choline magnesium trisalicylate	Tricosal, Trilisate	1–3 g/day in 2–3 divided doses			

(continued)

TABLE 9-2. CONTINUED

Classification	Drug	Brand name(s)	Dosage (PO, adult dose unless indicated)	Mechanism	Side effects	Contraindications and precautions
Carboxylic acid: acetic acids	Etodolac	Lodine, Lodine XL	Immediate release: 800–1200 mg/day in 2–4 divided doses Sustained release: 400–1000 mg once daily			
	Diclofenac	Cataflam, Voltaren, Voltaren XR	Immediate release: 100–200 mg/day in 2–3 divided doses Sustained release: 100–200 mg once daily			
	Diclofenac and misoprostol[b]	Arthrotec	150–200 mg/day (diclofenac) in 3 divided doses			
	Indomethacin	Indocin, Indocin SR	Immediate release: 50–200 mg/day in 2–3 divided doses Sustained release: 75 mg once or twice daily			
	Ketorolac[c]	Toradol	PO: 10 mg q4–6h; IM/IV: 30–60 mg × 1, followed by 15–30 mg q6h			
	Nabumetone	Relafen	1000–2000 mg in 1–2 divided doses			
Propionic acids	Fenoprofen	Nalfon	900–3200 mg/day in 3–4 divided doses			
	Flurbiprofen	Ansaid	200–300 mg/day in 2–4 divided doses			

	Drug	Brand	Dosing
	Ibuprofen	Motrin, Advil, Nuprin	OTC dose: 200–400 mg q4–6h; prescription dose: 1200–3200 mg/day in 3–4 divided doses
	Ketoprofen	Orudis KT (OTC), Actron (OTC), Orudis, Oruvail (extended release)	OTC dose: 12.5 mg q4–6h; prescription dose: 150–300 mg/day in 3–4 divided doses; Extended release: 200 mg once daily
	Naproxen	Naprosyn, Naprelan (extended release)	Immediate release: 500–1500 mg/day in 2–3 divided doses; Extended release: 750–1500 mg once daily
	Naproxen sodium	Aleve (OTC), Anaprox	OTC: 220 mg bid–tid; prescription: 550–1375 mg/day in 2–3 divided doses; may increase to 1650 mg/day for limited periods of time only
	Oxaprozin	Daypro	600–1800 mg/day; doses <1200 mg/day in 1–2 divided doses; doses >1200 mg/day in 2–3 divided doses
Fenamates	Meclofenamate	Meclomen	200–400 mg/day in 3–4 divided doses
	Mefenamic acid[a]	Ponstel	250 mg q6h
Oxicams	Meloxicam	Mobic	7.5–15 mg once daily
	Piroxicam	Feldene	10–20 mg/day

(continued)

TABLE 9-2. CONTINUED

Classification	Drug	Brand name(s)	Dosage (PO, adult dose unless indicated)	Mechanism	Side effects	Contraindications and precautions
Selective COX-2 inhibitors[e]	Celecoxib[e]	Celebrex	OA: 100–200 mg/day in 1–2 doses; RA: 200–400 mg/day in 2 divided doses	Preferential inhibition of COX-2 enzyme resulting in decreased prostaglandin production		
	Valdecoxib[e]	Bextra	10–20 mg once daily			
	Rofecoxib	Vioxx	12.5–25 mg once daily; 50 mg daily for acute pain up to 5 days			

OTC, over the counter.

[a]Salicylate level may be used to monitor therapy (target level is 15–30 mg/dL).

[b]Risk of gastric ulcer is decreased relative to other traditional NSAIDs.

[c]Not indicated for use exceeding 5 days due to increased risk of side effects including GI bleed; adjust dose based on weight and age.

[d]Not indicated for use exceeding 1 wk.

[e]Caution in patients with a history of hypersensitivity to sulfonamides.

Corticosteroids

Corticosteroids (Table 9-3) are often used in the treatment of rheumatic disease because of their profound antiinflammatory activity. However, they also have a significant side effect profile. The incidence of adverse effects increases with higher doses and prolonged use. Therefore, their use is often minimized when possible. Despite controversy over their long-term use and the risks involved with therapy, corticosteroids maintain a large role in the treatment of rheumatic diseases.

The dosage of individual agents depends on the condition treated. Refer to individual chapters for more specific dosing information. Regimens also vary depending on individual treatment history and response to therapy. Long-term, supraphysiologic doses may induce hypothalamic-pituitary-adrenal axis suppression. To reduce the risk of adrenal insufficiency, it is important to avoid abrupt discontinuation of therapy if a patient has been on supraphysiologic doses for more than a few days.

Disease-Modifying Antirheumatic Drugs

In treatment of RA, *disease-modifying antirheumatic drugs* (DMARDs) (Table 9-4) is a term used to describe a group of agents that exert antiinflammatory or immunosuppressant activity. These agents are generally started early in RA in an effort to prevent or slow disease progression. This group consists of agents that work by various mechanisms, exert different pharmacologic effects, and typically have a slow onset of action. These agents are often associated with severe toxicities, making appropriate monitoring essential. In addition to their use in RA, DMARDs are commonly used as "steroid-sparing drugs" for other diseases.

Biologic Agents

A newer group of agents, known as *biologic agents* (Table 9-5), has recently been introduced. Three new agents block the proinflammatory cytokine tumor necrosis factor (TNF)-alpha, thereby reducing inflammation and preventing structural damage to joints. Another biologic agent available is the interleukin (IL)-1 receptor antagonist Anakinra (Kineret). Further agents are under development.

Agents for Gout and Hyperuricemia

A variety of agents are available to treat gout and hyperuricemia (Table 9-6). It is important to identify the goal of treatment when selecting an agent. Some agents are used to treat acute gouty attacks, whereas others are used to prevent recurrent attacks or complications of hyperuricemia. In addition to the agents listed in Table 9-6, NSAIDs are commonly used to treat acute attacks. Refer to Table 9-2 for information on individual agents.

OSTEOPOROSIS

Patients with rheumatic disease are often at a higher risk for osteoporosis (Table 9-7), especially patients exposed to long-term corticosteroids. All patients should receive calcium and vitamin D supplementation. Other treatment options include hormone replacement therapy, bisphosphonates, and calcitonin. New agents directed at bone formation through the action of PTH are also now available.

TABLE 9-3. CORTICOSTEROIDS

Drug	Brand name(s)	Approximate equivalent doses (PO)	Mechanism	Side effects	Contraindications and precautions
Cortisone	Cortone acetate	25 mg	Inhibit inflammatory and immune cascade through multiple actions	HTN, increased appetite, GI upset, elevated blood glucose, psychosis, insomnia, immunosuppression, Cushing's syndrome (weight gain, buffalo hump, moon-face, thin skin), osteoporosis, cataracts	Infection, HTN, peptic ulcer disease, diabetes
Dexamethasone	Decadron, Dexameth, Hexadrol	0.75 mg			
Hydrocortisone[a]	Cortef, Hydrocortone	20 mg			
Methylprednisolone[a]	Medrol, Solu-Medrol, Depo-Medrol	4 mg			
Prednisolone[a]	Prelone, Pediapred	5 mg			
Prednisone	Deltasone, Orasone	5 mg			
Triamcinolone[a]	Artisocort, Kenalog	4 mg			

[a]May be given via intraarticular injection.

TABLE 9-4. DISEASE-MODIFYING ANTIRHEUMATIC DRUGS AND OTHER IMMUNOSUPPRESSANTS

Drug	Brand name(s)	Mechanism	Dosage	Side effects	Contraindications and precautions	Monitoring
Cyclophosphamide	Cytoxan	Interferes with DNA synthesis	PO: 1–2 mg/kg/day. IV: 0.5–1 g/m² (for lupus nephritis q1–3mos).	Hemorrhagic cystitis, infection, immunosuppression, malignancy, infertility	Renal or hepatic insufficiency, immunosuppression, infection. FDA pregnancy category: D	CBC and urinalysis weekly until dose is stable, then monthly. IV: check nadir 10–14 days post-dose
Hydroxychloroquine	Plaquenil	Inhibits lysosomal enzymes, impairs complement-dependent antigen–antibody reactions	PO: 6–7 mg/kg/day in 1–2 divided doses; max dose 400 mg/day.	Indigestion, skin rash, visual changes, retinopathy, neuromyopathy, bone marrow suppression	History of hypersensitivity or visual changes on related therapy, hepatic disease, G-6-PD deficiency, psoriasis, macular degeneration. FDA pregnancy category: C	Ophthalmologic exam q6–12mos
Leflunomide	Arava	Inhibits pyrimidine synthesis	PO: 10–20 mg/day.	LFT elevation, diarrhea, rash, alopecia	Pregnancy, hepatic disease, immunosuppression, renal impairment, infection. FDA pregnancy category: X	ALT monthly initially, then q4–8wks
Methotrexate	Rheumatrex, Trexall	Inhibits dihydrofolate reductase thereby inhibiting DNA synthesis; inhibits adenosine pathway	Oral/IM/SC: 7.5–25 mg weekly.	Anorexia, nausea, and mouth sores (incidence reduced by administration of 1 mg qd folic acid), LFT elevation	Renal or hepatic impairment, liver disease, chronic alcohol use, preexisting bone marrow suppression, pregnancy. FDA pregnancy category: D	Baseline CBC, creatinine, LFTs, and albumin, then q4–8wks. Liver biopsy if LFTs persistently elevated

(continued)

TABLE 9-4. CONTINUED

Drug	Brand name(s)	Mechanism	Dosage	Side effects	Contraindications and precautions	Monitoring
Sulfasalazine	Azulfidine	Reduces lymphocyte response	PO: 500 mg–3 g/day in 2 divided doses (start with 500 mg once daily, titrate to goal of 1 g bid; may increase to 3 g/d if needed).	Skin rash, nausea, abdominal pain, diarrhea, photosensitivity, headache, LFT abnormalities, blood dyscrasias	Hypersensitivity to sulfasalazine, sulfa, or salicylates, GI or GU obstruction, renal or hepatic insufficiency, G-6-PD deficiency FDA pregnancy category: B	CBC and LFT q2–4wks × 3 mos, q2–3mos thereafter
Azathioprine	Imuran	Interferes with DNA synthesis and cellular metabolism	PO: 1–2 mg/kg/day.	Nausea, vomiting, diarrhea, rash, bone marrow suppression, infection, hepatitis, malignancy	Pregnancy, renal or hepatic impairment, immunosuppression FDA pregnancy category: D	CBC and LFTs q1–2wks until dose is stable, then monthly
Cyclosporine	Sandimmune, Neoral, Gengraf	Inhibits production and release of cytokines (e.g., IL-2) from lymphocytes	Sandimmune: 2–5 mg/kg/day in 2 divided doses PO; Neoral: 2–4 mg/kg/day in 2 divided doses PO.	HTN, nephrotoxicity, hirsutism, gingivitis, tremor	Renal or hepatic insufficiency, HTN, concomitant use with other nephrotoxic agents FDA pregnancy category: C	CBC, serum creatinine, BP qwk until stable, then q2–4wks

Drug	Brand	Mechanism	Dose	Adverse effects	Contraindications / FDA pregnancy category	Monitoring
Gold[a]						
Injectable (IM)		Inhibits T- and B-cell activity				
Sodium thiomalate)	Myo-chrysine, Aurolate		Initial 10-mg test dose followed by 25-mg dose during wk 2. Subsequent doses are 25–50 mg/wk. Interval may be extended after several months or after total cumulative dose of 1 g.	Skin rash, stomatitis, gingivitis, metallic taste, blood dyscrasias, proteinuria		CBC and UA weekly initially, then before every 2nd or 3rd injection
Aurothioglucose	Solganal					
Oral						
Auranofin	Ridaura		3–9 mg/day in 1–3 divided doses.	Diarrhea, rash, proteinuria	FDA pregnancy category: C	CBC and UA q2–4 wks
Penicillamine	Cuprimine, Depen	Inhibits T-cell activity, impairs antigen presentation	PO: 125–250 mg daily, may increase by 125–250 mg q1–2mos (max 750 mg/day).	Skin rash, arthralgia, proteinuria, hematuria, neutropenia, thrombocytopenia, DIL	History of hypersensitivity to penicillamine, renal insufficiency, concomitant administration with other hematopoietic-depressant drugs, pregnancy FDA pregnancy category: D	CBC and urinalysis q2wks × 6 mos, monthly thereafter

(continued)

TABLE 9-4. CONTINUED

Drug	Brand name(s)	Mechanism	Dosage	Side effects	Contraindications and precautions	Monitoring
Mycopheno-late mofetil	CellCept	Inhibits B- and T-lymphocyte proliferation by blocking purine synthesis	PO: 500–2000 mg daily in two divided doses.	Thrombocytopenia, leukopenia, anemia, neutropenia, HTN, infections, diarrhea, abdominal pain, nausea and vomiting, tremor, insomnia, malignancy	Hypersensitivity to drug, pregnancy, caution with GI, renal, liver, bone marrow disorders FDA pregnancy category: D	CBC performed weekly for the first mo, 2×/mo for the 2nd and 3rd mos, then 1×/mo for the first year Creatinine, electrolytes; LFTs q3mos

G-6-PD, glucose-6-phosphate dehydrogenase; GU, genitourinary; IL, interleukin; LFT, liver function test.
^aAvailability of injectable gold products is limited.

TABLE 9-5. BIOLOGIC AGENTS

Class	Drug	Brand name(s)	Dosage	Mechanism	Side effects	Contraindications and precautions
TNF-alpha blockers	Etanercept	Enbrel	SC injection: 25 mg 2×/wk	Soluble TNF receptor—administration results in inhibition of TNF-alpha	Injection site reactions, infection (including TB[a], headache, demyelinating disease, optic neuritis, transverse myelitis, SLE	Active infection, immunosuppression, demyelinating disease, latent or active TB
	Infliximab	Remicade	IV infusion: 3–10 mg/kg repeated at wks 2 and 6, followed by once q4–8wks	Human:murine chimeric anti-TNF mAb—administration results in inhibition of TNF-alpha	Infusion reactions, infection (including TB[a]), demyelinating disease, SLE	Known hypersensitivity to murine antibodies, infection, immunosuppression, demyelinating disease, latent or active TB
	Adalimumab	Humira	40 mg SC q2wks	Human anti-TNF mAb—administration results in inhibition of TNF-alpha	Injection site reactions, infection (including TB[a]), demyelinating disease, SLE	Active infection, immunosuppression, demyelinating disease, latent or active TB
IL-1 blockers	Anakinra	Kineret	SC injection: 100 mg daily	IL-1 receptor antagonist	Injection site reactions, infections (pneumonia), decreased neutrophil count	Acute or chronic infection, asthma

IL, interleukin; TNF, tumor necrosis factor.
[a]Evaluate risk for TB before initiation of therapy.

TABLE 9-6. AGENTS FOR GOUT AND HYPERURICEMIA

Drug	Brand name(s)	Dosage	Mechanism	Side effects	Contraindications and precautions
Allopurinol	Lopurin, Zurinol, Zyloprim	PO: 100–600 mg/day; adjusted to achieve target uric acid level <6 mg/dL.	Inhibition of uric acid synthesis by inhibiting xanthine oxidase.	Rash, pruritus, nausea, vomiting, LFT elevation, agranulocytosis, aplastic anemia.	Renal dysfunction, history of hypersensitivity, pregnancy.
				Risk of acute gout attack may be minimized if taken with colchicine during initiation.	Do not start during acute attack.
Colchicine	No brand name available	Acute attacks: PO 0.5–0.6 mg bid; prevention: 0.5–1.2 mg/day in 1–2 divided doses.	Reduces deposition of urate crystals by decreasing leukocyte motility, phagocytosis in joints and lactic acid production.	Diarrhea, nausea, vomiting, abdominal pain.	Renal or hepatic dysfunction, gastrointestinal or cardiac disorders, blood dyscrasias, pregnancy.
Colchicine and probenecid	ColBenemid, Col-Probenecid, Proben-C	1 tablet (0.5 mg colchicine and 500 mg probenecid) daily × 7 days, followed by 1 tablet bid.	Refer to individual agents.	Refer to individual agents.	Refer to individual agents.
Probenecid	Benemid, Probalan	PO: 250 mg bid × 7 days, increase dose by 500 mg/day q2–4 wks if necessary to maintenance dose of 500–3000 mg/day in 2–3 divided doses.	Promotes excretion of uric acid by competitively inhibiting reabsorption in proximal convoluted renal tubule.	Headache, anorexia, nausea, precipitation of acute gouty attack, flushing.	Renal insufficiency, urolithiasis, history of hypersensitivity, increased bleeding risk.
					Do not start during acute attack.
Sulfinpyrazone	Anturane	PO: 100–800 mg/day in divided doses.	Increases urinary excretion of uric acid.	Nausea, vomiting, abdominal pain, anemia, leukopenia, decreased platelet aggregation.	Renal insufficiency, urolithiasis, peptic ulcer disease, blood dyscrasias.
					Do not start during acute attack.

LFT, liver function test.

TABLE 9-7. OSTEOPOROSIS

Drug	Brand name(s)	Dosage	Mechanism	Side effects	Contraindications and precautions
Alendronate	Fosamax	Prevention: 5 mg once daily or 35 mg/wk. Treatment: 10 mg once daily or 70 mg/wk.	Inhibits bone resorption via actions on osteoclasts and osteoclast precursors	Esophagitis,[a] acid reflux, nausea, headache, pain	Hypocalcemia, renal impairment, GI abnormalities that delay esophageal emptying time, inability to sit or stand upright for 30 mins after dose
Calcitonin	Calcimar (injection) Miacalcin (nasal spray)	Injection: 100 IUs daily or qod. Nasal: 200 IUs daily, alternating nostrils.	Inhibits osteoclastic bone resorption	Diarrhea, local irritation at injection site, nausea, vomiting, abdominal pain	History of hypersensitivity
Calcium	Various products	1000–1500 mg/day (elemental calcium).	Supplementation	Rarely constipation or nephrolithiasis	History of nephrolithiasis, concomitant use with digoxin
Estrogen: conjugated	Premarin, Premphase, Prempro, Cenestin (synthetic)	0.625 mg/day in 28-day cycles in combination with progesterone for women with an intact uterus. Unopposed estrogen may be given only to women who have had a hysterectomy.	Supplementation, mimics natural estrogen to prevent bone loss	Breast tenderness, vaginal bleeding or spotting, fluid retention, weight changes, elevated BP; breast cancer	High risk for or history of estrogen-dependent cancer; family history of breast cancer, thromboembolic disorders, undiagnosed vaginal bleeding, hepatic disease
Estrogen: esterified	Estratab, Estratest	0.3–1.25 mg/day (see Estrogen: conjugated for cyclic dosing information).			

(continued)

71

TABLE 9-7. CONTINUED

Drug	Brand name(s)	Dosage	Mechanism	Side effects	Contraindications and precautions
Raloxifene	Evista	60 mg daily.	Selective estrogen receptor modulator; mimics estrogen to prevent bone loss	Hot flashes, weight gain, nausea, abdominal pain	Pregnancy, premenopausal women, thromboembolic disorders, concurrent use of hormone replacement therapy
Risedronate	Actonel	Treatment and prevention: 5 mg once daily or 35 mg once weekly.	Inhibits bone resorption via actions on osteoclasts and osteoclast precursors	Esophagitis,[a] acid reflux, nausea, headache, pain	Hypocalcemia, renal impairment, GI abnormalities that delay esophageal emptying time, inability to sit or stand upright for 30 mins after dose
Teriparatide	Forteo	20 μg SC injection once daily.	Active PTH peptide supplementation; stimulates bone formation and remodeling	Nausea, leg cramps, hypercalcemia, osteosarcoma (in animals)	Hypercalcemia
Vitamin D	Various products	400–800 IU/day (vitamin D_3).	Supplementation	Rarely, nausea, vomiting, and diarrhea have been reported	Hypercalcemia

Note: All dosages PO unless otherwise specified.

[a]The importance of patient education to enhance efficacy and help reduce side effects cannot be overemphasized. Patients should take these medications first thing in the morning with a full 8 oz of water. It is important not to eat, drink, or take any other medications before or within 30 mins of administration to enhance absorption of the agent. Tell the patient to remain sitting or standing for 30 mins after administration to reduce GI side effects associated with the bisphosphonates.

KEY POINTS

- Due to the severity of illnesses and the toxicities of agents used to treat rheumatic diseases, careful monitoring is necessary.
- Evaluate comorbidities, such as renal, liver, cardiac, and pulmonary function, before initiation of any drug and adjust dosing and monitoring accordingly.

SUGGESTED READING

Ad Hoc Committee on Clinical Guidelines. Guidelines for monitoring drug therapy in rheumatoid arthritis. *Arthritis Rheum* 1996;39:723–731.

Boh LE. Osteoarthritis. In: Dipiro JT, Talbert RL, eds. *Pharmacotherapy: a pathophysiologic approach*, 4th ed. Stamford, CT: Appleton and Lange, 1999:1441–1457.

Drug Facts and Comparisons. St. Louis, MO: *Facts and comparisons*, 2001.

Drugdex Editorial Staff. Micromedex, Inc., 2001.

Dunkin MA. 2001 Drug Guide. *Arthritis Today* 2001;15(7)[Suppl].

Lacy CF, Armstrong LL, Goldman MP, Lance LL. *Drug information handbook*, 8th ed. Hudson, OH: Lexi-Comp, 2000.

Schuna AA, Schmidt MJ, Pigarelli DW. Rheumatoid arthritis. In: Dipiro JT, Talbert RL, eds. *Pharmacotherapy, a pathophysiologic approach*, 4th ed. Stamford, CT: Appleton and Lange, 1999:1427–1440.

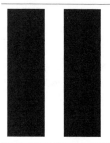

Common
Rheumatic
Diseases

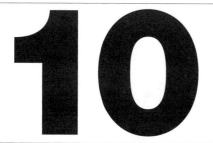

Rheumatoid Arthritis

Kevin M. Latinis

INTRODUCTION

RA is an *inflammatory arthritis* commonly presenting as a symmetric polyarthritis with significant morning stiffness. RA affects approximately 1% of the population and accounts for a significant degree of morbidity and increased mortality in affected patients. On rare occasions, RA is self-limiting but more often is chronic, disabling, and sometimes associated with systemic manifestations. RA occurs worldwide and increases in incidence with age. Women are affected approximately three times more often than men, and evidence supports a familial predisposition. Although the fundamental etiology of RA is still unknown, much has been elucidated in the understanding of how the inflammatory process leads to joint destruction. As a consequence, effective new therapies have been engineered to specifically target and disrupt end-organ damage.

CAUSES

Pathophysiology

The etiology of RA remains poorly understood. However, evidence supports an immune-mediated process leading to joint inflammation and destruction. Genetic studies have demonstrated links to major histocompatibility class II molecules, in particular HLA-DRB1. RA is characterized by synovial inflammation with hyperplasia and increased vascularity (pannus formation) in addition to leukocytic infiltration. Several cytokines, including IL-1, IL-6, and TNF-alpha, have been found to be associated with the inflammatory cascade and provide targets for antiinflammatory therapy [1].

The pathogenesis of joint destruction in RA includes initial T-cell activation, lymphocyte proliferation, and angiogenesis in the synovial membrane. Next, neutrophils infiltrate the synovial fluid, leading to synovial membrane proliferation. The synovial membrane enlarges to become the pannus and begins to invade the cartilage and bone. Finally, proliferation of the pannus leads to more profound cartilage destruction, subchondral bone erosions, and periarticular ligament laxity. Cytokine-stimulated osteoclast activity also likely contributes to erosions and periarticular osteoporosis found with RA.

Differential Diagnosis

The differential diagnosis of inflammatory polyarthritis includes RA, crystalline arthritis, lupus, seronegative spondyloarthropathies, infectious arthritis, endocrine arthropathies, and adult-onset Still's disease (AOSD).

PRESENTATION

History

The presentation and course of RA is variable. Typically, patients present with an insidious onset of **symmetric joint pain, swelling, and morning stiffness** worsening

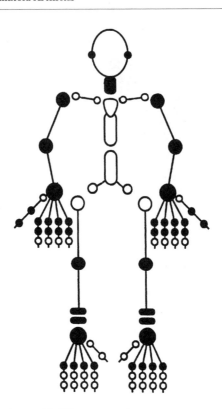

FIG. 10-1. Joint involvement in RA.

over several weeks. Less common presentations include acute, rapidly progressive polyarthritis and, more rarely, monoarthritis.

The most commonly involved joints include the **wrists, MCP joints, MTP joints, and PIP joints** (Fig. 10-1). Large joints can also be involved and include the shoulder, knee, ankle, elbow, and hip. The severity and duration of morning stiffness often correlate with the overall disease activity. Generalized malaise and fatigue also often accompany active inflammation.

Through the course of RA, patients often experience a waxing and waning pattern of synovitis coupled with progressive structural damage, leading to significant deformities and disabilities with advanced disease. Extensive joint damage can lead to functional limitations in joints as well as neurologic compromise, leading to symptoms of muscle weakness and atrophy.

Physical Exam

Physical findings in RA involve the identification of symmetric joint inflammation early in the course of the disease and manifestations of joint destruction with chronic disease. Active synovitis is characterized by warmth, swelling, pain, and palpable effusions. Range of motion can be restricted in joints with significant effusions, including deeper joints that may not demonstrate other signs of inflammation. Chronic joint destruction with significant degree of cartilage loss produces crepitus on palpation. Specific joint manifestations follow:

- The **wrists** are involved in most patients and, over time, can lead to radial-ulnar subluxation and subluxation of carpal bones with radial deviation. Synovitis at the wrist can lead to median nerve entrapment, resulting in CTS or, more rarely, ulnar nerve entrapment, resulting in Guyon's canal syndrome.
- In the **hands,** the MCPs are commonly involved and, with extensive damage, may lead to ulnar deviation of the hand. The PIP joints are often involved with sparing of DIP joints. Chronic inflammation with destruction of surrounding tendons can lead to Z-shaped thumb (hyperextension of first interphalangeal joint with palmar subluxation of first MCP), swan-neck (hyperextension at PIP, flexion at DIP), and boutonniere (flexion at PIP, hyperextension of DIP) deformities. Tenosynovitis of finger tendon sheaths can lead to nodule formation with subsequent catching or tendon rupture.
- **Elbow** involvement is evident by fullness at the radial-humeral joint with the tendency of patients to maintain the joint in flexion. Over time, this can lead to flexion contractures. Additionally, inflammation can lead to compressive neuropathy of the ulnar nerve with paresthesias and weakness in the ulnar distribution.
- Involvement of the **shoulder** usually manifests as loss of range of motion, with decreased abduction and limited rotation. Effusions are difficult to appreciate, because the shoulder joint lies underneath the rotator cuff. Pain in the shoulder can lead to limited range of motion, and adhesive capsulitis, or frozen shoulder, can develop rapidly.
- **Cervical spine** involvement with RA is common. Inflammation with involvement of the odontoid process, lateral masses, or tenosynovitis of the transverse ligament can lead to C1-C2 cervical instability. This may manifest with neck stiffness with decreased range of motion. Compression of cord, nerve roots, or vertebral arteries can occur, leading to neurologic compromise, and may require emergent stabilization. RA involvement of the thoracic and lumbar spine is rare.
- **Hip** involvement with RA is also common, but symptoms are often delayed. When present, exam findings include decreased range of motion and pain radiating to the groin, thigh, buttock, low back, or knee.
- Involvement of the **knee** includes detectable effusions and synovial thickening. Prolonged inflammation can lead to significant instability. Posterior herniation of the synovial capsule can result in a popliteal (Baker's) cyst, and rupture can mimic thrombophlebitis.
- Because of weight-bearing, RA involvement of the **foot and ankle** is often symptomatic. The joints most commonly affected include the MTP, talonavicular, and ankle joints. MTP joints can develop cocking-up deformities with subluxation of the MTP fat pads, causing pain with ambulation. Inflammation of the talonavicular joint and ankle joints results in eversion of the foot and can cause nerve entrapment, resulting in paresthesias of the sole.

With the discovery of more effective treatments, extraarticular manifestations of RA occur much less commonly than they did in previous decades. However, severe RA can manifest with sequelae of systemic inflammation, especially in RF-positive patients. Common extraarticular manifestations follow:

- **Skin** manifestations include formation of SC rheumatoid nodules and vasculitic skin ulcerations. Rheumatoid nodules typically form during active inflammation over pressure points in bursae and tendon sheaths. Common sites include the olecranon bursa, the extensor surface of the forearm, the Achilles tendon, and the tendons of the fingers.
- **Ocular** involvement usually involves sicca symptoms of dry eyes (and dry mouth) but can include episcleritis or a more concerning scleritis.
- **Pulmonary** involvement of RA may include interstitial fibrosis or pulmonary nodules. Interstitial fibrosis generally involves the lower lung fields and is often not clinically symptomatic, but it may be severely debilitating in some cases. Pleurisy and pleural effusions may also develop due to inflammation of the pleura.
- **Neurologic** manifestations of RA are usually related to nerve entrapment or cervical spine instability. Vasculitis of vasa vasorum can lead to symptoms of mononeuritis multiplex.

TABLE 10-1. AMERICAN COLLEGE OF RHEUMATOLOGY CRITERIA FOR THE DIAGNOSIS OF RA

1. Morning stiffness. Patients typically have morning stiffness lasting for >1 hr.
2. Swelling of ≥ 3 joints (observed by a physician).
3. Symmetric distribution.
4. Involvement of the hand joints, especially the wrist, MCPs, and PIPs, sparing the DIPs.
5. Positive RF (found in 80% of patients with RA).
6. Rheumatoid nodules on extensor tendon surfaces, especially the olecranon.
7. Radiographic changes (periarticular osteopenia and erosions).

Note: For the diagnosis of RA, a patient should have at least four of the seven criteria. Criteria 1–4 must be present for ≥ 6 wks.

- **Cardiac** involvement may include pericardial effusions, pericarditis, valvular lesions, conduction defects, or myocardiopathy.
- **GI** and **renal** manifestations of RA are rare. Amyloidosis can sometimes occur, affecting these organs.
- **Hematologic** effects of RA usually include a hypochromic-microcytic anemia. Felty's syndrome is the triad of RA with neutropenia and splenomegaly.

MANAGEMENT

Workup

Diagnosis of RA involves the accumulation of clinical, lab, and radiologic features that develop over the course of the disease. Early RA is often difficult to diagnose definitively, yet it can usually be confirmed as the disease progresses. The American College of Rheumatology has provided criteria for the diagnosis of RA [2] (Table 10-1). These criteria were designed for inclusion and monitoring of patients in clinical studies and not for routine clinical diagnosis. However, they can serve as diagnostic guidelines for evaluation of patients with suspected RA. *In practice, a patient with symmetric, inflammatory polyarthritis of the small joints of the hands with a positive RF most likely has RA.*

Factors associated with a poor prognosis in RA include positive RF, multiple joints involved at presentation, radiographic changes at presentation, and extraarticular features such as vasculitis, Felty's syndrome, interstitial lung disease, ocular involvement, or pericarditis [3].

According to the American College of Rheumatology, the baseline evaluation of patients with RA should include the following: assessment of the degree of joint pain, duration of morning stiffness, presence or absence of fatigue, and limitation of function. Physical exam should include documentation of actively inflamed joints, mechanical joint problems (loss of motion, crepitus, instability, malalignment, and deformity), and extraarticular manifestations. Lab evaluation should include a baseline CBC, electrolyte panel, creatinine, hepatic panel, UA, and stool occult blood to assess general organ function and comorbidities before initiating medications. Draw an RF (see Chap. 5, Lab Evaluation of Rheumatic Diseases) at baseline and repeat 6–12 mos later if initially negative; it is not necessary to monitor RF throughout the course of the disease. ESR and CRP are markers of inflammation and may be useful to monitor disease activity, although they are not specific for RA. Finally, perform radiographs of involved joints. These may be uninformative early in disease but can be used to monitor disease progression and treatment responses (refer to Chap. 6, Radiographic Evaluation of Rheumatic Diseases). Of note, x-rays of feet are more likely to show erosions with early RA than hands.

Treatment

The goals of treatment of RA are to alleviate pain, control inflammation, preserve and improve activities of daily living, and prevent progressive joint destruction. Early recognition of disease and pharmacologic treatment provide the cornerstone for management of RA. Medical treatment includes the use of NSAIDs, DMARDs, and corticosteroids. Equally important in the management of RA is nonpharmacologic treatment, including patient education, physical therapy, occupational therapy, orthotics, and surgery.

The use of **NSAIDs** in high doses can help alleviate symptoms from pain and inflammation in most patients with RA. Closely monitor toxicities, especially GI ulcerations and renal dysfunction. Some patients may benefit from selective COX-2 inhibitors that have documented reduced GI toxicities [4,5] or addition of GI prophylaxis in the form of misoprostol or proton pump inhibitors. NSAIDs do not prevent progression of bone and cartilage damage; therefore, current treatment strategies recommend NSAID use in combination with DMARDs for initial therapy. For details on dosing, toxicities, and monitoring of specific agents see Chap. 9, Drugs Used in the Treatment of Rheumatic Diseases.

DMARDs can slow or arrest the progression of RA. Institute DMARDs early (within the first few months of diagnosis). Evidence indicates that outcomes are improved for patients treated more aggressively at presentation. Therefore, initiation of therapy with NSAIDs and DMARDs simultaneously is recommended. Many of the DMARDs have significant potential toxicities and may take several months to attain optimal clinical benefit; therefore, careful monitoring for side effects and symptom relief is required. For severe disease flares, the use of oral corticosteroids may also be necessary while waiting for optimal benefit from DMARDs. Following is a list of commonly used DMARDs with associated toxicities and monitoring recommendations.

Oral **methotrexate** is considered to be the DMARD of choice for most patients. From a starting dose of 7.5–10 mg once/wk, the dose may be increased to 20–25 mg weekly over a period of 8–12 wks. If methotrexate is at least partially effective, continue it as other agents are added. Common side effects include stomatitis, nausea, and diarrhea. Supplementation with folic acid, 1–2 mg daily, can reduce such side effects without significantly reducing efficacy. Bone marrow suppression is uncommon, but it may occur at low doses in elderly patients. The risk of liver toxicity is increased by alcohol consumption, preexisting liver disease, and possibly by diabetes and obesity. Important contraindications to methotrexate therapy include liver disease, abnormal liver function tests, and regular alcohol consumption. Check liver function tests and blood counts every month until the dose is stable and every 2–3 mos thereafter. Perform a liver biopsy in patients with persistent elevation of liver transaminases or decrease in serum albumin to rule out methotrexate-induced hepatotoxicity.

Hydroxychloroquine is effective at doses of 400 mg/day, but do not give it to patients with renal or hepatic insufficiency. The risk of macular toxicity is extremely unusual if the dose does not exceed 6–7 mg/kg/day and rarely occurs before 6 yrs of treatment. Nonetheless, an ophthalmologist should perform a baseline exam and monitor the patient every 6–12 mos. Nausea and skin discoloration occur occasionally.

Initiate **sulfasalazine** at 500 mg twice daily and gradually increase to 2–3 g daily in divided doses. An enteric-coated preparation improves GI tolerability. Monitor for neutropenia and hepatotoxicity every 1–3 mos. GI intolerance due to nausea or abdominal pain may occur. Avoid sulfasalazine in patients with sulfa allergies or glucose-6-phosphate dehydrogenase deficiency.

Leflunomide is a pyrimidine synthesis inhibitor with efficacy comparable to methotrexate in treatment of RA [6]. Diarrhea, nausea, and hair loss are common side effects. Monitor liver functions every 1–3 mos. The effective starting dose is 20 mg/day. Loading doses are not necessary. Reduce the daily dose to 10 mg/day if the medication is not tolerated or if transaminase levels become elevated.

Cyclosporine is an inhibitor of T-cell activation with known clinical efficacy in treatment of RA. Efficacy is increased when used in combination with methotrexate. Cost and potential for severe renal toxicity, even in low doses, have limited its use to the treatment of severe, refractory RA. BP and renal function should be monitored closely.

TNF blockers are agents that inhibit the action of TNF-alpha and are emerging as potent medications for the treatment of RA. TNF blockers are well tolerated, and patients generally respond rapidly. They are typically administered in conjunction with methotrexate therapy. Serious infections have occurred rarely. Hence, do not give TNF blockers to patients with indolent chronic infections such as osteomyelitis or TB or to anyone with significant and active common infections. Temporarily suspend treatment with TNF inhibitors in patients undergoing surgery. Also, avoid or use TNF blockers with extreme caution in patients with congestive heart failure or significant coronary artery disease.

Etanercept is a genetically engineered human protein consisting of two molecules of the p75 TNF receptor. The usual dose is 25 mg SC twice/wk. Evidence suggests that treatment with etanercept alone is as effective as methotrexate in controlling symptoms and more effective in slowing the rate of bone erosion [7]. Rare cases of demyelinating disease, pancytopenia, SLE, congestive heart failure, TB, and atypical mycobacterial infections have been reported.

Infliximab is a chimeric human murine antibody specific for human TNF that is administered 3–10 mg/kg IV q1–2 mos. For RA, current recommendations are to co-administer infliximab with methotrexate. Cases of TB reactivation and development of demyelinating diseases have been reported.

Adalimumab is a fully human monoclonal antibody specific for TNF. It is administered at 40 mg SC q2wks. It has efficacy and toxicities similar to those of etanercept and infliximab. Studies support its use as monotherapy or with methotrexate.

Minocycline, a tetracycline antibiotic, has demonstrated moderate efficacy for the treatment of RA in several clinical trials. Its antiinflammatory effect is thought to be through inhibition of matrix metalloproteinases. From a starting dose of 50 mg bid, the dose can be increased to 100 mg bid. Dizziness is a common side effect.

Anakinra is an IL-1 receptor antagonist and is given daily in 100-mg SC injections. It has demonstrated favorable effects on limiting radiologic progression of RA and has shown dramatic clinical improvement in some patients [8]. Side effects include minor injection site reactions and respiratory infections.

Other DMARDs less commonly used to treat RA include **gold salts, azathioprine, penicillamine,** and **cyclophosphamide** (for rheumatoid vasculitis). For details on dosing, toxicities, and monitoring of specific agents see Chap. 9, Drugs Used in the Treatment of Rheumatic Diseases.

Combination regimens of multiple DMARDs or DMARDs plus biologic agents are increasingly popular treatment regimens. If tolerated, methotrexate should be part of every combination. Evidence indicates increased efficacy in the treatment of RA for the following combination regimens:

- Hydroxychloroquine, sulfasalazine, and methotrexate
- Cyclosporine and methotrexate
- Leflunomide and methotrexate [9]
- Etanercept and methotrexate [7]
- Infliximab and methotrexate [10]

Corticosteroids in low doses (prednisone, 5–10 mg) are extremely effective for promptly reducing the symptoms of RA and are useful in helping patients recover their previous functional status. Unfortunately, short courses of oral corticosteroids produce only interim benefit, and chronic therapy is often necessary to maintain symptom management. Corticosteroids are appropriate in patients with significant limitations in their activities of daily living, particularly early in the course of disease while awaiting the efficacy of slow-acting DMARDs. Make every effort to taper to the lowest possible dose and to eliminate steroid therapy when feasible. Toxicities of corticosteroids are well known and include weight gain, cushingoid features, osteoporosis (for details on treatment and prevention of osteoporosis related to corticosteroids, see

Chap. 50, Osteoporosis), AVN, infection, diabetes, HTN, and increases in serum cholesterol levels. Keeping the daily dose of prednisone at ≤5 mg can often reduce toxicities. Finally, avoid adrenal insufficiency by tapering corticosteroid doses slowly over several months.

Ancillary medical services can augment treatment strategies for patients with RA at any stage of disease. **Occupational therapy** usually focuses on the hand and wrist and can help patients with splinting, work simplification, activities of daily living, and assistive devices. **Physical therapy** assists in stretching and strengthening exercises for large joints such as the shoulder and knee, gait evaluation, and fitting with crutches and canes. Moderate exercise is appropriate for all patients and can help reduce stiffness and maintain joint range of motion. In general, an exercise program should not produce pain for >2 hrs after its completion. **Orthopedic surgery** to correct hand deformities and replace large joints such as the hip, knee, and shoulder may benefit patients with advanced disease. The primary indication for reconstructive hand surgery is refractory functional impairment limiting activities of daily living. Total joint arthroplasty to replace the knee or hip should also be considered when pain cannot be controlled adequately with medications or joint instability causes significant fall risk.

Follow-Up

The course of RA differs between patients. Whereas some patients may experience mild disease and have spontaneous remission, most suffer a chronic course with intermittent disease flares and progressive joint destruction. Monitor patients clinically on a frequent basis for disease progression or remission, response to therapy, and drug toxicities. Adjust drug therapies to attain the minimal effective doses with an emphasis on limiting use of chronic steroids. Mortality rates have been documented to be increased in RA patients with death related to comorbidities and drug toxicities, including infections, pulmonary and renal disease, and GI bleeding.

RELATED CONDITIONS

Palindromic rheumatism is a condition similar to RA in which patients develop recurrent onsets of acute, self-limited arthritis. Attacks usually last hours to a few days and may involve any set of joints. Lab tests are nonspecific, and synovial fluid analysis reveals an inflammatory reaction. Joint damage and systemic manifestations are rare. Diagnosis is based on the presence of a relapsing and remitting course of arthritis. Many patients with palindromic rheumatism later progress to develop RA. Treatment is similar to that for RA. NSAIDs may provide pain relief. Corticosteroids and some DMARDs may also be beneficial.

Relapsing seronegative symmetrical synovitis with pitting edema (RS3PE) is a condition usually characterized by sudden onset of polyarthritis associated with pitting edema of the hands and/or feet. Lab markers of inflammation are variable, and RF is absent. Synovitis is commonly present but rarely leads to joint destruction. Treatment involves the use of low-dose corticosteroids (prednisone, 5–10 mg), typically with dramatic improvement of symptoms. NSAIDs and hydroxychloroquine may also provide symptomatic relief and may be useful as steroid-sparing agents. RS3PE may be related to polymyalgia rheumatica and sometimes occurs in association with malignancies.

KEY POINTS TO REMEMBER

- Early diagnosis of RA and treatment with DMARDs is the current standard of care for RA.
- The goal of treatment of RA is clinical remission: absence of pain and synovitis and normalization of acute phase reactants.
- RA primarily affects the MCP and PIP joints of the hands in a symmetric distribution.
- RF, rheumatoid nodules, HLA-DR4, and extraarticular manifestations of RA predict a more severe disease course.

SUGGESTED READING

Guerne PA, Weisman MH. Palindromic rheumatism: part of or apart from the spectrum of rheumatoid arthritis. *Am J Med* 1992;93:451–460.

Guidelines for the management of rheumatoid arthritis 2002 Update. American College of Rheumatology Subcommittee on Rheumatoid Arthritis Guidelines. *Arthritis Rheum* 2002;46:328–346.

Harris ED Jr. Rheumatoid arthritis: pathophysiology and implications for therapy. *New Engl J Med* 1990;322:1277–1289.

Kremer JM. Rational use of new and existing disease-modifying agents in rheumatoid arthritis. *Ann Intern Med* 2001;134:695–706.

Olivieri I, Salvarani C, Cantini F. RS3PE syndrome: an overview. *Clin Exp Rheumatol* 2000;18:S53–S55.

REFERENCES

1. Choy HS, Panayi GS. Cytokine pathways and joint inflammation in rheumatoid arthritis. *N Engl J Med* 2001;344:907–916.
2. Arnett FC, Edworthy SM, Bloch DA, et al. The American Rheumatism Association 1987 revised criteria for the classification of rheumatoid arthritis. *Arthritis Rheum* 1988;31:315–324.
3. Pincus T, Callahan LF. Early mortality in RA predicted by poor clinical status. *Bull Rheum Dis* 1992;41:1–4.
4. Bombardier C, Laine L, Reicin A, et al. Comparison of upper gastrointestinal toxicity of rofecoxib and naproxen in patients with rheumatoid arthritis. VIGOR Study Group. *N Engl J Med* 2000;343:1520–1528.
5. Silverstein FE, Faich G, Goldstein JL, et al. Gastrointestinal toxicity with celecoxib vs nonsteroidal anti-inflammatory drugs for osteoarthritis and rheumatoid arthritis: the CLASS study: a randomized controlled trial. Celecoxib Long-term Arthritis Safety Study. *JAMA* 2000;284:1247–1255.
6. Strand V, Tugwell P, Bombardier C, et al. Function and health-related quality of life: results from a randomized controlled trial of leflunomide versus methotrexate or placebo in patients with active rheumatoid arthritis. Leflunomide Rheumatoid Arthritis Investigators Group. *Arthritis Rheum* 1999;42:1870–1878.
7. Martin JM, Fleischmann RW, Tesser RM, et al. A comparison of etanercept and methotrexate in patients with early rheumatoid arthritis. *N Engl J Med* 2000;343:1586–1593.
8. Jiang Y, Genant HK, Watt I, et al. A multicenter, double-blind, dose-ranging, randomized, placebo-controlled study of recombinant human interleukin-1 receptor antagonist in patients with rheumatoid arthritis: radiologic progression and correlation of Genant and Larsen scores. *Arthritis Rheum* 2000;43:1001–1009.
9. Cohen S, Cannon GW, Schiff M, et al. Two-year, blinded, randomized, controlled trial of treatment of active rheumatoid arthritis with leflunomide compared with methotrexate. *Arthritis Rheum* 2001;44(9):1984–1992.
10. Lipsky PE, van der Heijde DM, St. Clair EW, et al. Infliximab and methotrexate in the treatment of rheumatoid arthritis. Anti-Tumor Necrosis Factor Trial in Rheumatoid Arthritis with Concomitant Therapy Study Group. *N Engl J Med* 2000;343:1594–1602.

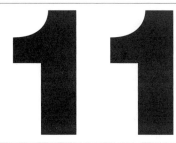

Osteoarthritis

Rebecca M. Shepherd

INTRODUCTION

OA was previously thought of as part of the natural aging process—hence the term "degenerative joint disease." Now it is known to be caused by multiple factors including genetics, biochemistry, inflammation, and mechanical forces. In 1995, 21 million people reported having OA. This number is an increase from that reported in 1985 and is thought to be secondary to the aging population rather than the change in definition. Arthritis is named the second leading cause for adults receiving Social Security Disability payments. The prevalence of OA increases with age so that, in men and women aged >60 yrs, the prevalence is 17% and 29.6%, respectively. The prevalence of knee OA as defined by radiographic exam of the tibiofemoral compartment was 33% in adults aged 63–93. An estimated 59.4 million Americans will be affected by some type of arthritis by the year 2020.

CAUSES

Pathophysiology

A list of types of OA follows:

- **Primary idiopathic:** either localized or generalized. The localized form affects one to two joint groups: DIP, PIP, or CMC joints of hands; cervical or lumbar spine; first MTP of feet; knees; and hips (Fig. 11-1). The generalized form involves three or more joint groups and is frequently associated with Heberden's nodes, which are bony enlargements of the DIP joints.
- **Secondary:** consider if patient develops OA in atypical joints, such as MCP joints of the hands, wrists, ankles, shoulders, or elbows (see Risk Factors).
- **Erosive OA:** also known as inflammatory OA; a severe form of OA or an entity of its own. Affects the DIP and PIP joints of the hand, with negative RF.

Cartilage failure in OA is caused by an imbalance of the dynamic degradative and repair processes within the cartilage, synovium, and bone. The contributing factors are multiple and complex. The most common instigating factor is macrotrauma or repeated microtrauma to normal cartilage. As a result of injury, chondrocytes release degradative cytokines and proteases; repair efforts in response are inadequate. Also contributing are multiple factors such as genetically defective cartilage, obesity, age, and secondary causes of OA such as endocrinopathies.

Differential Diagnosis

The following diagnoses must be considered when diagnosing OA: RA; seronegative spondyloarthropathies (e.g., PsA, ReA, AS, and enteropathic arthritis); crystalline arthropathies; infectious arthritis, including bacterial and viral etiologies; neoplastic synovitis (most common with blood dyscrasias); periarticular bursitis and tendonitis; and referred pain from a different joint.

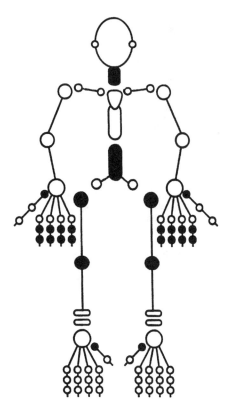

FIG. 11-1. Joint involvement in OA.

PRESENTATION

Risk Factors

Following is a list of risk factors for primary OA:

- Age: The prevalence of OA greatly increases with age.
- Gender: Women suffer from OA more often than men.
- Obesity: Association is present with knee, hand, and hip.
- High bone mass: Women with osteoporosis are less likely to have OA.
- Mechanical factors: Repeated use of the joint leads to degeneration of the joint. This is evident in previous joint injury; repeated movement in occupational OA, such as bending and squatting; and sports-related OA.
- Genetic: There is a genetic component in subsets of OA. Knee, hip, and hand OA are particularly susceptible to genetic influence. For example, "nodal" arthritis, such as Heberden's and Bouchard's nodes, has been associated with HLA-A1 and HLA-B8, although further supportive data are needed. Research suggests that collagen genes and genes encoding for extracellular matrix proteins may contribute to the development of OA. Stickler syndrome (premature OA associated with retinal and vitreous degeneration) is a known autosomal dominant form of early OA; familial chondrocalcinosis is also an autosomal dominant premature form of OA associated with deposition of calcium-containing crystals in the joint space.

Following is a list of risk factors for secondary OA:

- **Mechanical:** Posttraumatic and postsurgical joints are apt to develop OA more frequently; congenital anomalies are also a predisposing factor, with hip dysplasia accounting for up to 25% of OA cases in white patients.
- **Inflammatory diseases:** Joints affected by rheumatoid and infectious arthritis are at increased risk.
- **Metabolic disease:** Acromegaly, Paget's disease, Cushing's syndrome, crystal arthropathies, ochronosis, hemochromatosis, Wilson's disease, and steroid injections are predisposing factors.
- **Bleeding dyscrasias:** Pathologic causes, such as hemophilia, or iatrogenic causes, such as warfarin use, can lead to hemarthrosis.
- **Neuropathic joints:** as seen in diabetes, syphilis, spinal cord trauma, and Charcot's joint.

History and Physical Exam

Patients generally present after the age of 40. The most common presenting complaint in OA is pain. **The pain is mechanical in nature;** it is worse with activity, such as walking, and alleviated with rest. As disease progresses, stiffness can become a manifestation. Stiffness can occur after a period of inactivity, called a "gel" effect, and is alleviated within 30 mins; this is unlike RA, in which morning stiffness lasting >60 mins is a prominent symptom. Patients may complain of joints "locking," particularly the knees, which is due to loose material within the joint. Exam of the suspected joint may demonstrate tenderness to palpation, usually without evidence of inflammation. Crepitus, bony enlargement, decreased range of motion, joint effusion, and osteophytes along the periphery of the joint may be found. The joints most commonly involved are DIP and PIP joints, knees, hips, and spine. Consider secondary OA or another disease process if other joints are involved.

A list of specific joints follows:

- **Hands:** Hand involvement is common in OA and occurs in women more than in men. There is also a familial association. OA enlargements of the DIP and PIP joints are referred to as *Heberden's* and *Bouchard's nodes*, respectively. The first CMC joint is also commonly affected in OA and causes a squared-off appearance to the hand. Soft cysts can form on the dorsal aspect of DIP joints.
- **Feet:** The first MTP joint is often affected. Bursal inflammation occurs at the medial side of the metatarsal head, called a *bunion*. Hallux rigidus occurs with limitation of dorsiflexion of the big toe, which may impede ambulation. Involvement of the subtalar joint also causes difficulty with walking.
- **Knees:** Tenderness along the joint line may be present, as well as crepitus on placing a hand over the patella during range of motion. Osteophytes may be palpable. The medial and lateral compartments are most often affected in OA, with cartilage loss beginning in the medial aspect of the tibiofemoral joint. Medial and lateral compartment narrowing, called *genu varus* ("bow-legged") and *genu valgus* ("knock-kneed"), respectively, occurs secondary to malalignment. The patella may also be involved, with pain and tenderness anteriorly. Patients with chondromalacia patellae (patients aged 15–30 with patellar cartilage derangement) have a higher incidence of patellar OA.
- **Hips:** OA of the hips is most common in older patients and is present in men more than in women. Patients describe pain in the outer groin or inner thigh area; it may also radiate to the medial knee or distal thigh, buttocks, or sciatic region. OA pain must be differentiated from that of trochanteric bursitis, lumbosacral or knee OA, lumbar radiculopathy, herniation, and vascular insufficiency. On exam, internal rotation is diminished, with eventual loss of extension, abduction, and flexion. Contractures occur, and shortening of the limb may occur. A limp and, eventually, lordosis of the spine may develop in an effort to reduce hip pain on walking.
- **Spine:** Spinal involvement in OA is most common at spinal levels C5, T8, and L3, which represent the areas of greatest spinal flexibility. It is classified as OA or

spondylosis, which is OA that develops in conjunction with degenerative disk disease. OA occurs in the posterior apophyseal joints, with resultant joint space narrowing, sclerosis, and osteophyte formation. Spondylosis is characterized by degenerative changes of the disks and vertebral bodies. Pain occurs from local paraspinal ligament and muscle spasm or from radicular symptoms. Radicular symptoms of the cervical spine include neck pain with radiation to the shoulders, back, and extremities, and weakness and paresthesias of the upper extremities. Lumbar spine symptoms include low back pain with radiation down to the buttocks, legs, and feet. This pain increases with exertion. The physical exam in spinal OA is often unrevealing but may demonstrate decreased range of motion or local tenderness. Careful neurologic exam is important to detect radicular involvement.

- **Shoulder:** OA involvement of the shoulder is infrequent. When present, OA ranges from mild discomfort to complete joint destruction. Osteophytes located along the undersurface of the acromioclavicular joint may result in rotator cuff tendonitis or tears due to the juxtaposition of tendons with the inferior portion of the acromioclavicular joint.

MANAGEMENT

Diagnostic Workup

Radiographic evidence of OA is very common and does not necessarily correlate with symptomatic disease. The following features are often seen on radiographs of OA joints: joint space narrowing, subchondral sclerosis, osteophytes at the periphery of joints, and subchondral cysts.

There are no serologic markers for primary OA. Obtain blood work to rule out secondary causes of OA or differentiate between other arthritides, such as RA. RF, ESR, and CBC should all be normal; the RF may be mildly positive in elderly patients.

Synovial fluid is noninflammatory, clear, and transparent, with few WBCs (<2000 WBCs/μL).

The diagnosis of OA is based on the clinical picture and supported by radiologic and lab data. The American College of Rheumatology created guidelines that were originally designed as guidelines for clinical studies but are used to assist in the diagnosis of OA. There are limitations to these guidelines in that they pertain only to certain joints, the correlation between radiographic findings and clinical presentation is highly variable, and only patients with *idiopathic OA* are included.

- **Knee:** knee pain and osteophytes and one of the following: age >50, crepitus on motion, and stiffness lasting <30 mins.
- **Hand:** hand pain, aching, or stiffness, and at least three of the following: hard tissue enlargement of more than one of the selected joints (2nd and 3rd DIP or PIP; the 1st CMC joint of each hand), hard tissue enlargement of more than one DIP joint, deformity of at least one of ten selected joints, and fewer than three swollen MCP joints.
- **Hip:** hip pain and at least two of the following: ESR <20 mm/hr, radiographic acetabular or femoral osteophytes, and radiographic joint space narrowing.

Treatment and Follow-Up

The treatment of OA should be a multimodal approach to reduce pain and disability and improve quality of life. Treatment is not necessary during the asymptomatic phase of OA.

A **nonpharmacologic** approach includes

- Reduction of stress and load on the joint.
- Strengthening of surrounding periarticular muscles and maintaining joint stability and flexibility; patients can accomplish this with the aid of a trained physical therapist. Occupational therapy may be useful in symptomatic OA of the hand.

- Weight reduction.
- Patient education and self-help groups: Arthritis Foundation, 1-800-283-7800; www.arthritis.org.

Pharmaceutical therapies are addressed in the following sections.

Analgesics

Topical analgesics, such as capsaicin and salicylate, are effective in reducing pain in specific joints such as the knee, shoulder, elbow, and hand. They are most effective when used for intermittent isolated flares in those who cannot tolerate oral agents. **Acetaminophen** is indicated for pain control in those for whom nonpharmacologic agents have not worked. Dosing is safe at <4000 mg/day (or <2000 mg in patients with liver failure or alcohol use). This analgesic has no antiinflammatory effects. Many studies have confirmed the benefit of acetaminophen in treating OA, but whether it is equivalent to NSAIDs is controversial. Some studies demonstrate equivalent results in patient satisfaction, whereas others show a patient preference for NSAIDs. Hepatotoxicity is the most common side effect and occurs in those with concurrent liver damage from other processes (e.g., alcohol and infection with hepatitis C virus).

NSAIDs

Nonselective NSAIDs have had a long-standing, invaluable role in the treatment of OA. NSAIDs are given to those patients who cannot tolerate or who fail simple analgesic therapy. At low doses (e.g., ibuprofen 1200 mg daily), NSAIDs act as analgesics by inhibiting prostaglandin sensitization of peripheral pain receptors. At higher doses (e.g., ibuprofen, 2400 mg/day), NSAIDs inhibit the function of COX, which catalyzes the production of prostaglandins from arachidonic acid. Many different NSAIDs are used to control pain in patients with OA. Choosing an appropriate NSAID depends on such factors as efficacy, cost, frequency of dosing, prior adverse reactions, and comorbidities such as peptic ulcer disease or renal dysfunction. No specific class of NSAID is known to be superior to the others.

The following considerations may be helpful in prescribing an effective NSAID:

- A short-acting NSAID taken as needed is appropriate for episodic pain. Continuous therapy is indicated if prn dosing does not control the pain.
- If pain control is not adequate, maximize the dose of a specific NSAID before declaring treatment failure; 2–4 wks is a sufficient trial period.
- Be wary of the toxicity of NSAIDs such as
  - GI upset and bleed
  - Renal impairment in those with renal disease, heart failure, or diuretic use
  - Neurologic dysfunction, especially in the elderly population

Protection against GI toxicity. Several trials have recently investigated the use of gastroprotective agents in patients who take NSAIDs. In the OMNIUM study, treatment outcomes for ulcers, erosions, and gastric symptoms were similar between the group using misoprostol (Cytotec) and those using 20-mg and 40-mg omeprazole (Prilosec). Secondary prevention or "maintenance" was more successful with the omeprazole arm. The ASTRONAUT study demonstrated that omeprazole healed and prevented relapse in patients with both gastric and duodenal ulcers. Two previous trials demonstrated reduction in duodenal, but not gastric, ulcers with the use of ranitidine. The trials can be used to guide primary preventive therapy in high-risk patients, although large, controlled trials to date focus on secondary prevention.

Selective Cyclooxygenase-2 Inhibitors

Selective COX-2 inhibitors spare COX-1, which accounts for decreased GI toxicity. Celecoxib (Celebrex), rofecoxib (Vioxx), and valdecoxib (Bextra) are approved for the treatment of OA. Studies such as the VIGOR and CLASS trials demonstrate fewer GI complications of selective COX-2 inhibitors compared to those associated with nonselective inhibitors. Do not use COX-2 inhibitors in cases of renal disease, heart failure, or volume depletion.

Opiates

Although not routinely used as first-line agents, opiates can give significant relief to patients for whom NSAIDs are contraindicated or ineffective and surgery is not an option.

Corticosteroids

There is no indication for oral corticosteroid use in OA. Intraarticular steroid injections are indicated in patients who have pain in one or two joints and inadequate response to or inability to take NSAIDs. Steroids reduce biochemical turnover of the cartilage and osteophyte formation in animal models. Give injections only when infection is not suspected. Corticosteroids are frequently mixed with lidocaine and injected in crystalline form. The amount of steroid injected depends on the size of the joint. Generally, do not undertake intraarticular injections of the hips unless under fluoroscopic guidance. Give injections only 3–4 times yearly per joint.

Hyaluronic Acid

Intraarticular injection of hyaluronate into the knee joint can be effective in decreasing pain for several months. Two forms are currently available, Hyagen and Synvisc, for injecting intraarticularly in weekly doses for 3 and 5 wks, respectively. Intraarticular hyaluronate is FDA approved for knee OA.

Arthroscopic Irrigation

Arthroscopic irrigation may be indicated in patients who have OA of the knee or shoulder that is not controlled with NSAIDs or intraarticular corticosteroids. The procedure involves irrigating the joint with sterile normal saline to remove debris and crystalline material. The procedure is best performed with visual guidance to irrigate all compartments of the knee.

Surgical Intervention

When conservative measures are no longer effective at relieving pain or the joint becomes unstable, refer patients to surgical subspecialists. The aim of surgical intervention is to relieve pain and improve function of the joint via fusion or replacement of the joint with prostheses. Arthroplasty, or total joint replacement, provides significant pain relief; undertake it only in those patients who are medically stable enough to undergo surgical intervention and strenuous rehabilitation. Prostheses are expected to last 15 yrs, although obesity and higher activity levels increase the chance of prosthetic failure.

KEY POINTS TO REMEMBER

- OA is very prevalent and manifests with symptoms of mechanical joint pain.
- OA affects PIP, DIP, and first CMC joints of hands.
- Surgical referral is indicated with uncontrollable pain or joint instability.
- Nonpharmacologic approaches are useful and should be reinforced at each patient encounter.

SUGGESTED READING

Altman R, et al. The American College of Rheumatology criteria for the classification and reporting of osteoarthritis of the hip. *Arthritis Rheum* 1991;34:505.

Altman R, et al. The American College of Rheumatology criteria for the classification and reporting of osteoarthritis of the hand. *Arthritis Rheum* 1990;33:1601.

Bombardier C, et al. Comparison of upper gastrointestinal toxicity of rofecoxib and naproxen in patients with rheumatoid arthritis. *N Engl J Med* 2000;343:1520.

Creamer P, Hochberg MC. Osteoarthritis. *Lancet* 1997;350:503.

Hawkey CJ, et al. Omeprazole compared with misoprostol for ulcers associated with nonsteroidal antiinflammatory drugs. *N Engl J Med* 1998;338:727.

Moskowitz RW. Clinical and laboratory findings in osteoarthritis. In: Koopman WJ, ed. *Arthritis and allied conditions*. Baltimore: Williams & Wilkins, 1997:1985–2011.

National Arthritis Data Workgroup. Arthritis prevalence and activity limitation— United States, 1990. *MMWR Morb Mortal Wkly Rep* 1994;43:433.

Recommendations for the medical management of osteoarthritis of the hip and knee 2000 update. American College of Rheumatology subcommittee on osteoarthritis guidelines. *Arthritis Rheum* 2000;43:1905–1915.

Solomon L. Clinical features of osteoarthritis. In: Kelley WN, Hams ED, Ruddy S, Sledge CB, eds. *Textbook of rheumatology*. Philadelphia: WB Saunders, 1996: 1383.

Yeomans ND, et al. A comparison of omeprazole with ranitidine for ulcers associated with nonsteroidal antiinflammatory drugs. *N Engl J Med* 1998;338:719.

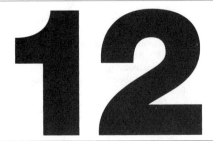

Systemic Lupus Erythematosus

Celso R. Velázquez

INTRODUCTION

SLE is a multisystem disease of unknown etiology. Clinical manifestations cover a spectrum from mild to life-threatening, and the course may be characterized by acute or chronic exacerbations and remissions. Patients with SLE have humoral and cellular immune abnormalities. Multiple autoantibodies, particularly ANAs, are present in the serum.

SLE occurs at any age but most commonly between 15 and 40 yrs. It is more frequent in women, with a female to male ratio of 8:1 in adults. Prevalence is approximately 1 case/1000 population, but it varies with race, ethnicity, and socioeconomic background.

CAUSES

Etiology and Pathophysiology

The etiology of SLE is unknown. Genetic, hormonal, immune, and environmental factors may play a role. There is a 50% concordance in monozygotic twins, and first-degree relatives have an increased frequency of autoantibodies. SLE may be associated with HLA-DR2 and -DR3. Hereditary deficiencies of C4 and C1q/r/s are strongly associated with susceptibility to the disease. The fact that SLE is much more common in women in their child-bearing years suggests a hormonal role. Abnormalities in the immune system include B- and T-lymphocyte hyperactivity and defects in immune system regulation, but they are incompletely understood. Exposure to ultraviolet light may increase disease activity in many patients. Tissue damage is mediated by autoantibodies (e.g., antibodies to cell-surface antigens causing cytopenias), by immune complex deposition with complement activation (as occurs in glomerulonephritis), and by thrombosis associated with antiphospholipid antibodies.

PRESENTATION

History and Physical Exam

SLE is highly variable in onset and in course. Early symptoms are frequently nonspecific (e.g., fatigue, malaise, arthralgias or arthritis, and fever). Severe manifestations (e.g., seizures or renal dysfunction) usually occur within the first few years after diagnosis or may appear at disease onset. Signs and symptoms in patients with SLE may be due to SLE, medication side effects, or unrelated intercurrent illnesses.

General Signs and Symptoms

Fatigue occurs in almost all patients with SLE. It may persist even in patients who are otherwise doing well. Fatigue may be due to anemia, infections, medications, or fibromyalgia. Weight loss is common before SLE is diagnosed. **Lymphadenopathy** is common and may increase with disease exacerbations. **Fever** is common in SLE and may be due to infection or disease activity. Fever as high as 41°C may be seen with active SLE. Always evaluate patients with SLE and fever for infection.

Musculoskeletal Signs and Symptoms

Arthralgias and arthritis are the most common presenting manifestations of SLE. Arthritis may involve any joint, but a symmetric arthritis of the small joints of hands, wrists, and knees is typical. "Swan neck" and "boutonniere" deformities are seen (see Chap. 2, Rheumatologic Joint Exam). Deformities are initially reducible but may become fixed. Joint erosions are rare. **AVN** is an important cause of disability in late SLE and may affect the hip, shoulder, and knee (see Chap. 51, Avascular Necrosis). AVN is usually painful and may be bilateral. Corticosteroid use is a risk factor for AVN. Early radiographs may be normal, but MRI is diagnostic. **Osteoporosis** is common and is worsened by steroid use (see Chap. 50, Osteoporosis). Myositis is rare, but myopathy secondary to corticosteroids or hydroxychloroquine can occur. **Fibromyalgia** is common in SLE (see Chap. 36, Fibromyalgia Syndrome).

Mucocutaneous Signs and Symptoms

Approximately half of patients are **photosensitive,** with skin and systemic manifestations exacerbated by sunlight. The classic **butterfly rash** develops in approximately 50% of patients and occurs in a malar distribution, sparing the nasolabial folds. The rash is usually erythematous but may be elevated and with fine scaling. Healing is generally without scarring. The **differential diagnosis** of a malar rash includes acne rosacea, seborrheic dermatitis, polymorphous light eruption, and contact dermatitis. **Subacute cutaneous lupus erythematosus** is an erythematous, papulosquamous, or annular lesion that commonly occurs on sun-exposed skin. It occurs in 10% of patients and is nonscarring. **Discoid lupus** begins as erythematous papules or plaques that become infiltrated and have an adherent scale. Follicular plugging is prominent. The lesions expand, leaving central hypopigmentation, atrophic scarring, and permanent alopecia. Some patients with discoid lupus lesions have positive ANA but have only a 10% chance of developing systemic lupus. **Mucous membrane** lesions include oral, vaginal, and nasal septal ulcers that may or may not be painful. **Alopecia** is common and may be diffuse or patchy. Livedo reticularis and vasculitis with palpable purpura and ulcerations may be present.

Renal Signs and Symptoms

The kidney is clinically involved in more than half of SLE patients during their disease course and is an important cause of morbidity. Patients may have asymptomatic abnormalities on urinalysis or present with nephritic or nephrotic syndromes. The **WHO classification** (Table 12-1) is based on findings on kidney biopsy. The clinical manifestations may overlap, but in general, classes III and IV have more severe nephritis and a poorer prognosis. These patients may benefit from aggressive immunosuppressive therapy. Decreased C3 levels and increased levels of double-stranded

TABLE 12-1. WHO CLASSIFICATION OF LUPUS NEPHRITIS

WHO classification	Clinical manifestations
I. Normal glomeruli	Asymptomatic
II. Mesangial disease	Low-grade hematuria or proteinuria
III. Focal proliferative glomerulonephritis	Nephritic urinary sediment (hematuria, casts), variable proteinuria (usually non-nephrotic)
IV. Diffuse proliferative glomerulo-nephritis	Nephritic and nephrotic syndromes, hypertension, variable renal insufficiency
V. Membranous nephropathy	Nephrotic syndrome
VI. Sclerosing nephropathy	Inactive urinary sediment, azotemia

DNA (DS-DNA) antibodies often correlate with lupus nephritis activity. **Kidney biopsies** are performed to assess disease activity and establish prognosis when the clinical picture is unclear and in patients with abnormal urinary sediments or proteinuria. Consider NSAID toxicity, uncontrolled HTN, and thrombotic thrombocytopenic purpura in patients with worsening renal function. SLE often becomes quiescent when patients develop renal failure. Manage end-stage lupus nephropathy with dialysis and transplantation. Recurrence of nephritis in allograft transplantation occurs in 5% of patients.

GI Signs and Symptoms
Symptoms such as anorexia, nausea, and vomiting are common. **Abdominal pain** may be due to peritoneal inflammation, but other causes of abdominal pain, including infection, thrombosis, medication side effects, appendicitis, peptic ulcer disease, and gastroenteritis, are more common. Mesenteric vasculitis presents with insidious abdominal pain or with infarction, bowel perforation, and peritonitis. Symptoms of peritonitis may be masked by corticosteroids. NSAIDs, azathioprine, and corticosteroids may cause pancreatitis. NSAIDs occasionally cause liver enzyme elevations.

Cardiovascular Signs and Symptoms
Pericarditis is the most common cardiac manifestation and presents with substernal chest pain and a rub. Pleuritis, CAD, and costochondritis can also cause chest pain. Silent pericardial effusions are common. Tamponade is rare. **Myocarditis** usually occurs in the setting of active systemic disease and may cause tachycardia and congestive heart failure. **Murmurs** are common and are due to anemia, infection, or valvular abnormalities. **Libman-Sacks endocarditis** refers to nonbacterial verrucous lesions that may be asymptomatic. Bacterial endocarditis may develop on damaged valves. Valvular abnormalities also occur in patients with APAs. Conduction abnormalities may also occur. **CAD** occurs more frequently in SLE patients and is a major cause of mortality. CAD risk factors are common; treat them aggressively. **Raynaud's phenomenon** is common in SLE.

Pulmonary Signs and Symptoms
Pleuritis is the most common manifestation and causes inspiratory chest pain. Small, asymptomatic pleural effusions are often seen on chest x-rays. Pleural fluid is typically an exudate with 3000–5000 WBCs/mm^3, normal glucose, decreased complement levels, and positive ANA. Acute lupus pneumonitis presents with fever, dyspnea, cough, and, occasionally, hemoptysis. Rarely, SLE can be associated with an interstitial lung disease.

Neuropsychiatric Signs and Symptoms
Neuropsychiatric symptoms are common in SLE, covering a spectrum from mild to life-threatening, and may occur at onset or during the course of the disease (Table 12-2). Consider conditions such as infections, uremia, severe HTN, and medication side effects in the differential diagnosis. **Seizures** occur most commonly in patients with active systemic disease. An **organic brain syndrome** usually manifests with varying degrees of cognitive impairment, but agitation, delirium, or coma may occur. **Psychosis** may be an initial manifestation of SLE. Corticosteroids may cause psychosis, and differentiation from SLE psychosis is difficult and may require a trial of increasing the corticosteroid dose. Improvement suggests that psychosis is due to SLE. **Stroke** may be due to HTN, atherosclerosis, APAs, cardiac embolism, or thrombocytopenia. Vasculitis is an uncommon cause of neuropsychiatric SLE. **Transverse myelitis** is rare but catastrophic and presents with rapidly ascending paralysis or paraparesis, sphincter tone loss, and numbness (see Chap. 7, Rheumatologic Emergencies). CSF shows increased protein and pleocytosis. Urgent imaging with MRI is essential. Evaluation of neuropsychiatric lupus includes routine blood tests, CSF analysis, imaging, and EEG in cases of seizures. CSF analysis can exclude infection and may show pleocytosis and increased protein. Antineuronal antibodies in the CSF suggest neuropsychiatric SLE. MRI is more sensitive than CT for detecting mild changes. Antineuronal antibodies and antiribosomal P pro-

TABLE 12-2. NEUROPSYCHIATRIC MANIFESTATIONS OF SLE

Diffuse manifestations (antineuronal antibodies and antiribosomal P protein antibodies found in the serum)

Organic brain syndrome (cognitive dysfunction, dementia, altered consciousness) (20%)

Psychosis (15%)

Depression

Aseptic meningitis

Focal manifestations (often associated with antiphospholipid antibodies)

Stroke

Transverse myelitis (rare)

Movement disorders (rare)

Seizures (15%)

Generalized

Focal

Peripheral neuropathies

Symmetric, sensorimotor neuropathy

Mononeuritis multiplex

Cranial neuropathies (rare)

Guillain-Barré syndrome (rare)

tein antibodies can be found in the serum of patients with diffuse neuropsychiatric symptoms. APAs are often detected in patients with focal symptoms. Patients with APAs may require anticoagulation in addition to corticosteroids or immunosuppressives.

Hematologic Signs and Symptoms

Anemia is the most common abnormality in SLE. Anemia of chronic disease is more common than autoimmune hemolytic anemia. Other causes of anemia are iron deficiency and renal disease. A positive Coombs' test may be found without evidence of hemolysis. **Leukopenia** with WBC counts of 2500–4000/mm^3 and **lymphocytopenia** with counts <1500/mm^3 are common. Leukopenia often correlates with disease activity. **Thrombocytopenia** with platelet counts <50,000/mm^3 is found in 10% of patients but rarely causes symptomatic bleeding. Idiopathic thrombocytopenic purpura may be an initial manifestation of SLE. Thrombotic thrombocytopenic purpura can also occur in SLE patients and should be treated urgently with plasmapheresis. Cytopenias may also be caused by medications used in patients with SLE. The ESR and CRP levels are frequently elevated but are not reliable indicators of disease activity or superimposed infection. The **antiphospholipid syndrome (APS)** may occur in patients with SLE (see Chap. 39, Antiphospholipid Syndrome). Patients have arterial and venous thrombosis and may have increased pregnancy morbidity. APAs are detected with the lupus anticoagulant test, by aCL assays, or by the finding of a false-positive VDRL test for syphilis.

Serologic Abnormalities

SLE is characterized by the presence of multiple autoantibodies. **ANA** is positive in virtually all SLE patients. Antibodies to DS-DNA and anti-Sm are specific for SLE but much less sensitive than ANA. Antibodies to other antigens (SSA/Ro, SSB/La, RNP) are also seen and often denote characteristic subsets of disease.

MANAGEMENT

Diagnosis and Differential Diagnosis

Lupus can affect numerous organ systems alone or in combination, and each clinical manifestation may have its own broad differential diagnosis. There is no definitive diagnostic test, so the diagnosis must be made by careful history, physical exam, and lab tests. The diagnosis of lupus requires multiple organ system involvement and evidence of autoimmunity. **ANAs are present in >99% of patients with SLE;** their absence practically rules out the diagnosis. ANAs are nonspecific and are also present in other rheumatic diseases, infections, and in healthy individuals. The American College of Rheumatology criteria (Table 12-3) were developed for classification purposes for clinical studies and should be used only as a guideline to aid the diagnostic workup. Four or more criteria, present serially or simultaneously, are needed for diagnosis. The differential diagnosis should include DIL and CTDs such as RA, vasculitis, and MCTD. Older patients presenting with SLE tend to have less renal impairment and more serositis and sicca symptoms (dry eyes and dry mouth).

Drug-Induced Lupus

Some medications can induce a lupuslike syndrome (Table 12-4). DIL can occur after several months or years of use. Patients typically present with fever, arthralgias or arthritis, and serositis. Renal and neurologic manifestations are very unusual. ANAs are present in most patients, as are antihistone antibodies. Symptoms resolve days to weeks after stopping the drug. Drugs that cause DIL may be used safely in patients with SLE. Some medications may also induce ANAs without causing clinical manifestations of DIL. In these cases, medications need not be stopped.

Treatment and Follow-Up

SLE is a chronic disease with a highly variable course. Most patients spend more time dealing with chronic mild disease and medication side effects than with severe manifestations. Patients are usually not familiar with the disease when they are diagnosed, so education and psychosocial intervention are important. Make patients aware of the importance of prompt evaluation of fever and advise them regarding birth control.

    General measures include avoiding sun exposure and using sunscreens and appropriate clothing to prevent photosensitivity. Naps and adjustments at work may decrease fatigue. A regular exercise program helps prevent deconditioning, weight gain, and osteoporosis.

    Medications: The type and severity of clinical manifestations should guide drug treatment. Minimize side effects using the lowest effective dose of medication (see Chap. 9, Drugs Used in the Treatment of Rheumatic Diseases).

    NSAIDs are used for treatment of arthralgias, arthritis, fever, and serositis. Low-dose aspirin is often used for prophylaxis in patients with APAs.

    Antimalarial drugs: Hydroxychloroquine (Plaquenil) is the most frequently used antimalarial drug in SLE. Hydroxychloroquine is useful for cutaneous manifestations (rashes, alopecia, photosensitivity) and for arthritis and fatigue. The dosage is 200–400 mg PO qd after meals. Chloroquine (Aralen, Aralen HCl) and quinacrine (Mepacrine) are other antimalarials sometimes used for refractory skin disease.

    Corticosteroids are used for treatment when NSAIDs or antimalarials are not effective and for severe manifestations. Prednisone is the preferred drug. Use the minimum effective dose to decrease adverse effects. Use topical or intralesional corticosteroids for cutaneous manifestations. High-strength (fluorinated) preparations cause skin atrophy and should not be used on the face. Intraarticular corticosteroids are useful to avoid systemic effects when there is a small number of swollen joints. **Moderate doses of prednisone** (0.5 mg/kg PO qd) are used for arthritis, serositis, high fever, and mild nephritis. **High-dose prednisone** (1 mg/kg PO qd, may be bid or tid) is used for life-threatening disease such as disseminated vasculitis, pneumonitis, severe nephritis, severe thrombocytopenia, severe hemolytic anemia, myocarditis, or CNS involvement. **IV (bolus) methylprednisolone (SoluMedrol)** (1 g IV qd in divided doses for 3–5 days) is used

TABLE 12-3. THE 1997 REVISED AMERICAN COLLEGE OF RHEUMATOLOGY CRITERIA FOR THE CLASSIFICATION OF SLE

Criteria	Definition	Frequency (%)
Malar rash	Fixed malar erythema, flat or raised.	50
Discoid rash	Erythematous raised patches with scaling and follicular plugging; atrophic scarring may occur in older lesions.	25
Photosensitivity	Skin rash as an unusual reaction to sunlight, by patient history or physician observation.	50
Oral ulcers	Oral or nasopharyngeal ulcers, usually painless, observed by physician.	25
Arthritis	Nonerosive arthritis of two or more peripheral joints.	88
Serositis	Pleuritis (history of pleuritic pain or rub heard by physician or evidence of pleural effusion) *or*	50
	Pericarditis (documented by ECG or rub or evidence of pericardial effusion).	30
Renal disorder	Persistent proteinuria (>0.5 g/day or $>3+$) *or*	50
	Cellular casts of any type.	
Neurologic disorder	Seizures (in the absence of other causes) *or*	15
	Psychosis (in the absence of other causes).	15
Hematologic disorder	Hemolytic anemia *or*	15
	Leukopenia ($<4000/mm^3$ on two or more occasions) *or*	42
	Lymphopenia ($<1500/mm^3$ on two or more occasions) *or*	10
	Thrombocytopenia ($<100,000/mm^3$ on two or more occasions in the absence of offending drugs).	10
Immunologic disorder	Anti–double-stranded DNA *or*	40
	Anti-Sm *or*	25
	Positive finding of APAs based on:	40
	An abnormal serum level of IgG or IgM anticardiolipin antibodies *or*	
	A positive test result for lupus anticoagulant using a standard method *or*	
	A false-positive serologic test for syphilis known to be positive for at least 6 mos and confirmed by *Treponema pallidum* immobilization or fluorescent antibody absorption test.	
ANA	An abnormal titer of ANA by immunofluorescence or an equivalent assay in the absence of drugs associated with DIL.	>99

Note: Other common manifestations not included in the current criteria are fever (60%), alopecia (26%), Raynaud's phenomenon (23%), and organic brain syndrome (20%).

TABLE 12-4. DRUGS ASSOCIATED WITH DIL

Atenolol	Methyldopa
Biologic inhibitors of TNF	Minocycline
Captopril	Minoxidil
Carbamazepine	Phenytoin
Chlorpromazine	Primidone
Enalapril	Procainamide[a]
Ethosuximide	Quinidine[a]
Hydralazine[a]	Statins
Hydrochlorothiazide	Sulfasalazine
Isoniazid	Trimethadione
Lithium	

[a]The risk of DIL is higher with these medications.

occasionally for severe manifestations (e.g., rapidly progressive renal failure, transverse myelitis, or psychosis). High-dose oral prednisone follows IV therapy. Slowly taper corticosteroids after disease is controlled. Do not reduce the dosage by >10% every week. Patients should be monitored for relapse during tapering. Some patients are unable to taper below a certain dose without relapse. Corticosteroid side effects are related to dosage and duration and are common causes of morbidity, and even mortality, in SLE patients. Corticosteroids increase susceptibility to infection and may mask signs of inflammation, requiring a high index of suspicion for conditions such as infections in patients with SLE. **Osteoporosis** is common in SLE patients on corticosteroids (see Chap. 50, Osteoporosis).

Immunosuppressives are used in patients who do not respond to high-dose corticosteroids or as "steroid-sparing" agents. Azathioprine (Imuran), CYC (Cytoxan, Neosar), and methotrexate are commonly used.

Azathioprine is less effective but safer than CYC in nephritis and is also used as a steroid-sparing agent for other manifestations. Initial dose is 1 mg/kg/day PO qd or bid and can be increased to 3 mg/kg/day to achieve a nadir WBC count of 3500–4500/ mm^3. The most common side effects are GI intolerance and bone marrow toxicity.

CYC is used for severe nephritis and other life-threatening manifestations (neuropsychiatric SLE, interstitial lung disease). IV bolus regimens are used more commonly and may be less toxic, but also less effective, than daily oral therapy. IV doses of 0.5–1 g/m^2 are given q1–3mos and are adjusted to a WBC >2000/mm^3 and a neutrophil count >1000/mm^3 10–14 days after infusion. Monthly doses for 6 mos are followed by doses q3mos for 18 mos. **CYC has severe toxicities** and should be used by experienced practitioners.

Methotrexate is used for arthritis and serositis. Dosage is 7.5–20 mg PO once weekly. Oral ulcerations and GI intolerance are common. Bone marrow and liver toxicity can occur.

Dapsone is used in cutaneous lupus, including subacute cutaneous lupus erythematosus and discoid lupus. Starting dosage is 50 mg PO qd. Patients with glucose-6-phosphate dehydrogenase deficiency are at increased risk for hemolysis, so measure hemoglobin regularly.

Hormonal therapies may have a role in SLE. Danazol (Danocrine) is useful in autoimmune thrombocytopenia. Dehydroepiandrosterone is a weakly androgenic steroid that reduces SLE activity.

Other therapies: Mycophenolate mofetil (CellCept) is beneficial in lupus nephritis. Dosage is 1 g PO bid. IV immunoglobulins and plasma exchange are sometimes used for severe unresponsive thrombocytopenia.

Approach to the Lupus Flare

Flares are episodic increases in disease activity that occur in most patients with SLE. New symptoms or worsening of previous organ system involvement is possible, and it is important to determine whether the manifestations are due to SLE activity, medication side effects, or other diseases (e.g., infections and pulmonary embolism). Lupus flares are an important reason for hospitalization. Patients with flares present most commonly with fatigue, arthritis, and worsening mucocutaneous manifestations. Fever may occur, but always rule out infections. Renal and neuropsychiatric deterioration and serositis are also seen. Flares often occur in a set pattern, and many patients are able to tell when their symptoms are due to lupus activity. Identify precipitating factors (UV exposure, missed medications, infections, pregnancy). Leukocytosis suggests infection rather than SLE activity. Decreased C3 and C4 levels and elevated DS-DNA antibodies are useful in identifying a flare in those patients in whom a relation between these serologic abnormalities and disease activity was established in the past. ANA testing is of no value in patients with known SLE, as the titer does not correlate with disease activity. In the absence of life-threatening manifestations, consider increasing the corticosteroid dose only after the initial evaluation is complete. Taper the corticosteroid dose after the flare has subsided.

Pregnancy in Systemic Lupus Erythematosus

Fertility is normal in patients with SLE. Although contraceptives containing estrogen may be safe, progesterone-only or barrier methods may be preferred, particularly in women with APAs, due to concerns of increased risk of thrombotic disorders. SLE may flare during pregnancy and postpartum, but most flares are mild. The frequency of flares is lower in women whose disease was well controlled at conception. Prematurity, in utero fetal death, and spontaneous abortion are more common in SLE. Patients with nephritis may have severe exacerbations with acute renal failure, preeclampsia, and maternal death. The children of patients with anti-Ro/SSA positivity are at increased risk for congenital heart block and neonatal lupus. Patients with APAs may have an increased risk of preeclampsia, fetal wastage, and miscarriage. Corticosteroids are safe in pregnancy. Avoid NSAIDs in the last weeks of pregnancy. Close monitoring is essential for good outcomes.

KEY POINTS TO REMEMBER

- Testing for ANA is not useful in patients with established SLE presenting with a flare.
- Diagnosis of lupus requires multiple organ system involvement and evidence of autoimmunity.
- Most patients with lupus have a relatively benign clinical course.

SUGGESTED READING

Boumpas DT, Austin HA 3rd, Fessler BJ, et al. Systemic lupus erythematosus: emerging concepts. Part 1. *Ann Intern Med* 1995;122:940–950.

Chan TM, Li FK, Tang CSO, et al. Efficacy of mycophenolate mofetil in patients with diffuse proliferative lupus nephritis. *N Engl J Med* 2000;343:1156–1162.

Rubin RL. Etiology and mechanisms of drug-induced lupus. *Curr Opin Rheumatol* 1999;11:357–363.

Ruiz-Irastorza G, Khamashta MA, Castellino G, Hughes GRV. Systemic lupus erythematosus. *Lancet* 2001;357:1027–1032.

Traynor AE, Schroeder J, Rosa RM, et al. Treatment of severe systemic lupus erythematosus with high dose chemotherapy and hematopoietic stem-cell transplantation: a phase I study. *Lancet* 2000;356:701–707.

Wallace DJ, Hahn B, eds. *Dubois' lupus erythematosus*, 5th ed. Baltimore: Williams & Wilkins, 1997.

West SG. Neuropsychiatric lupus. *Rheum Dis Clin North Am* 1994;20:129–158.

Crystalline Arthritis

13

Gout

Shannon C. Lynn

INTRODUCTION

Gout is a metabolic disease related to abnormal uric acid metabolism. Overproduction or, more commonly, undersecretion of uric acid leads to the deposition of monosodium urate crystals in the joint and soft tissues. Gout is characterized by severe acute inflammation, usually of a single joint. The natural history of gout classically has three stages. **Asymptomatic hyperuricemia** usually exists for years before the initial acute attack. **Acute intermittent gout** then develops. Patients have acute attacks followed by symptom-free periods. The attacks become more frequent until **chronic gouty arthritis** ensues. In these patients, the intercritical periods are no longer asymptomatic, and joint pain persists. Tophi (uric acid deposits) are often seen in these patients. Gout may also involve the kidneys (causing gouty nephropathy) and urinary tract (uric acid stones). 90% of gout occurs in men between the ages of 30 and 50. Gout is very uncommon in premenopausal women.

CAUSES

Pathophysiology

Gout may be a primary disorder due to an enzyme deficiency or may be due to secondary causes leading to increased uric acid levels. **Secondary causes** are common and include medications (diuretics, cyclosporine, low-dose aspirin, niacin), myeloproliferative disorders, multiple myeloma, hemoglobinopathies, chronic renal disease, hypothyroidism, and lead poisoning. Acute gout is an inflammatory response to monosodium urate crystal deposition in the joint space. This is more likely to happen in patients with high uric acid levels. It is not clear what initiates the inflammatory process, as crystals can be present in the joint space during asymptomatic periods without inflammation. Uric acid is produced by the degradation of purines by xanthine dehydrogenase or xanthine oxidase. Normal uric acid levels are <6.5 mg/dL in men and 6 mg/dL in premenopausal women. In postmenopausal women, the uric acid levels are equal to those of men because of the loss of the uricosuric effects of estrogen. Two-thirds of uric acid excretion is via the kidney, with a small portion of uric acid excretion by the GI tract.

PRESENTATION

History and Physical Exam

The sudden onset of **severe pain, erythema, swelling, and disability of a single distal lower extremity joint** characterizes an acute gout attack. The erythema and swelling can be accompanied by pruritus, desquamation, and fever. Inflammation often extends beyond the affected joint. An acute attack involves more than one joint in only 20% of cases, but when it does, it is usually in an asymmetric distribution. A polyarticular distribution occurs more frequently with recurrent attacks or gout attributed to secondary causes (e.g., myeloproliferative disease, lymphoproliferative disease, or transplant recipient). Gout most commonly involves the MTP joint of the great toe (podagra). Other common sites are the ankle, knee, and wrist. Gout rarely involves the hips or shoulders. Tophi in the external ears, hands, feet, and olecranon and prepatellar bursa can exist in patients with long-standing gout. *Intercritical gout* describes the asymptomatic periods between acute attacks. Without treatment, the patient can expect a recurrent attack within 2 yrs. Recurrent attacks are usually more severe and more likely to be polyarticular. Left untreated, the disease progresses to chronic gouty arthritis in approximately 12 yrs (range, 5–40 yrs). Tophi occur most commonly at the base of the great toe, fingers, wrists, hands, olecranon bursa, and Achilles tendon. Higher uric acid levels are associated with more tophi. Complications of tophi include pain, deformity, joint destruction, and nerve compression.

MANAGEMENT

Diagnostic Workup

The diagnosis is based primarily on history, physical exam, and the presence of **urate crystals** in joint fluid. Patients with gout almost invariably have hyperuricemia, but uric acid levels may be normal during an attack. Attacks are also associated with an increased ESR and leukocyte count. Aspiration of the joint is essential for diagnosis and reveals intracellular monosodium urate crystals. Monosodium urate crystals are needle-shaped and demonstrate negative birefringence with polarized microscopy. Leukocyte counts are elevated in the joint fluid. Crystals can also be identified during the intercritical period. Radiographs early in the course of the disease are normal, but as the disease progresses, punched-out erosions with overhanging edges ("rat-bite lesions") in the bone are evident.

The **differential diagnosis** of gout includes cellulitis, septic arthritis, pseudogout, and RA. Gout mimics cellulitis in that the affected area is swollen, erythematous, and painful and is accompanied by fever and leukocytosis. Joint aspiration is critical to rule out bacterial infection; treat suspicious cases with antibiotics until cultures are negative.

Treatment

First and foremost, one should treat the acute attack; later, consider the need for treating hyperuricemia.

Acute Gouty Attack

- **NSAIDs:** Any NSAID can be used, but most studies use indomethacin (see Chap. 9, Drugs Used in the Treatment of Rheumatic Diseases). Contraindications include peptic ulcer disease, chronic renal insufficiency, and drug allergy. COX-2 inhibitors may also be used. Use aspirin with caution, as it impairs uric acid secretion.
- **Colchicine** inhibits phagocytosis of urate crystals by neutrophils and also modifies chemotactic factors. It is most effective if started within the first 12–24 hrs of the attack. Oral dosing is limited by GI side effects, most predominately diarrhea with cramping that may be severe. Classically, oral dosing is started with 1 mg followed by 0.5 mg q2h until the patient develops abdominal discomfort, diarrhea, or reaches the 8-mg/day maximal dose. Most patients do not tolerate the classic dosing regimen due to severe GI side effects. Lower oral doses (e.g., 0.6 mg bid) are a reasonable alternative. The patient should respond within 48 hrs. The GI side effects may also be avoided with IV colchicine. Traditionally, IV colchicine is reserved for polyarticular attacks or hospitalized patients who failed first-line therapy with NSAIDs. **Contraindications to IV colchicine** include leukopenia, hepatic disease, chronic renal insufficiency, and recent use of oral colchicine. The initial dose is 1–2 mg IV, followed by 1 mg IV in 6–12 hrs if needed. Do not exceed 4 mg IV qd. Do not use further parenteral or oral colchicine for 7 days. IV extravasation can cause local tissue necrosis, so use a secure IV line. Colchicine administered parenterally can cause severe reactions such as aplastic anemia, thrombocytopenia, and neutropenia.

Deaths have occurred. Due to these problems and the availability of other agents, IV colchicine is avoided by many practitioners and banned in some countries in Europe.

- **Corticosteroids:** Intraarticular steroid injections are used frequently. They are a safe, local treatment for consideration in all patients once septic arthritis has been ruled out. Intraarticular injection of corticosteroids (Aristocort, Atolone, Depo-Medrol, Kenalog) (10–40 mg) may be used. Oral corticosteroid therapy is reserved for patients who have failed or have a contraindication to NSAIDs or colchicine or are experiencing a polyarticular attack. Prednisone is started at 40–60 mg PO qd and tapered over 7 days. A rebound attack may occur with tapering of corticosteroids. **Rule out septic arthritis before initiating oral corticosteroid therapy.**
- **ACTH/Corticotropin** is a good option in patients who cannot tolerate colchicine or who have coexisting disease that precludes the use of colchicine or NSAIDs. Dose is 40–80 USP units SC or IM.
- **Analgesia:** Acute attacks usually resolve spontaneously within 5–7 days. Patients with contraindications to the above therapies or complicating factors (e.g., postop patients with NPO orders, renal failure, and coagulopathy) may require opioid analgesics.
- **Ice** applied to affected joints for at least 30 mins 4× daily for 6 days can decrease pain and swelling with acute attacks.

After the initial attack, educate patients about weight loss and decreasing alcohol intake. In addition, reevaluate the patient's drug regimen. For example, if the patient is being treated with niacin for hypercholesterolemia or diuretics (especially thiazides) for HTN, make substitutions. Low-dose aspirin is commonly used in patients with coronary artery disease but may increase the risk of recurrent gout attacks.

Prophylactic Therapy

The goal of prophylactic therapy is to prevent recurrent attacks. Give prophylactic therapy before the initiation of treatment to lower uric acid levels, as changes in uric acid levels (increases or decreases) may precipitate acute attacks.

The dose of colchicine is 0.6 mg PO bid or 0.6 mg PO daily if the patient has renal or hepatic disease. Possible side effects of long-term colchicine therapy include myositis and mixed peripheral neuropathy.

Daily indomethacin or other NSAIDs are useful. Use with caution in the elderly because of the risk of peptic ulcer disease and chronic renal insufficiency.

Treatment of Hyperuricemia

Consider therapy if the patient is at high risk for recurrence based on level of hyperuricemia (5% yearly incidence of acute gout in patients with uric acid levels >9 mg/dL), alcohol consumption, diet, obesity, and diuretic therapy. **Asymptomatic hyperuricemia does not require treatment.** Hyperuricemia is highly prevalent among hypertensive patients. Almost 75% of patients with HTN and chronic renal insufficiency have increased uric acid levels. Hyperuricemia is independently associated with increased mortality in patients with cardiovascular disease, especially in women, but it is not clear whether treatment of hyperuricemia in these patients is beneficial. Treatment of hyperuricemia aims to reduce serum uric acid levels and prevent progression of disease to chronic gouty arthritis. The uric acid level goal is approximately 5 mg/dL. Consider treatment of hyperuricemia if the patient has tophaceous gout, gouty nephropathy, uric acid kidney stones, or repeated attacks (generally, >three/year). **Do not start these agents during an acute attack:** rather, start them 6–8 wks after the attack subsides. Continue therapy to lower uric acid levels indefinitely. A common mistake is stopping treatment when uric acid levels have normalized, which usually precipitates another attack.

Uricosuric Agents

Probenecid (Benemid, Probalan) and **sulfinpyrazone** (Anturane) inhibit tubular reabsorption of urate. These agents are ineffective if the serum creatinine level is >2 mg/dL; do not use them if the patient has a history of uric acid kidney stones, low urinary flow (<1 mL/min), or high levels of urine uric acid at baseline (>800 mg/24 hrs). Perform a 24-hr urine collection for creatinine and uric acid before initiation of therapy. Advise the patient to maintain a daily urine output >2 L to avoid precipitation of uric acid stones. To decrease this risk, alkalinizing agents (potassium citrate) may be added. Start probenecid at 500 mg PO bid and increase to 1000 mg PO bid if necessary. Sulfinpyrazone also inhibits platelet function.

Xanthine Oxidase Inhibitor

Allopurinol (Lopurin, Zyloprim) is currently the preferred agent for lowering uric acid levels in patients with arthritis and/or kidney involvement. It is useful in patients with both underexcretion and overproduction of uric acid and is also beneficial for tophaceous gout. It decreases urate production by inhibiting the final step of urate synthesis and, thus, decreases uric acid levels, facilitating tophus mobilization. Allopurinol may also precipitate acute attacks when started; therefore, continue prophylactic colchicine or NSAIDs for ≥2 wks after initiation of allopurinol. The initial dose is 100 mg PO qd. After 2 wks, if uric acid is still elevated, increase the dose to 300 mg qd. Multiple drug interactions may occur with allopurinol (i.e., azathioprine, probenecid, ampicillin, and cyclosporine). The most common side effects of allopurinol are rash, diarrhea, nausea, liver dysfunction, and pruritus. If a rash develops, stop or decrease the dose of allopurinol. A more severe but rare (<1 case/1000 patients treated) reaction is exfoliative dermatitis, which can be accompanied by vasculitis, fever, liver dysfunction, eosinophilia, and acute interstitial nephritis. 20% of patients with this syndrome respond to discontinuation of allopurinol; however, 80% have a more severe course.

KEY POINTS TO REMEMBER

- Gout and RA rarely coexist.
- Gout is uncommon in premenopausal women.
- Uric acid–lowering therapy is indicated in patients with multiple gout attacks.

SUGGESTED READING

Emmerson BT. The management of gout. *N Engl J Med* 1996;334:445–451.
Pittman JR, Bross MH. Diagnosis and management of gout. *Am Fam Physician* 1999;59:1799–1806.
Schlesinger N, Detry MA, Holland BK, Baker DG, et al. Local ice therapy during bouts of acute gouty arthritis. *J Rheumatol* 2002; 29:331–334.
Simkin PA. Gout and hyperuricemia. *Curr Op Rheum* 1997;9:268–273.
Taylor CT, Brooks NC, Kelley KW. Corticotropin for acute management of gout. *Ann Pharmacother* 2001;35:365–368.

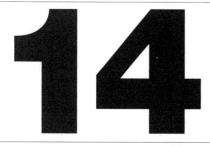

Pseudogout: Calcium Pyrophosphate Dihydrate Crystal Deposition Disease

Shannon C. Lynn

INTRODUCTION

Calcium pyrophosphate dihydrate **(CPPD)** crystal deposition disease is characterized by an inflammatory reaction to CPPD crystals in connective tissues. CPPD may be asymptomatic or manifest with acute or chronic arthropathy. The acute form of CPPD is also known as *pseudogout*. CPPD is a disease of the elderly (average age, 72 yrs). >50% of patients over the age of 85 have radiographic evidence of CPPD deposition.

CAUSES

Pathophysiology

The pathophysiology of CPPD is not clearly understood. It is believed to be secondary to high levels of calcium or inorganic pyrophosphate that, given the right matrix conditions, precipitate to form crystals. Crystal formation may be related to abnormal metabolism of pyrophosphate by cartilage. Crystals are potent activators of cytokine production and the inflammatory pathway. However, crystals can be present in synovial fluid between acute attacks in patients with no evidence of inflammation. Crystal load or the size of crystals may play a role in the inflammatory reaction.

CPPD can be idiopathic or **secondary** to a large number of other diseases including hypothyroidism, hyperparathyroidism, X-linked hypophosphatemic rickets, ochronosis, familial hypocalciuric hypercalcemia, gout, hemochromatosis, and hypomagnesemia. Predisposing factors to early onset of CPPD include joint trauma, familial chondrocalcinosis, and hemochromatosis. CPPD can affect ligaments, tendons, articular cartilage, and synovium.

PRESENTATION

History and Physical Exam

Acute CPPD (pseudogout) manifests as severe, sudden-onset mono- or oligoarthritis with erythema, swelling, and pain, much like acute gout. Pseudogout can be associated with fever, leukocytosis, and an increased ESR. Attacks may be precipitated by severe illness, trauma, or surgery. It is more common in men and can involve any joint but most frequently affects the knee (50% of cases). Subacute attacks can involve more than one joint.

Chronic CPPD may mimic different arthropathies. Some patients (more commonly women) have slowly progressive joint pain similar to that of OA ("pseudo-OA") with attacks similar to gout. Multiple joints may be affected. Involvement of joints that are not usually involved in OA (e.g., wrists, shoulders, ankles) suggests the diagnosis of CPPD. Another form of chronic CPPD is a "pseudorheumatoid" presentation that is only seen in <5% of patients with CPPD. These patients have symmetric joint involvement and prominent systemic signs (e.g., morning stiffness, fatigue) as well as local joint changes with synovial thickening, local edema, flexion contractures, and decreased range of motion. Differentiation of the two syndromes may be made radiographically: RA has typical bony erosions and osteopenia that are not seen in CPPD.

Some patients also develop joint degeneration that is similar to that seen in patients with neuropathies ("pseudoneuropathic" form of CPPD). CPPD is most frequently **asymptomatic,** with calcium pyrophosphate crystals deposited in cartilage seen incidentally on x-rays (**chondrocalcinosis**).

MANAGEMENT

Diagnostic Workup

Diagnosis is based on history, physical exam, and the presence of intracellular crystals in synovial fluid or radiographic evidence of CPPD. In an acute attack, the typical synovial leukocyte count is 15,000–30,000 cells/mm^3, with a neutrophilic predominance. CPPD crystals **show positive birefringence,** are smaller than urate crystals, and are usually more difficult to identify. Even if crystals are seen, send synovial fluid for culture to rule out co-infection. Chondrocalcinosis is usually seen on radiographs in cartilage (knee menisci, triangular ligament of the wrist, symphysis pubis, glenohumeral joint) and tendon insertion sites (Achilles, quadriceps). Chondrocalcinosis is common in elderly patients, and it may be a misleading finding in patients who have other causes of joint pain. Screening for the metabolic diseases mentioned above may be appropriate, particularly in young patients or patients with severe arthritis. Check calcium, phosphorus, magnesium, alkaline phosphatase, ferritin, iron, total iron-binding capacity, and TSH levels.

Treatment

Joint aspiration usually provides some pain relief in acute cases. If only one joint is involved, an intraarticular corticosteroid injection is very beneficial. **NSAIDs** are also used. Oral **colchicine,** dosed similarly to gout flare management dosage, may be helpful in acute cases. Systemic corticosteroids are sometimes needed for severe cases, but hold them until infection is ruled out. There is no therapy proven to eliminate the CPPD crystals or to prevent attacks. Treatment of coexisting diseases may lead to improvement of joint symptoms.

BASIC CALCIUM PHOSPHATE CRYSTAL–ASSOCIATED ARTHRITIS

Much like uric acid crystals and CPPD, basic calcium phosphate (BCP) crystal deposition in joint spaces can stimulate an inflammatory response. BCP arthritis can occur as either an acute monoarthritis or cause destructive arthritis. The acute presentation of BCP deposition may mimic that of a septic joint; however, the peripheral WBC count and ESR are normal. The inflammation is usually self-limited, with resolution within 5 days. Diagnosis of BCP deposition is made clinically, as BCP crystals are visible only with electron microscopy. Management is similar to that for CPPD.

KEY POINTS TO REMEMBER

- Pseudogout can often mimic RA.
- CPPD crystal deposition disease is a common cause of monoarthritis in the elderly.

SUGGESTED READING

Doherty M, Dieppe P. Clinical aspects of calcium pyrophosphate dihydrate crystal deposition. *Rheum Dis Clin North Am* 1988;14:395–414.

Rosenthal AK. Calcium crystal-associated arthritides. *Curr Op Rheum* 1998;10:273–277.

Rull M. Calcium crystal-associated diseases and miscellaneous crystals. *Curr Op Rheum* 1997;9:274–279.

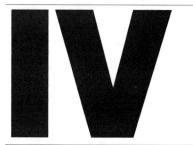

IV

Seronegative Spondyloarthropathies

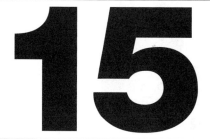

Undifferentiated Spondyloarthropathy

Kevin M. Latinis

INTRODUCTION

The seronegative spondyloarthropathies are a group of disorders characterized by axial skeletal inflammation and negative rheumatoid factor serologies. This group of diseases includes AS, PsA, ReA, enteropathic arthritis, and undifferentiated spondyloarthropathy.

Although not well studied, a few reports suggest that the prevalence of the spondyloarthropathies approach 1–2% in the general population. A 20-fold increased risk occurs in **HLA-B27**–positive individuals. The actual numbers of diagnoses of spondyloarthropathies is much lower than 1–2% of the population, primarily because many of the cases are subclinical or misdiagnosed or remit before formal diagnosis. These diseases tend to occur more often in men and younger populations (<45 yrs) and demonstrate familial aggregation.

CAUSES

Differential Diagnosis

The differential diagnosis of seronegative spondyloarthropathies includes forms of polyarticular inflammatory arthritis (see Chap. 1, Approach to the Rheumatology Consult), including SLE, RA, and infectious arthritis.

PRESENTATION

History and Physical Exam

The seronegative spondyloarthropathies all have in common a history of **inflammatory arthritis,** often including symptoms of axial skeletal pain, which is classically low back pain deriving from sacroiliitis or spondylitis (Fig. 15-1). Symptoms are worse in the morning and with rest and are improved with activity and stretching. Symptom onset is usually gradual, increasing over several months. When peripheral joint involvement occurs, it typically is asymmetric and oligoarticular and most often involves the lower extremities. Enthesopathy, or inflammation at insertions of tendons or ligaments to bone, is another common feature. When present, it can lead to the formation of dactylitis (sausage digits), plantar fasciitis, and Achilles tendonitis. Additional extraarticular features associated with the seronegative spondyloarthropathies include skin and mucous membrane lesions, ocular inflammation (uveitis more commonly than conjunctivitis), aortic root dilatation, and bowel inflammation. Seronegative spondyloarthropathies are generally familial and variably associated with the HLA-B27 major histocompatibility complex class I allele.

MANAGEMENT

Diagnostic Workup

Several criteria exist for the general diagnosis of seronegative spondyloarthropathies. Two of the more commonly used broad classifications are the European Spondyloarthropathy Study Group (Table 15-1) and the Amor classification (Table 15-2). These

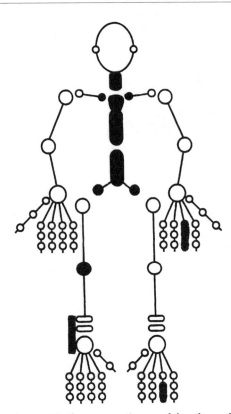

FIG. 15-1. Joint involvement in the seronegative spondyloarthropathies.

classifications both have moderate sensitivity (75%, 85%) and specificity (87%, 90%). They originally were developed for classification purposes but are often useful to guide diagnostic workups. The specific spondyloarthropathies, some of which have their own diagnostic criteria, are discussed in Chap. 16, Ankylosing Spondylitis; Chap. 17, Psoriatic Arthritis; Chap. 18, Reactive Arthritis; and Chap. 19, Enteropathic Arthritis. Spondyloarthropathies that do not fit into any known disease category, yet fit the European Spondyloarthropathy Study Group or Amor criteria, are classified as undifferentiated spondyloarthropathies.

MANAGEMENT

Treatment and Follow-Up

The goal of therapy for all spondyloarthropathies is to *control symptoms of pain and stiffness and avoid loss of mobility and range of motion*. Physical therapy and patient education are important for all seronegative spondyloarthropathies. NSAIDs, often in high doses, generally work well for inflammatory pain. Manage pain and stiffness resistant to NSAIDs by the addition of steroid-sparing antirheumatic drugs (e.g., methotrexate), sulfasalazine, or TNF blockers (see Chap. 9, Drugs Used in the Treatment of Rheumatic Diseases). For acute arthritic flares, intraarticular or systemic corticosteroids may prove beneficial. For details about the treatment of specific spondyloarthropathies, see Chap. 16, Ankylosing Spondylitis; Chap. 17, Psoriatic Arthritis; Chap. 18, Reactive Arthritis; and Chap. 19, Enteropathic Arthritis.

TABLE 15-1. TWO ENTRY CRITERIA (EUROPEAN SPONDYLOARTHROPATHY STUDY GROUP)

Inflammatory spinal pain *or*

Synovitis (asymmetric or predominantly in the lower limbs)

and

One or more of the following:

    Positive family history

    Psoriasis

    Inflammatory bowel disease

    Urethritis, cervicitis, or acute diarrhea within 1 mo before arthritis

    Alternating buttock pain

    Enthesopathy

    Sacroiliitis

TABLE 15-2. MULTIPLE ENTRY CRITERIA (AMOR)

Criterion	Grade
1. Lumbar or dorsal pain during the night or morning stiffness of lumbar or dorsal spine	1
2. Asymmetric oligoarthritis	2
3. Buttock pain	1
If affecting alternately the right or the left buttock	2
4. Sausagelike toe or digit	2
5. Heel pain	2
6. Iritis	2
7. Nongonococcal urethritis or cervicitis accompanying, *or* within 1 mo before, the onset of arthritis	1
8. Acute diarrhea accompanying, *or* within 1 mo before, the onset of arthritis	1
9. Presence or history of psoriasis, balanitis, or inflammatory bowel disease (ulcerative colitis or Crohn's disease)	2
10. Sacroiliitis (grade ~2 if bilateral; grade ~3 if unilateral)	3
11. Presence of HLA-B27 or familial history of AS, ReA, uveitis, psoriasis, or chronic enterocolopathies	2
12. Clear-cut improvement of rheumatic complaints with NSAIDs in less than 48 hrs or relapse of the pain in less than 48 hrs if NSAIDs discontinued	2

Note: A patient will be considered as suffering from a spondyloarthropathy if the sum of the applicable criteria is at least six.

KEY POINTS TO REMEMBER

- Consider seronegative spondyloarthropathies in the differential diagnosis of younger patients with chronic low back pain.
- Seronegative spondyloarthropathies are characterized by spinal involvement and varying degrees of peripheral joint involvement (primarily asymmetric lower extremity) and variable degrees of extraarticular manifestations.

SUGGESTED READING

Alvarez I, Lopez de Castro JA. HLA-B27 and immunogenetics of spondyloarthropathies. *Curr Opin Rheumatol* 2000;12:248–253.

Amor B, Dougados M, Mijiyawa M. [Criteria of the classification of spondylarthropathies]. *Revue du Rhumatisme et des Maladies Osteo-Articulaires* 1999;57:85–89.

Braun J, Bollow M, Remlinger G, et al. Prevalence of spondylarthropathies in HLA-B27 positive and negative blood donors. *Arthritis Rheum* 1998;41:58–67.

Dougados M, van der Linden S, Juhlin R, et al. The European Spondylarthropathy Study Group preliminary criteria for the classification of spondylarthropathy. *Arthritis Rheum* 1991;34:1218–1227.

Gladman DD. Clinical aspects of the spondyloarthropathies. *Am J Med Sci* 1998;316:234–238.

Kerr HE, Sturrock RD. Clinical aspects, outcome assessment, disease course, and extra-articular features of spondyloarthropathies. *Curr Opin Rheumatol* 1999; 11:235–237.

Khan MA. Spondyloarthropathies. *Curr Opin Rheumatol* 1999;11:233–234.

Koehler L, Kuipers JG, Zeidler H. Managing seronegative spondarthritides. *Rheumatology (Oxford)* 2000;39:360–368.

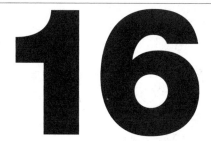

Ankylosing Spondylitis

Kevin M. Latinis

INTRODUCTION

AS is a chronic **inflammatory arthritis of the back,** involving the SI joints and articular joints of the spine. Additionally, AS may be associated with peripheral arthritis of the knees, hips, and shoulders as well as extraarticular manifestations involving the eyes, heart, and lungs.

AS occurs with a male to female ratio of approximately 3:1 to 9:1. The age of onset is most often <40 yrs, with peak incidence between the ages of 20 and 30. The prevalence of AS ranges from 0 to 1.4%, with a wide variation noted in different ethnic populations. The primary reason for ethnic variation relates to the expression of HLA-B27. In the United States, HLA-B27 is more common in whites of Northern European descent and less common in blacks. In white males, AS has an HLA-B27 expression of 80–95%. The prevalence of AS in HLA-B27–positive individuals is estimated to be 10–20%. Like all of the seronegative spondyloarthropathies, AS has a strong familial aggregation.

CAUSES

Pathophysiology

The etiology of AS is unknown. However, recent evidence supports the role of inflammatory cytokines in disease pathogenesis. The strong association with **HLA-B27** also suggests an immune-dependent component. Histologically, synovitis and enthesitis in AS are difficult to distinguish from synovitis of RA.

Differential Diagnosis

The differential diagnosis of AS includes noninflammatory causes of low back pain, other seronegative spondyloarthropathies, and diffuse idiopathic skeletal hyperostosis.

PRESENTATION

History and Physical Exam

Patients typically complain of low back pain and stiffness with inflammatory characteristics (Fig. 16-1) (e.g., exacerbation of pain with rest and improvement with activity). The pain can often wake the patient at night. A warm shower, exercise, and antiinflammatories usually provide some relief. Symptoms progress gradually over a period of months to years and, over time, may lead to significant spinal deformities, leading to loss of range of motion of the lower back. Significant morbidity and physical disability result from flattening of the lumbar lordosis, kyphosis of the thoracic spine, flexion of the cervical spine, and flexion contractures in the pelvis and knee joints.

The physical exam should include evaluation of range of motion of the spine. This is first assessed by performing a modified **Schober's test:** Make marks 10 cm above and 5 cm below the level of the sacral dimples. Next, have the patient reach for the floor without bending his or her knees. The distance between these two marks should increase from 15 cm to ≥19 cm if normal spinal motion is present. Evaluate lateral rotation and lateral flexion in both directions as well. Evaluate chest expansion by

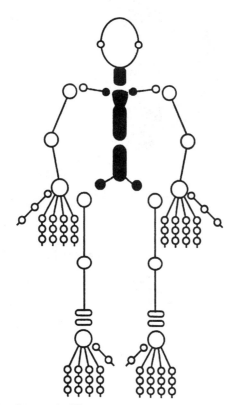

FIG. 16-1. Joint involvement in AS.

measuring the circumference of the chest at the level of T4 at the end of both maximal inspiration and maximal expiration. Expansion should be >2.5 cm. Clinical exam for sacroiliitis is variable and generally does not contribute to the diagnosis.

Extraarticular manifestations of AS include anterior uveitis, increased risk of fracture of fused spine, C1-2 subluxation, and restrictive lung disease (mostly from stiffness of the chest wall, but these patients can also develop pulmonary fibrosis). Less common manifestations include cardiac abnormalities (including conduction abnormalities, myocardial dysfunction, or aortitis leading to aortic regurgitation), renal disease from NSAIDs or amyloid deposition, and bowel mucosa ulcerations.

MANAGEMENT

Diagnostic Workup

The New York criteria for AS, last revised in 1984, are commonly used to diagnose AS. The criteria rely on both clinical and radiologic criteria. The clinical criteria consist of the following three components:

- Low back pain and stiffness of >3 mos' duration, improving with exercise but not relieved with rest.
- Limitation of motion of the lumbar spine in both the sagittal and frontal planes.
- Limitation of chest expansion relative to normal values corrected for age and gender.

The radiologic criteria consist of the following two components:

- Sacroiliitis with more than minimum abnormality bilaterally.
- Sacroiliitis of unequivocal abnormality unilaterally.

A patient is designated as having *definite AS* if at least one radiologic criterion and one clinical criterion are present. A patient is designated as having *probable AS* if three clinical criteria are present or if one of the radiologic criteria is present without any signs or symptoms of the clinical criteria. In practice, these criteria are highly specific for AS, but they lack sensitivity to serve as a reliable screening tool. Therefore, AS is likely to be underdiagnosed if these criteria are strictly followed. Furthermore, these criteria fail to address the presence of familial associations, HLA-B27, or extraarticular manifestations of AS.

The key to diagnosing AS is having a high index of suspicion in young to middle-aged patients who complain of inflammatory-type back pain. Direct further history and physical exam at pursuing this diagnosis. Family history of similar complaints or rheumatologic diseases is important.

Most lab tests for AS are nonspecific. Indicators of inflammation (e.g., elevated ESR or CRP) support the diagnosis but may not correlate with disease severity. Measurement of HLA-B27 may support the diagnosis and provide evidence of heritability, but in clinical practice it is only useful for ruling out the diagnosis if absent in white males.

Radiographs play an important role in the diagnosis of AS. Anterior-posterior x-rays of the SI joints and other affected joints, including the spine or peripheral joints, are usually adequate and should be performed initially. Additionally, the modified Ferguson view of the SI joints may be useful (a posterior-anterior x-ray taken of the SI joints with the patient in the prone position and the x-ray tube angled 30 degrees obliquely). Standardization of scoring systems for sacroiliitis has increased the reliability of x-rays for diagnosis. However, x-rays are less sensitive in early disease. CT is more sensitive for detection of sacroiliitis while offering the same degree of specificity. If the clinical suspicion for AS is high and x-rays are negative or unequivocal for sacroiliitis, perform a CT scan of the pelvis. MRI can also be performed and has an even higher sensitivity for sacroiliitis, but it has a higher rate of false positives and is limited by cost. MRI is currently not recommended in the diagnostic evaluation of AS. In severe AS, radiographs of the spine may demonstrate ankylosis of the spine with syndesmophytes (osseous formations that attach to ligaments) and a "bamboo spine" appearance.

MANAGEMENT

Treatment and Follow-Up

Refer all patients diagnosed with AS for **physical therapy** to initiate treatment with range of motion exercises and postural training. Studies show that physical therapy can limit pain and improve functional status in most patients with AS.

Specific pharmacologic therapy for AS is limited. The first-line therapy for patients with AS is **NSAIDs** to limit symptoms of inflammatory arthritis. Classically, AS is treated with high doses of either indomethacin (Indochron E-R, Indocin) or naproxen (Aleve, Anaprox, Naprelan, Naprosyn), but patient satisfaction should ultimately dictate which NSAID works best. Maximum doses of NSAIDs are generally required. Monitor NSAID-associated toxicities closely (see Chap. 9, Drugs Used in the Treatment of Rheumatic Diseases). Patients at risk for GI toxicity may benefit from selective COX-2 inhibitors.

Steroid-sparing agents may be used to treat more severe and refractory AS. Most success has been with escalating doses of sulfasalazine (Azulfidine, Azulfidine EN-tabs). Sulfasalazine is initiated at a dose of 500 mg PO bid and is doubled each week until a daily dose of 3 g is reached or toxicities prevent escalation. At maximum tolerated doses, sulfasalazine has been shown to improve peripheral joint symptoms but has limited effects on axial symptoms. Discontinue sulfasalazine if no response has been attained by 4 mos or if severe toxicities occur. Monitor patients periodically (at least every 3 mos) for leukopenia and neutropenia. Mesalamine (5-aminosalicylic acid), in doses of 1500–4000 mg/day, has demonstrated similar benefit in early trials but may be better tolerated. Oral methotrexate (Rheumatrex) initiated at doses of 12.5 mg/wk has also shown some success in relieving symptoms from peripheral arthritis but has limited effect on axial symptoms (monitoring and dosing recommendations are outlined in Chap. 9, Drugs Used in the Treatment of Rheumatic Diseases).

Systemic and intraarticular steroids have been used to control severe symptoms in AS. High-dose pulse steroids [e.g., methylprednisolone (Solu-Medrol) IV at 1–2 mg/kg/day] can provide rapid symptomatic relief. However, complications of long-term steroid usage limit their use as maintenance therapy. Local injections of depot steroids can provide symptomatic relief to patients with otherwise poorly controlled joint pain. Either blind injections of SI joints or radiographically guided injections can be used.

Recent studies have demonstrated promising results in the use of biologic modifying agents to control symptoms of AS. Specifically, the anti-TNF agents, infliximab (Remicade) and etanercept (Enbrel), have been shown to significantly limit disease activity and signs of inflammation in early AS.

Finally, surgery may be beneficial for progressive or refractory AS with significant morbidity from skeletal deformities. Total hip and knee replacements, hip arthroplasty, and spinal fusion (for unstable vertebral articulations) have all been demonstrated to provide durable symptomatic benefit.

Most patients with AS have mild to moderately severe disease, usually characterized by a chronic relapsing and remitting course. AS has not been associated with an increase in mortality but can produce significant morbidity if not recognized and treated appropriately. Severe AS occurs less commonly but produces significant morbidity related to axial skeletal fusion. One study has correlated seven prognostic indicators with more severe disease. These include *hip arthritis, ESR >30 mm/hr, dactylitis, oligoarthritis, decreased range of motion of the lumbar spine, limited efficacy of NSAIDs, and onset before age 16.* More severe disease is associated with hip involvement or with the presence of any three factors at the time of diagnosis. Two functional indexes shown to be sensitive in detecting improvement or deterioration in clinical disease include the Bath Ankylosing Spondylitis Functional Index and the Dougados Functional Index.

KEY POINTS TO REMEMBER

- AS spinal involvement usually progresses from lower spine to upper spine.
- Spinal involvement is more common than peripheral arthritis in AS.
- Evaluate patients with AS for extraarticular features such as ocular disease.

SUGGESTED READING

Braun J, Brandt J, Listing J, et al. Treatment of active ankylosing spondylitis with infliximab: a randomised controlled multicentre trial. *Lancet* 2002;359:1187–1193.

Calin A, Elswood J. A prospective nationwide cross-sectional study of NSAID usage in 1331 patients with ankylosing spondylitis. *J Rheumatol* 1990;17:801–803.

Clegg DO, Reda DJ, Abdellatif M. Comparison of sulfasalazine and placebo for the treatment of axial and peripheral articular manifestations of the seronegative spondylarthropathies: a Department of Veterans Affairs cooperative study. *Arthritis Rheum* 1999;42:2325–2329.

Dougados M, Behier JM, Jolchine I, et al. Efficacy of celecoxib, a cyclooxygenase 2–specific inhibitor, in the treatment of ankylosing spondylitis: a six-week controlled study with comparison against placebo and against a conventional nonsteroidal antiinflammatory drug. *Arthritis Rheum* 2001;44:180–185.

Gorman JD, Sack KE, Davis JC. Treatment of ankylosing spondylitis by inhibition of tumor necrosis factor-alpha. *N Engl J Med* 2002;346:1349–1356.

Gran JT, Husby G. Clinical, epidemiologic, and therapeutic aspects of ankylosing spondylitis. *Curr Opin Rheumatol* 1998;10:292–298.

Ruof J, Sangha O, Stucki G. Comparative responsiveness of 3 functional indices in ankylosing spondylitis. *J Rheumatol* 1999;26:1959–1963.

Spoorenberg A, van der Heijde D, de Klerk E, et al. A comparative study of the usefulness of the Bath Ankylosing Spondylitis Functional Index and the Dougados Functional Index in the assessment of ankylosing spondylitis. *J Rheumatol* 1999;26:961–965.

van der Linden S, Valkenburg HA, Cats A. Evaluation of diagnostic criteria for ankylosing spondylitis. A proposal for modification of the New York criteria. *Arthritis Rheum* 1984;27:361–368.

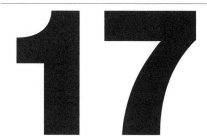

Psoriatic Arthritis

Kevin M. Latinis

INTRODUCTION

PsA is an **inflammatory arthritis** associated with psoriasis. The disease ranges from asymptomatic to severely debilitating. PsA can resemble RA, but many features differentiate these diseases.

PsA occurs equally in men and women, with a mean age of onset between 35 and 45. PsA occurs with an annual incidence of approximately 6 per 100,000 and a prevalence in the United States of approximately 100 per 100,000. It occurs in approximately 4–10% of patients with psoriasis (psoriasis has a prevalence of approximately 0.1–2%). As with all of the seronegative spondyloarthropathies, PsA demonstrates familial aggregation. Yet, unlike AS or ReA, the association with HLA-B27 is less common (approximately 40%).

CAUSES

Pathophysiology

The etiology of PsA is poorly understood. Genetic, environmental, and immunologic mechanisms likely contribute to the disease. PsA has a familial association and has been linked to several human major histocompatibility complex class I and II loci. The immune system appears to play an active role in the pathogenesis of this disease, as evidenced by the accumulation of immune cells at sites of disease and the production of inflammatory cytokines in both the skin and synovium. Further, treatments aimed at blocking TNF have improved disease activity. Finally, bacterial and viral infections and localized trauma have all been implicated in contributing to disease. However, evidence does not yet support these claims.

PRESENTATION

History and Physical Exam

Patients with PsA classically present with inflammatory arthritis symptoms of pain and stiffness in affected joints (Fig. 17-1) that is worsened with immobility and improved with activity and NSAIDs. Most patients already have psoriasis when the arthritis develops; however, a small percentage of patients develop arthritis before skin changes. Furthermore, skin disease activity does not correlate with arthritis.

PsA has been subclassified according to *five* different patterns of arthritis. (Numbers in parentheses represent relative occurrence of each pattern.)

- Asymmetric oligoarthritis: At least five joints are affected in an asymmetric distribution (30–50%).
- Symmetric polyarthritis: multiple symmetric joints involved. This is sometimes difficult to distinguish from RA (30–50%).
- Spondyloarthropathy: including sacroiliitis and spondylitis (5–30%).
- Distal arthritis: involving the DIP joints (10%).
- Arthritis mutilans: severe destructive arthritis leading to significant joint deformities (rare).

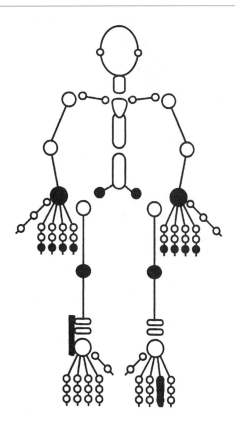

FIG. 17-1. Joint involvement in PsA.

Additional features of PsA include **enthesitis, dactylitis, and skin and nail changes.** Enthesitis is commonly manifested as pain in the heel and sole of the foot. Dactylitis occurs secondary to inflammation at tendon insertions, along the tendon sheaths, and in the joint spaces of the fingers and toes. It commonly causes the appearance of "sausage digits." Skin changes of psoriasis include salmon-colored hyperkeratotic scaling plaques commonly located on extensor surfaces. Seek occult psoriasis in the external auditory canal, umbilicus, intergluteal cleft, and axilla. Nail changes include pitting and onycholysis. Pitting is sometimes subtle; examine nails carefully in a patient suspected of PsA. Onycholysis is commonly mistaken for onychomycosis; examine nail scrapings for fungal elements and culture. Nail lesions occur in up to 90% of patients with PsA. Severity of skin involvement, nail disease, and arthritis are independent of each other.

MANAGEMENT

Diagnostic Workup

There are no formal diagnostic criteria for PsA. Rather, the diagnosis is made through a compilation of clinical and radiologic findings (the diagnosis of seronegative spondyloarthropathies is addressed in Chap. 15, Undifferentiated Spondyloarthropathy). Highly suspect PsA in a patient with asymmetric inflammatory arthritis and psoriasis. However, variable presentations can sometimes make this distinction difficult. Obtain x-rays of affected joints. Classic findings supporting the diagnosis of PsA include erosive changes and new bone growth in distal joints, "pencil-in-cup" erosions, lysis of terminal phalanges, periostitis, and new bone growth at sites of enthesitis. MRI may be useful to identify subclinical enthesitis, arthritis, and periarthritis, but cost precludes its routine use in diagnosis. Lab tests are not routinely useful in the diagnosis of PsA. ESR is variably elevated, and anemia associated with chronic inflammation can occur. PsA usually occurs in the absence of RF or ANA, but these tests may be positive in a small percentage of cases.

Treatment and Follow-Up

The goals of treatment are to *provide symptomatic relief of arthritis and skin disease* and *limit disease progression*. As with all seronegative spondyloarthropathies, therapy should include consultation with physical and occupational therapists. For severe skin involvement, consultation with a dermatologist is recommended.

The treatment of PsA is largely extrapolated from therapies known to be effective for RA. Symptomatic relief can often be attained with the use of NSAIDs. For patients at risk for GI toxicities, selective COX-2 inhibitors may be more appropriate.

For more aggressive disease or symptoms refractory to NSAIDs, treatment includes the use of steriod-sparing antirheumatic drugs. Commonly used drugs include sulfasalazine (Azulfidine; Azulfidine EN-tabs), methotrexate (Rheumatrex), azathioprine (Imuran), and TNF blockers. Initiate sulfasalazine at 500 mg PO twice daily, and gradually increase to 2–3 g daily in divided doses. Dose escalation is often limited by GI side effects. Initiate oral methotrexate at 7.5 mg weekly and escalate to a maximum of 25 mg weekly. Monitor methotrexate treatment for associated toxicities (see Chap. 9, Drugs Used in the Treatment of Rheumatic Diseases). It is commonly believed that PsA patients have a higher incidence and risk for hepatic toxicity with methotrexate use; however, no formal recommendations are available to guide monitoring and use of routine liver biopsies. Follow liver function tests carefully; consideration of liver biopsy every 2–3 g cumulative dose may be prudent, as cirrhosis can occur without liver function abnormalities. Azathioprine in doses similar to those used to treat RA has also been shown to be effective and is usually well tolerated.

Recent studies have shown encouraging results with the use of TNF-alpha inhibitors. As with RA, TNF-alpha has been found in elevated concentrations in joints affected by PsA. Treatment with etanercept (Enbrel) (25 mg SC twice weekly)—alone or in combination with NSAIDs, methotrexate, or steroids—significantly improves symptoms. Further, etanercept is generally well tolerated. Infliximab (Remicade), an IV TNF blocker, has similar efficacy. See Chap. 9, Drugs Used in the Treatment of Rheumatic Diseases for monitoring recommendations of TNF blockers.

Other regimens that treat both skin and joint symptoms include psoralen and ultraviolet A irradiation, cyclosporine, gold salts, and retinoic acid derivatives. Treatment with oral retinoic acid (25–100 mg/day) may take 4 mos to attain a response. Oral cyclosporine in doses between 2.5 and 5 mg/kg/day also takes several months to take effect. Even at these low doses, cyclosporin has significant potential to cause renal toxicity.

Corticosteroid treatment is currently not recommended for long-term treatment of PsA. However, steroids may provide symptomatic relief while the patient waits for the delayed action of steroid-sparing antirheumatic drugs to take effect. Intraarticular injections of steroids may also provide symptomatic relief but are contraindicated if psoriatic skin lesions overlie access to joint spaces due to risk of intraarticular seeding with gram-positive bacteria.

In severely disabled patients with significant joint deformities, surgery with joint replacements or arthroplasties may provide functional benefit and symptomatic relief.

KEY POINTS TO REMEMBER

- PsA occurs in up to 10% of patients with psoriasis.
- PsA is one of the few inflammatory arthritides that can affect the DIP joints.
- Enthesitis may present as heel and sole of foot pain.

SUGGESTED READING

Gladman DD, Brockbank J. Psoriatic arthritis. *Expert Opin Investig Drugs* 2000;9: 1511–1522.

Jones G, Crotty M, Brooks P. Interventions for treating psoriatic arthritis (Cochrane Review). In: *The Cochrane library*. Oxford: Update Software, Issue 1, 2002.

McGonagle D, Conaghan PG, Emery P. Psoriatic arthritis: a unified concept twenty years on. *Arthritis Rheum* 1999;42:1080–1086.

Mease PJ, Goffe BS, Metz J, et al. Etanercept in the treatment of psoriatic arthritis and psoriasis: a randomised trial. *Lancet* 2000;356:385–390.

Van den Bosch F, Kruithof E, Baeten D, et al. Effects of a loading dose regimen of three infusions of chimeric monoclonal antibody to tumour necrosis factor alpha (infliximab) in spondyloarthropathy: an open pilot study. *Ann Rheum Dis* 2000;59:428–433.

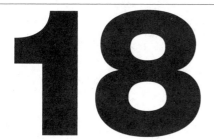

Reactive Arthritis

Kevin M. Latinis

INTRODUCTION

ReA is a syndrome that includes *noninfectious arthritis occurring after a prior genitourinary (GU) or enteric infection* and associated with extraarticular manifestations (e.g., conjunctivitis, uveitis, and various skin lesions). This syndrome includes the previously described Reiter's syndrome, which is defined as the triad of urethritis, arthritis, and uveitis that is classically associated with a recent GU chlamydial infection (although this is frequently absent).

The true prevalence and incidence of ReA are not well known. However, it is less common relative to the other spondyloarthropathies. ReA tends to have a familial association and, similar to AS, ReA is strongly associated with **HLA-B27** expression, which is present in approximately 80% of the confirmed cases. HLA-B27 is present in up to 50% of Native Americans, 3–8% of people in the United States, and 9% of Europeans, and is low to absent in certain native populations of South America, Australia, and South Africa. The prevalence of ReA varies accordingly. ReA occurs more commonly in men, with an 8:1 gender ratio, and is a disease of the young and middle aged, with an average age of onset in the 20s.

CAUSES

Pathophysiology

The pathogenesis of ReA is still poorly understood. However, it is known to have strong clinical associations with specific bacterial infections and the expression of HLA-B27. The link between these associations is still unknown. The bacterium responsible for the GU disease is usually *Chlamydia trachomatis*. The bacteria responsible for the enteric disease include *Shigella, Salmonella, Campylobacter*, and *Yersinia* species. These infections tend to occur within 1 mo of the development of arthritis. Even with available advanced techniques, it is difficult to recover these organisms from affected joints. It is hypothesized that association of antigenic determinants from these organisms with HLA-B27 alters the immune system in a way that causes an inflammatory response in the affected joints and entheses.

PRESENTATION

History and Physical Exam

Acute onset of asymmetric lower extremity oligoarthritis within 2–4 wks of a GU chlamydial infection or infectious diarrhea is a common presentation. The joints most commonly affected include knees, ankles, and feet. Enthesopathy is a common complaint, with Achilles tendonitis and plantar fasciitis often causing presenting symptoms. Additionally, enthesitis can lead to the development of sausage digits (i.e., dactylitis). Inflammatory low back pain occurs, with symptoms consistent with sacroiliitis or spondylitis. Other symptoms associated with ReA include conjunctivitis and, in more severe instances, uveitis. Skin manifestations include *circinate balanitis*, a discrete shallow ulcer on the glans penis, and *keratoderma blennorrhagicum*, hyperkeratotic pustular lesions found on the palms and soles that are histologically identical to pustular psoriasis. Further, pitting nail changes and onycholysis can mimic psoriatic changes. On rare occasions, ReA can lead to pathology of the heart valves, in particular causing aortic insufficiency.

MANAGEMENT

Diagnostic Workup

ReA is a clinical diagnosis. There are no criteria to differentiate ReA from the other seronegative spondyloarthropathies; however, patients should fulfill the criteria outlined previously for the general diagnosis of seronegative spondyloarthropathy (see Chap. 15, Undifferentiated Spondyloarthropathy). The diagnosis is supported by microbiologic evidence of either chlamydial GU infection or infectious gastroenteritis preceding joint or extraarticular symptoms. Nonspecific tests of inflammation (e.g., ESR or CRP) may be elevated but are not useful diagnostically. HLA-B27 studies are not necessary if there is a strong clinical suspicion but may prove useful if diagnosis is equivocal. Obtain radiographs of involved joints, as sacroiliitis and enthesitis are often evident. Additional findings such as fluffy erosions at the calcaneus or pencil-in-cup erosions of the digits support the diagnosis. Syndesmophytes (ossified ligaments) of the spine may also be evident.

Treatment and Follow-Up

ReA is usually self-limited and abates spontaneously after several months. However, an estimated 15–50% of cases are recurrent, and 15–30% become chronic, with symptoms lasting 10–20 yrs. Cases of either recurrent or chronic ReA can lead to significant joint destruction and disability. Disease activity can be monitored primarily by clinical signs and symptoms. ESR can also be monitored, as this also tends to correlate with disease activity.

In most cases of ReA, symptomatic relief can be provided with **NSAID** therapy. For limited joint involvement, intraarticular steroids may provide symptomatic relief of inflamed joints. For more severe or relapsing and chronic disease states, use of steroid-sparing antirheumatic drugs [e.g., sulfasalazine (Azulfidine, Azulfidine EN-tabs) or methotrexate (Rheumatrex)] may be helpful. Chronic use of steroids should be avoided, but short courses may provide symptomatic relief until steroid-sparing antirheumatic drug therapy becomes effective. Limited studies are available to guide current pharmacologic treatment strategies. Despite the link with an infectious etiology, antibiotics have shown limited utility in treatment of ReA. Physical therapy may be beneficial, especially to prevent contractures and muscle atrophy in patients with spinal involvement.

KEY POINTS TO REMEMBER

- ReA often presents with symptoms of isolated heel pain.
- ReA classically follows a recent GI or GU infection.

SUGGESTED READING

Clegg DO, Reda DJ, Weisman MH, et al. Comparison of sulfasalazine and placebo in the treatment of reactive arthritis (Reiter's syndrome). A Department of Veterans Affairs Cooperative Study. *Arthritis Rheum* 1996;39:2021–2027.

Toivanen P, Toivanen A. Two forms of reactive arthritis? *Ann Rheum Dis* 1999;58:737–741.

Wallace DJ, Weisman M. Should a war criminal be rewarded with eponymous distinction? The double life of Hans Reiter (1881–1969). *J Clin Rheumatol* 2000;6:49–54.

Wollenhaupt J, Zeidler H. Undifferentiated arthritis and reactive arthritis. *Curr Opin Rheumatol* 1998;10:306–313.

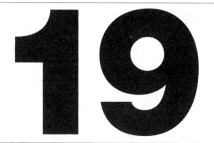

Enteropathic Arthritis

Kevin M. Latinis

INTRODUCTION

Crohn's disease and ulcerative colitis are associated with the extraintestinal manifestation of peripheral arthritis in approximately 10–20% of cases. In some instances, the arthritis may clinically predate the onset of the inflammatory bowel symptoms.

Arthritis associated with inflammatory bowel disease (IBD) occurs most often in children and young adults and has no gender predilection. It commonly demonstrates a familial association. Yet, unlike most of the other seronegative spondyloarthropathies, it has only an approximately 30% association with HLA-B27 expression (more frequently in patients with symptoms of spondylitis and sacroiliitis).

CAUSES

Pathophysiology

The etiology of enteropathic arthritis is poorly understood. Interestingly, disease activity of the peripheral arthritis is thought to reflect the state of the enteritis. In contrast, spondylitis and sacroiliitis may occur independently of the enteritis. Immune activation and inflammatory cytokines likely contribute to the pathogenesis, as inhibition of TNF activity is effective in relieving symptoms of both the enteritis and its associated arthritis.

PRESENTATION

History and Physical Exam

Bowel pathology usually occurs before extraintestinal associations; however, arthritis can sometimes be the presenting symptom of IBD. The arthritis associated with IBD is typically **oligoarticular, migratory, and asymmetric,** and it generally affects the lower limbs. The inflammatory arthritis may lead to large joint effusions, especially in the knees. Other associated conditions include uveitis, aortic regurgitation, and skin manifestations. Erythema nodosum and pyoderma gangrenosum are associated with Crohn's disease and ulcerative colitis, respectively. Spondyloarthropathy accounts for approximately 10–20% of the arthritis associated with IBD. Clinically, it is similar to AS (see Chap. 16, Ankylosing Spondylitis), except that the sacroiliitis may be unilateral.

MANAGEMENT

Diagnostic Workup

No diagnostic criteria exist to confirm the diagnosis of enteropathic arthritis; however, the general diagnostic guidelines for seronegative spondyloarthropathies may be useful (see Chap. 15, Undifferentiated Spondyloarthropathy). In general, a clinical diagnosis is made in patients with IBD who present with typical lower extremity arthritis, spondylitis, or other extraarticular manifestations. Anemia and elevated CRP and ESR are non-specific indicators of inflammation and may be present. HLA-B27 is less frequently associated with enteropathic arthritis and, thus, is not clinically useful. ANAs and RF are typically negative. Synovial fluid is generally consistent with an inflammatory arthritis (see Chap. 4, Synovial Fluid Analysis).

Treatment and Follow-Up

As the disease activity of the arthritis typically parallels the IBD, treatment is aimed at controlling GI symptoms and disease progression. Medications commonly used include sulfasalazine (Azulfidine, Azulfidine EN-tabs), 5-ASA, methotrexate (Rheumatrex), and azathioprine (Imuran) and usually benefit both the enteritis and the arthritis. Steroids may be used to control severe flares. Newer evidence supports the use of TNF-alpha inhibitors (specifically, infliximab), at least in the treatment of active Crohn's disease. In patients with associated arthritis, this practice has also proved effective to relieve joint complaints. Avoid NSAIDs if possible in patients with IBD and arthritis, as these medications can have adverse effects on the GI tract, including precipitating flares of the enteritis.

KEY POINTS TO REMEMBER

- Evaluate patients with persistent arthritis and GI symptoms (especially excessive diarrhea) for IBD.
- Joint symptoms of enteropathic arthritis typically parallel activity of IBD.

SUGGESTED READING

De Keyser F, Van Damme N, De Vos M, et al. Opportunities for immune modulation in the spondyloarthropathies with special reference to gut inflammation. *Inflammation Research* 2000;49:47–54.

Fornaciari G, Salvarani C, Beltrami M, et al. Musculoskeletal manifestations in inflammatory bowel disease. *Canadian J Gastroenterol* 2001;15:399–403.

Leirisalo-Repo M. Enteropathic arthritis, Whipple's disease, juvenile spondyloarthropathy, and uveitis. *Curr Opin Rheumatol* 1994;6:385–390.

Mielants H, Veys EM. Clinical and radiographic features of Reiter's syndrome and inflammatory bowel disease related to arthritis. *Curr Opin Rheumatol* 1990;6:570–576.

V

Vasculitis

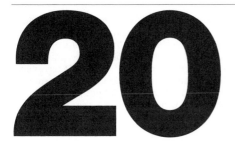

Introduction to Vasculitis

Ernesto Gutierrez

The vasculitides are group of disorders characterized by **inflammation of blood vessel** walls. Vasculitis is often considered in patients when nonspecific symptoms of inflammation (e.g., unexplained fever, weight loss, arthralgias, and myalgias) are coupled with signs and symptoms of end-organ hypoperfusion or dysfunction.

Vasculitides are commonly classified according to the *size of vessels* that are predominantly affected. Temporal arteritis and Takayasu's arteritis (TA) are considered large-vessel vasculitides; polyarteritis nodosa (PAN) and Kawasaki disease are grouped under medium-vessel vasculitides; and WG, microscopic polyangiitis, CSS, HSP, cryoglobulinemic vasculitis, and leukocytoclastic angiitis are considered small-vessel vasculitides. Behçet's syndrome is unique among the vasculitides in its ability to affect vessels of any size.

Although other classification systems exist and not every individual vasculitis fits neatly into its assigned category, this classification allows a diagnostic approach to patients with suspected vasculitis. The first step in this approach is to assign a vessel size category to the observed clinical signs, symptoms, and lab data. The next step is to emphasize the characteristic patterns of each vasculitis within the chosen category and determine whether the patient's pattern of disease fits into one of the primary vasculitides. The final step is the use of specialized lab tests or diagnostic procedures to define the extent of disease and to elucidate any other characteristic features.

When determining a predominant vessel size category, certain clues are helpful. Palpable purpura, superficial ulceration, mononeuritis multiplex, and RBC casts in the urine are signs of *small-vessel* vasculitis. Cutaneous nodules, livedo reticularis, papulonecrotic lesions, and digital infarction are signs of *medium-vessel* involvement. Pulse deficits or bruits are signs of *large-vessel* disease. Although organ failure is not specific for any particular vessel size, the clinical and lab pattern of organ dysfunction may help. For example, renal failure may be a manifestation of small-vessel disease (e.g., glomerulonephritis) or may be caused by medium- or large-vessel disease, resulting in chronic renal ischemia or acute renal infarction; renal artery bruits, abdominal ultrasound with vascular Doppler studies, and urine studies differentiate the two. Similarly, hemoptysis may be caused by life-threatening alveolar hemorrhage consistent with small-vessel vasculitis or by a ruptured bronchial artery aneurysm consistent with medium-vessel vasculitis.

Once a vessel size category is assigned, the characteristics of each vasculitis within the size category should be emphasized. For example, WG, microscopic polyangiitis, and CSS are considered pauciimmune small-vessel vasculitides (i.e., immune complex deposition and complement consumption are not features of disease). Therefore, low complement levels in someone with small-vessel vasculitis argue against any of these. Similarly, IgA-dominant immune complex deposition is characteristic of HSP. CSS occurs only in patients with preexisting asthma. Do further specialized testing to exploit these differences and to define the extent of disease.

The American College of Rheumatology (see www.rheumatology.org) has established classification criteria for several primary vasculitides. These criteria were developed using prospective data from patients with the diagnosis of an individual vasculitis and were intended as guidelines to assure accurate diagnosis in patients taking part in clinical investigations. They are not intended as definite diagnostic criteria that accurately predict the presence of any particular vasculitis in an individual patient. With these caveats, use each criterion as a general guideline when approaching individual patients and not as diagnostic criteria. **The Chapel Hill Consensus Conference** has developed definitions for the most common and well-recognized vasculitides. They are intended to provide a standardized system of diagnostic terms and definitions with regard to the vasculitides. Rather than provide a set of clinical and lab features, these definitions provide a descriptive term that defines the abnormalities in a patient that merit a particular diagnostic term.

SUGGESTED READING

Jennette JC, Falk RJ, Andrassy K, et al. Nomenclature of systemic vasculitides: proposal of an international consensus conference. *Arthritis Rheum* 1994;37:187–192.

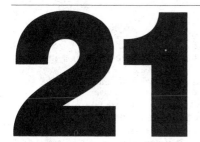

Takayasu's Arteritis

Ernesto Gutierrez

INTRODUCTION

The Chapel Hill Consensus Conference defines TA as a **granulomatous inflammation of the aorta and its major branches,** usually in patients <50 yrs. TA may also affect the pulmonary and coronary arteries. TA is most common in Asian countries. The incidence is highest in Japan, with 150 new cases per year. Sweden and Olmsted County in Minnesota have incidence rates of 1.2 and 2.6 cases per million per year, respectively. In Japan, TA characteristically affects women more than men (8:1 ratio), with peak onset in the third decade. The average time between onset of symptoms and diagnosis is 19 mos.

CAUSES

Pathophysiology

TA is a focal panarteritis affecting large vessels and their major branches, with subsequent occlusion, thrombosis, and aneurysm formation. On gross exam, the affected vessels are thick and rigid. The lumen is affected in a characteristic "skipped" fashion, with normal lumen alternating with occlusions or aneurysms. Microscopic exam of active aortic inflammation reveals infiltration around the vasa vasorum by lymphocytes and plasma cells, neovascularization of the media, and fibroblast and smooth muscle cell proliferation in the intima. Chronic aortitis is characterized by fibrosis in all three layers. Both types of inflammation are typically seen in the same patient at the same time, implying a recurrent process. The manifestations of TA are related either to the systemic effects of chronic inflammation or the effects of localized occlusion or aneurysm formation on organ function.

The cause of TA is unknown. In Japan and Korea, HLA associations and linkage analyses suggest that a TA susceptibility gene exists between the HLA-B locus and the HLA-DR, DQ loci, but studies in other countries support either the existence of other HLA associations or fail to show any HLA association. The association of TA with other autoimmune diseases suggests an autoimmune etiology. A murine model of large-vessel vasculitis suggests that active infection of large vessels with a herpes family virus may be involved in the pathogenesis.

Differential Diagnosis

The differential diagnosis of TA includes the infectious aortitides (e.g., tuberculous, mycotic, and syphilitic aortitis); Ehlers-Danlos syndrome; Marfan syndrome; seronegative spondyloarthropathies with aortic root involvement; GCA; sarcoid vasculopathy; and fibromuscular dysplasia.

PRESENTATION

History and Physical Exam

The clinical features of TA have been divided into three phases. Phase one is the "prepulseless" inflammatory phase characterized by nonspecific **constitutional symp-**

toms such as fever, arthralgias, and weight loss. Phase two is characterized by **vessel inflammation** manifesting as vessel pain and tenderness, most commonly carotodynia (i.e., pain on palpation of the carotid artery). Phase three is called the "burnt-out" or *fibrotic stage* and is characterized by **ischemic symptoms and signs.** It is important to realize the oversimplification of this scheme. As few as 16% of patients may have constitutional symptoms, and many patients have both inflammatory and fibrotic manifestations at the same time.

The classically described presentation of TA is that of a young woman with signs and symptoms of **abnormal cerebral or upper extremity blood flow.** The signs and symptoms are lightheadedness, headache, **pulselessness, subclavian bruits,** and **carotodynia.** These manifestations are attributed to ascending aorta and aortic arch involvement with resultant stenoses of their major branches and distal organ hyperperfusion. Other signs and symptoms include arm claudication, aortic regurgitation, heart failure, arrhythmia, syncope, transient ischemic attacks, stroke, and retinopathy. Ischemic heart disease secondary to coronary artery stenosis can also occur.

Further comparative studies show that, whereas TA most commonly affects the ascending aorta and aortic arch in Japan, TA tends to affect the thoracic and abdominal aortas more frequently in other countries. In Mexico and India, **renovascular disease** from either suprarenal abdominal aortic aneurysm or renal artery stenosis causes renovascular HTN in >70% of patients with TA. Studies also demonstrate **pulmonary artery involvement** with frequent pulmonary HTN. **Cutaneous involvement** occurs in approximately 15% of patients. Erythema nodosum tends to occur in the acute stage and is the predominant finding in Europe and North America, whereas pyoderma gangrenosum tends to occur in the fibrotic stage and is more common in Japan.

MANAGEMENT

Diagnostic Workup

The American College of Rheumatology 1990 classification criteria for TA require that at least three of the following six criteria be met for diagnosis:

- Age of disease onset <40 yrs
- Claudication of the extremities, especially the upper extremities
- Decreased pulses in one or both brachial arteries
- Blood pressure difference of >10 mm Hg between arms
- Bruit over the one or both subclavian arteries or abdominal aorta
- Arteriogram showing narrowing or occlusion, usually focal or segmental, of the aorta, its primary branches, or large arteries in the proximal upper or lower extremities not due to arteriosclerosis or fibromuscular dysplasia

Angiography is the gold standard for detecting diseased vessels. It defines the nature and extent of luminal involvement and provides measurement of the arterial pressures across stenoses. Perform full aortography on all patients as part of the initial evaluation of TA. Classification schemes exist for the distribution of aortic disease. Ultrasound can be used to evaluate for carotid and abdominal disease. CT with three-dimensional reconstruction and magnetic resonance angiography are gaining favor in diagnosing and managing TA, but proper evaluation and interpretation requires expertise unavailable in most centers.

Lab data in TA are nonspecific. Normochromic normocytic anemia of chronic inflammation, mild to moderate thrombocytosis, hypergammaglobulinemia, and elevated ESRs are common.

Treatment

The treatment of TA is both medical and surgical. Active inflammatory TA is treated initially with **oral corticosteroids.** The NIH protocol uses oral **prednisone,** 1 mg/kg qd for 3 mos, after which tapering to an alternate day regimen over 1–2 mos is started if disease improves. The Systemic Vascular Disorders Research Committee, Ministry of

Health and Welfare of Japan, recommends oral prednisone, 30 mg qd, for at least 2 wks after subjective symptoms are controlled and acute phase reactants normalize. The dose is then tapered over 4 mos. If disease fails to improve, the NIH recommends starting a **cytotoxic agent** [e.g., **daily oral cyclophosphamide (Cytoxan, Neosar),** 2 mg/kg qd, or **weekly oral methotrexate (Rheumatrex),** 0.15–0.3 mg/kg]. As many as 40% of patients need a cytotoxic agent. If steroids cannot be tapered to an alternate day regimen within 6 mos or cannot be discontinued within 12 mos of initiating a cytotoxic agent, the agent is considered a failure and is stopped. The long-term risk of cystitis, as well as bladder and other malignancies, with oral cyclophosphamide has led to the subsequent recommendation to use methotrexate. The Systemic Vascular Disorders Research Committee recommends a cytotoxic medication such as azathioprine (Imuran), 6-mercaptopurine (Purinethol), or cyclophosphamide only if the disease does not respond to steroids.

Renovascular HTN is the main cause of death. Unfortunately, the treatment of HTN is difficult, as the risk of ischemia across stenotic vessels caused by antihypertensive agents must be weighed against the risk of prolonged HTN. Furthermore, although limb BP readings are useful in detecting occlusive disease (either pulselessness and BP differences in patients with aortic arch disease or HTN in patients with renovascular disease) and in monitoring the progression of stenoses and limb ischemia, they are inadequate in monitoring the treatment of HTN. Studies have shown discordant readings between central invasive pressures and peripheral cuff pressures. Beta-blockers and ACE inhibitors are not contraindicated in TA.

Surgery is required in up to 50% of patients. The NIH indications for surgery are (a) HTN associated with renal artery stenosis, (b) extremity ischemia that limits activities of daily living, (c) severe (>70%) stenosis of at least three cerebral vessels, (d) symptoms of cerebral ischemia, (e) moderate aortic regurgitation, or (f) cardiac ischemia with proven coronary artery stenosis. 5-yr patency rates for revascularization procedures are highest in those patients who have inactive disease by histology at the time of operation. Angioplasty and endovascular stenting may also be used for stenosis—most commonly, renal artery stenosis—although there is increasing experience with angioplasty and stenting of subclavian, coronary, and aortic stenoses.

Difficulty arises in defining active disease. The NIH protocol defines active TA as the onset or worsening of any two of the following: (a) systemic features (e.g., fever, myalgias, or arthralgias), (b) elevated ESR, (c) features of vascular ischemia (e.g., claudication, pulse deficits, bruits, vascular pain, or asymmetric blood pressure readings), and (d) typical angiographic features. Unfortunately, pathologic specimens fail to correlate inflammatory activity with any of the four criteria. Newer imaging modalities, such as spiral CT and magnetic resonance angiography, may give information about the vessel wall that correlates with active inflammation, but further study is needed.

Follow-Up

For most patients, TA is a chronic disease; few patients experience a monophasic course. Current markers of active disease, as defined by the NIH protocol, are recognized as inadequate indicators of inflammation. As many as 60% of patients with clinically inactive disease may have angiographic evidence of new lesions, and 44% of patients undergoing surgery who have clinical remission may have active disease on histology. Reevaluate patients with recurring or relapsing symptoms and signs of systemic vascular inflammation as described above; however, the follow-up of patients who are in clinical remission has yet to be defined, as serial aortography is expensive and associated with risks, the role of other imaging modalities has yet to be defined, and pathologic exam is difficult to perform.

KEY POINTS TO REMEMBER

- TA may present with asymmetry of pulses in young to middle-aged patients with ongoing constitutional symptoms.
- Onset of TA is often accompanied by constitutional symptoms.

SUGGESTED READING

Arend WP, Michel BA, Bloch DA, et al. The American College of Rheumatology 1990 criteria for the classification of Takayasu arteritis. *Arthritis Rheum* 1990;33:1129–1132.

Giordino JM. Surgical treatment of Takayasu's arteritis. *Int J Cardiol* 2000;75 [suppl]:S123–S128.

Gravanis MB. Giant cell arteritis and Takayasu aortitis: morphological, pathologic, and pathogenetic and etiologic factors. *Int J Cardiol* 2000;75[suppl]:S21–S33.

Jennette JC, Falk RJ, Andrassy K, et al. Nomenclature of systemic vasculitides: proposal of an international consensus conference. *Arthritis Rheum* 1994;37:187–192.

Kerr GS. Takayasu's arteritis. *Rheum Dis Clin North Am* 1995;4:1041–1058.

Kerr GS, Hallahan CW, Giordano J, et al. Takayasu arteritis. *Ann Intern Med* 1994;120:919–929.

Numano F. Differences in clinical presentation and outcome in different countries for Takayasu's arteritis. *Curr Opin Rheumatol* 1997;9:12–15.

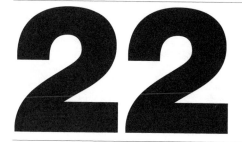

Giant Cell Arteritis and Polymyalgia Rheumatica

Ulker Tok

INTRODUCTION

GCA, or temporal arteritis, is defined by the Chapel Hill Consensus conference as a **granulomatous arteritis of the aorta and its major branches,** with a predilection for the extracranial branches of the carotid artery. It often involves the temporal artery and usually occurs in individuals >50 yrs. PMR is a syndrome classically character-ized by symmetric aching and morning stiffness in the shoulder and hip girdles, neck, and torso in patients >50. **A close relationship exists between PMR and GCA.** Although the precise nature of the association is not fully understood, they are considered by some investigators to be different phases of the same disease. PMR occurs in 50% of patients with GCA, whereas approximately 15% of patients with PMR develop GCA.

GCA is relatively common in Europe and the United States, with annual incidence of 0.49–27.3 per 100,000 persons ≥ 50. Autopsy studies have suggested a more com-mon occurrence of GCA. The incidence of PMR was 52.5 per 100,000 persons >50 in one study. Women are affected twice as often as men. Both GCA and PMR are more common in those with northern European ancestry.

CAUSES

Pathophysiology

Increased incidence of the two disorders after age 50 implies a relationship to aging. Reports on familial aggregation and an apparent increased incidence in persons from northern Europe and the United States suggest a genetic predisposition. Patients with PMR and GCA share a sequence polymorphism in the HLA-DRB1 gene, which may be linked to antigen selection and presentation. Both humoral and the cellular immune systems have been implicated in pathogenesis. Whether one develops PMR or GCA may depend on the cytokines that are activated. There is evidence that patients with PMR also have vascular involvement. Increased amounts of endothelial leuko-cyte adhesion molecules, IL-6, and immune complexes have been found in the sera of patients with GCA and PMR. Reduced levels of cytotoxic T cells occur in some patients.

The vasculitis in GCA tends to be patchy. The most severely affected arteries are the superficial temporal, vertebral, ophthalmic, and posterior ciliary arteries. Intimal thickening, with prominent cellular infiltration, is usually present. Necrosis of arte-rial walls and granulomas may also exist. The predominant cells are lymphocytes and multinucleated giant cells; neutrophils are rare.

Pathologic exam of joints with PMR may show lymphocytic synovitis. Synovial fluid analysis may be consistent with mild inflammation.

Differential Diagnosis

A few patients with findings of PMR develop persistent joint pain and swelling that mimics seronegative RA. PMR may also mimic hypothyroidism, fibromyalgia, poly-myositis, or other chronic inflammatory states (e.g., bacterial endocarditis).

The differential diagnosis of GCA includes TA. TA begins at a young age, does not commonly involve branches of the external carotid artery, and has not been demonstrated to involve the temporal artery. In rare cases, PAN or WG may involve the temporal artery. Occasionally, amyloidosis affects the temporal arteries and causes jaw and arm claudication.

PRESENTATION

History and Physical Exam

Onset for both GCA and PMR may be abrupt or insidious; symptoms are usually present for weeks or months before the diagnosis is established. PMR is classically characterized by **symmetric aching and morning stiffness in the shoulder and hip girdles, neck, and torso.** Fatigue, malaise, anorexia, weight loss, and low-grade fever may also occur. Synovitis in peripheral joints that promptly resolves with steroid treatment may be seen, making PMR difficult to distinguish from RA. CTS and swelling and pitting edema over the hands, wrists, ankles, and top of the feet may also be present. Joint exam shows decreased active range of motion of the shoulders, neck, and hips due to pain. Muscle strength is usually normal.

Headache is the most common initial symptom of GCA. The severity and location are variable. **Scalp tenderness** is also common and may be localized to temporal or occipital arteries or may be diffuse. The temporal arteries may be thickened, erythematous, and tender. **Vision loss** occurs in approximately 15% of patients and may be an early symptom. It results from ischemic optic neuropathy secondary to the involvement of ophthalmic and posterior ciliary arteries. It is abrupt and painless; once established, the visual deficit is usually permanent. Fundoscopy shows a pale disc with blurred margins consistent with ischemic optic neuropathy. Involvement of the facial artery may result in pain and spasm with mastication known as **jaw claudication.**

Involvement of the aortic arch and its branches occurs in 10–15% of patients and may cause reduced BP in one or both arms, arm claudication, and focal cerebral ischemia. Peripheral neuropathy or involvement of the skin, intracranial vessels, kidneys, or lungs rarely occurs.

MANAGEMENT

Diagnostic Workup

The American College of Rheumatology criteria for the classification of GCA require that three of the following five criteria be met for diagnosis:

- Age of onset >50 yrs
- New headache
- Temporal artery tenderness or decreased pulsation unrelated to atherosclerotic disease
- ESR >50 mm/hr
- Arterial biopsy specimen showing vasculitis with mononuclear cell infiltration, granulomatous inflammation, or multinucleated giant cells.

Suspect GCA in patients >50 who develop a new type of headache, jaw claudication, transient or sudden loss of vision, unexplained prolonged fever or anemia, high ESR, and PMR. Perform temporal artery biopsies in patients with suspected GCA or those with PMR who have symptoms or signs suggestive of GCA. To increase the chances that a biopsy will demonstrate vasculitis, the biopsy should be several centimeters long and include a section of a palpable abnormality if present. If the biopsy of one temporal artery is negative, perform contralateral biopsy if the clinical suspicion is high. Clinical and lab data are rarely helpful in predicting the results of a biopsy. A properly performed temporal artery biopsy defines the need for corticosteroid therapy in 90% of cases.

The American College of Rheumatology does not have a set of classification criteria for PMR. *The diagnosis of PMR is clinical and should be considered in elderly patients with symmetric aching and morning stiffness in the shoulder and hip girdles, neck, and torso.* The ESR is classically elevated and can exceed 100 mm/hr, but values <40 mm/hr may be seen in a few patients. Elevated CRP levels may be more sensitive than the ESR. Normocytic normochromic anemia of chronic inflammation and thrombocytosis may be seen; leukocyte and differential counts are generally normal. RF and ANAs are usually negative. Elevated hepatic enzymes occur in 20–30% of patients. Serum creatine kinase is normal. Tissue diagnosis of PMR is not necessary.

Treatment and Follow-Up

PMR is characterized by a prompt response to low-dose steroids. Depending on a patient's weight and symptoms, try **oral prednisone,** 7.5–20 mg qd. Increase the dose to a maximum of 20 mg qd if symptoms are not well controlled within 1 wk. Maintain the effective dose for 4 wks after the aching and stiffness have resolved. Then reduce the dose by 10% q2–4wks until the minimum dose that suppresses symptoms is reached. Once the dose is ≤10 mg qd, reduce it no faster than 1 mg/mo. **NSAIDs** may be used for mild disease. Initial ESR and CRP, as well as initial responses to therapy, provide useful prognostic information. Those patients with initial and persistently elevated ESR and CRP levels after 1 mo of therapy are likely to require therapy for extended periods of time. Steroids may be tapered successfully in some patients within a year. Most require treatment for 3–4 yrs, but withdrawal of steroids after 2 yrs is worth attempting. In most patients, PMR improves, and steroid therapy can eventually be discontinued. There is no evidence that patients with PMR have increased mortality compared to the general population.

Start patients strongly suspected of having GCA, especially those with impending vascular complications (e.g., vision loss), on corticosteroids. **Oral prednisone,** 40–60 mg qd in single or divided doses, is adequate. Inflammatory changes on biopsy specimens may be present for 1 wk after steroids are started. Use **pulse IV methylprednisolone (Solu-Medrol),** 1000 mg qd for 3 days, followed by **daily oral prednisone,** in patients with vision loss. 1 mo after symptoms resolve, begin steroid tapering as outlined above for PMR. ESR may not return to normal; do not use it as the only measure of disease activity. It may be necessary to continue prednisone, 10–20 mg qd, for several months before further reductions are tried. GCA tends to last several months to years, and steroids can eventually be reduced or discontinued. Some patients may require a longer duration of therapy.

Steroid-sparing drugs such as **methotrexate (Rheumatrex)** or **azathioprine (Imuran)** may be used in those patients at increased risk for steroid-related side effects, but strong evidence of efficacy is lacking.

Follow-up of GCA requires assessment of extracranial large-vessel involvement and its sequela (e.g., aortic dissection, renal artery stenosis, HTN, coronary artery disease, and subclavian, iliac, or femoral artery stenosis). Evaluate and observe patients with PMR for evidence of GCA.

KEY POINTS TO REMEMBER

- GCA is unusual in patients <50 yrs.
- PMR may be difficult to distinguish from RA.
- GCA may be a cause of fever of unknown origin in the elderly.
- PMR and GCA most often produce elevated ESR.

SUGGESTED READING

Barilla-LaBarca ML, Lenschow DJ, Brasington RD. Polymyalgia rheumatica/temporal arteritis: recent advances. *Curr Rheumatol Rep* 2002;4:39–46.

Gonzalez-Gay MA, Garcia-Porrua C, Salvarini C, et al. Diagnostic approach in a patient with polymyalgia. *Clin Exp Rheumatol* 1999;17:276–278.

Hunder GC. Giant cell arteritis and polymyalgia rheumatica. *Med Clin North Am* 1997;81:195–219.

Hunder GC, Bloch DA, Michel BA, et al. The American College of Rheumatology 1990 criteria for the classification of giant cell arteritis. *Arthritis Rheum* 1990;33:1122–1128.

Jennette JC, Falk RJ, Andrassy K. Nomenclature of systemic vasculitides: proposal of an international consensus conference. *Arthritis Rheum* 1994;37:187–192.

Salvarini C, Macchioni P, Bioardi L. Polymyalgia rheumatica. *Lancet* 1997;350:43–47.

Smetana GW, Shmerling RH. Does this patient have temporal arteritis? *JAMA* 2002;287:92–101.

Weyand CM. The pathogenesis of giant cell arteritis. *J Rheumatol* 2000;27:517–522.

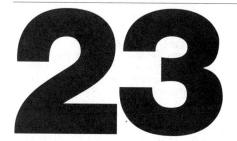

Polyarteritis Nodosa

Ernesto Gutierrez

INTRODUCTION

PAN is defined by the Chapel Hill Consensus Conference as a **necrotizing inflammation of medium- or small-sized arteries** without glomerulonephritis or vasculitis in arterioles, capillaries, or venules. PAN affects men and women ages 40–60 yrs equally. The annual incidence and prevalence are 0.7/100,000 and 6.3/100,000 people, respectively. PAN is caused by hepatitis B virus (HBV) infection in a minority of cases; most cases are idiopathic. Consequently, the widespread use of HBV vaccines has decreased the rates of HBV-related PAN, and the prevalence rates of PAN are higher in populations with endemic HBV infection.

CAUSES

Pathophysiology

The pathogenic mechanisms of PAN are not well understood, but they appear to involve immune-complex–mediated damage to vessel walls. In those patients with HBV-related PAN, hepatitis B surface antigen is believed to trigger the activation of the complement cascade. The clinical symptoms of PAN result from either systemic manifestations of cytokine activation or from local disruption of vessels. The pathologic lesions are focal segmental necrotizing vasculitis of medium- and small-sized arteries and, occasionally, arterioles. This inflammation commonly leads to vessel wall weakening with formation of microaneurysms, stenoses, endothelial dysfunction, and/or thrombotic formation.

Differential Diagnosis

Secondary causes of PAN include viral infections (e.g., HIV, CMV, parvovirus B19, human T-cell lymphotropic virus 1, and hepatitis B or C virus). The vasculitides of connective tissue diseases (e.g., SLE and RA) can present like PAN. Bacterial endocarditis, cholesterol embolization, sepsis, and malignancy can mimic PAN. MPA may have signs and symptoms similar to PAN but is distinguished by small-vessel vasculitis in the pulmonary and renal vasculature, normal angiography, and the tendency to relapse (see Chap. 26, Microscopic Polyangiitis).

PRESENTATION

History and Physical Exam

The signs and symptoms of PAN can be nonspecific. The majority of patients present with **systemic symptoms of inflammation** (e.g., malaise, arthralgias, myalgias, fever, or weight loss) along with **localized signs and symptoms of vasculitis** (e.g., peripheral neuropathy and GI, testicular, or cutaneous manifestations). Although the spectrum of disease encompasses limited disease to multiorgan dysfunction, the majority of patients present with acute illness and severe manifestations.

The most common symptom is **mononeuritis multiplex,** present in >70% of patients. It may be the initial presenting symptom. The lower limbs, especially the sciatic nerve and its peroneal and tibial branches, are most commonly affected. Hypoesthesia or hyperesthesia and pain are present in the areas of motor deficits. The motor deficits may be abrupt and may precede the sensory symptoms. Cranial nerve and CNS involvement are rare but may include cranial nerve palsies and hemorrhagic or ischemic strokes. The **cutaneous manifestations** of PAN are variable and include palpable purpura, which is usually papulopetechial and sometimes bullous or vesicular; livedo reticularis; subcutaneous nodules; and distal gangrene. **GI involvement** is one of the most severe manifestations of PAN. Mesenteric vasculitis with bowel wall ischemia, ulceration, or perforation is more common in the small bowel than in the stomach or colon. It usually presents with abdominal pain and GI bleeding. Hepatobiliary involvement in the absence of HBV infection is also possible and includes cholecystitis and liver hematoma or infarction. **Renal vasculitis** with subsequent vascular insufficiency, renal infarction, and HTN is a common manifestation. By definition, the renal manifestations of PAN cannot include glomerulonephritis; the presence of glomerulonephritis or pulmonary hemorrhage in a patient with symptoms of PAN merits the consideration of MPA. **Orchitis** is a classic manifestation of PAN.

Patients with HBV-related PAN tend to be <40 yrs and have a more acute and fulminant form of PAN than those with PAN without HBV. Malignant HTN, renal infarction, and orchitis are more common in HBV-related PAN. PAN tends to precede hepatitis, which tends to be silent. Seroconversion often leads to the remission of PAN.

Reports of limited forms of PAN exist in the literature. These reports refer to microaneurysms and stenoses limited to single organs without systemic involvement. Cutaneous PAN refers to a chronic cutaneous vasculitis of medium vessels with cutaneous and histologic features similar to PAN without systemic involvement.

MANAGEMENT

Diagnostic Workup

The American College of Rheumatology 1990 criteria for the classification of PAN require the presence of *three* of the following ten:

- Unintentional weight loss >4 kg since the start of illness
- Livedo reticularis
- Testicular pain or tenderness not due to infection, trauma, or other causes
- Diffuse myalgias, weakness, or leg tenderness
- Mononeuropathy or polyneuropathy
- Diastolic BP >90 mm Hg
- BUN >40 mg/dL or creatinine >1.5 mg/dL not due to dehydration or obstruction
- HBV infection
- Abnormal angiogram showing aneurysms or occlusions of visceral arteries not due to atherosclerosis, fibromuscular dysplasia, or noninflammatory disease
- Biopsy of small- or medium-sized vessels demonstrating granulocytes with or without mononuclear leukocytes in the vessel wall

Lab data supporting PAN include ESR >60 mm/hr, leukocytosis, hypereosinophilia, and normocytic normochromic anemia of chronic inflammation. Draw hepatitis serologies and investigate other causes of PAN appropriately. Positive tests for ANCA are uncommon with PAN. Seek biopsies of affected organ. Biopsies of skin lesions may demonstrate vasculitis of small-sized vessels and capillaries and should include the dermis to detect medium-sized muscular artery involvement. Other potential sites to biopsy include affected sural nerves, testicles, liver, and rectum. Visceral angiography may be used to demonstrate the presence of microaneurysms and stenoses in medium-sized vessels, usually in the renal, mesenteric, or hepatic arterial systems. Angiography may also be used before hepatic or renal biopsies to identify microaneurysms and minimize the risk of visceral bleeding. Measurement of urine protein and plasma creatinine and assessment of cardiac function provide prognostic information and help guide therapy.

Treatment and Follow-Up

Treatment depends on the presence of HBV as well as the assessment of disease activity. The **French Cooperative Study Group** (FCSG) for PAN has devised a five-factor score for determining prognosis. The five parameters predicting higher mortality are (a) proteinuria >1 g/day, (b) serum creatinine >140 μmol/L (1.58 mg/dL), (c) cardiomyopathy, (d) GI involvement, and (e) CNS involvement.

PAN without HBV and with none of the five factors above at the time of diagnosis can be treated with **oral prednisone, 1 mg/kg qd**. Treat the patient with one or more of the five factors with **pulse IV methylprednisolone (Medrol), 1000 mg qd for 3–5 days**, followed by **oral prednisone, 1 mg/kg qd**, and with **pulse IV cyclophosphamide** (Cytoxan, Neosar), 0.5–2.5 g every week to every month depending on the patient's condition, renal function, response to previous therapy, and hematologic data. The FCSG uses an initial dose of 0.6 g/m². Reserve **oral cyclophosphamide** for patients failing IV cyclophosphamide or for those with initial fulminant manifestations. Taper prednisone doses slowly after ESR returns to normal and the patient's clinical status improves, usually in 1 mo. The FCSG has used the following prednisone tapering scheme: Decrease the dose by 2.5 mg q10days for 1 mo, then decrease the dose every week until the dose is one-half the initial dose. Maintain this dose for 3 wks and then decrease it by 2.5 mg every wk until 20 mg qd is reached. Next, decrease the dose by 1 mg q2wks until 10 mg qd is reached; maintain that dose for 3 wks. Then decrease the dose by 1 mg/mo until it is stopped. Cyclophosphamide therapy should not exceed 1 yr. Patients receiving cyclophosphamide should receive **prophylaxis for *Pneumocystis carinii* pneumonia** with **oral trimethoprim 160 mg/sulfamethoxazole 800 mg 3×/wk (Bactrim, Septra)**. Consider **plasma exchange** only in refractory cases.

Treatment of HBV-related PAN involves treatment of both vasculitis and HBV infection. **Pulse IV methylprednisolone** as described above is used only if there are severe, life-threatening manifestations of vasculitis. Use steroids only in the first few weeks to control the vasculitis, then stop them abruptly to enhance viral clearance. Use plasma exchange after corticosteroids are withdrawn to control the symptoms of PAN. Continued steroids and the use of other immunosuppressants jeopardize viral clearance. **Standard anti-HBV agents** [e.g., **interferon alfa-2b** or **vidarabine (Vira-A)**] are used in conjunction. Consultation with a hepatologist is strongly advised.

PAN tends to be monophasic. Prognosis depends on the number of five-factor score risk factors. Patients with no risk factors have 88% 5-yr survival rates, patients with 1 risk factor have 74% survival, and patients with ≥ 2 risk factors have 54% survival. Follow-up involves clinical and lab assessment of disease status and monitoring of medication side effects and toxicities. In patients with HBV-related PAN, follow-up includes documentation of viral clearance.

KEY POINTS TO REMEMBER

- Classic PAN spares the lungs and glomeruli.
- Mesenteric angiography is sensitive and specific for PAN with GI involvement.
- Formal diagnosis of PAN requires the presence of 3 out of 10 specific criteria. Of these criteria, a biopsy or angiogram demonstrating vasculitis of small to medium-sized vessels helps solidify the diagnosis.

SUGGESTED READING

Gayraud M, Guillevin L, Cohen P, et al. Treatment of good-prognosis polyarteritis nodosa and Churg-Strauss syndrome: comparison of steroids and oral or pulse cyclophosphamide in 25 patients. French Cooperative Study Group for Vasculitides. *Br J Rheumatol* 1997;36:1290–1297.

Gayraud M, Guillevin L, le Toumelin P, et al. Long-term followup of polyarteritis nodosa, microscopic polyangiitis, and Churg-Strauss syndrome: analysis of four prospective trials including 278 patients. *Arthritis Rheum* 2001;44:666–675.

Guillevin L, Lhote F. Distinguishing polyarteritis nodosa from microscopic polyangiitis and implications for treatment. *Curr Opin Rheumatol* 1995;7:20–24.

Guillevin L, Lhote F. Treatment of polyarteritis nodosa and microscopic polyangiitis. *Arthritis Rheum* 1998;41:2100–2105.

Guillevin L, Lhote F, Cohen P, et al. Corticosteroids plus pulse cyclophosphamide and plasma exchanges versus corticosteroids plus pulse cyclophosphamide alone in the treatment of polyarteritis nodosa and Churg-Strauss syndrome in patients with factors predicting poor prognosis: a prospective, randomized trial in sixty-two patients. *Arthritis Rheum* 1995;38:1638–45.

Guillevin L, Lhote F, Gayroud M, et al. Prognostic factors in polyarteritis nodosa and Churg-Strauss syndrome: a prospective study in 342 patients. *Medicine (Baltimore)* 1996;75:17–28.

Guillevin L, Lhote F, Gherardi R. Polyarteritis nodosa, microscopic polyangiitis, and Churg-Strauss syndrome: clinical aspects, neurological manifestations, and treatment. *Neurol Clin* 1997;15:865–886.

Jennette JC, Falk RJ, Andrassy K, et al. Nomenclature of systemic vasculitides: proposal of an international consensus conference. *Arthritis Rheum* 1994;37:187–192.

Lhote F, Cohen P, Guillevin L. Polyarteritis nodosa, microscopic polyangiitis, and Churg-Strauss syndrome. *Lupus* 1998;7:238–258.

Lightfoot RW Jr, Michel BA, Bloch DA. The American College of Rheumatology 1990 criteria for the classification of polyarteritis nodosa. *Arthritis Rheum* 1990;33:1088–1093.

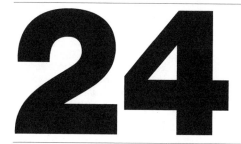

Wegener's Granulomatosis

Ernesto Gutierrez

INTRODUCTION

WG is defined by the Chapel Hill Consensus Conference as a **granulomatous inflammation** involving the **respiratory tract** and necrotizing vasculitis affecting small- to medium-sized vessels, commonly with necrotizing **glomerulonephritis.** Before the use of immunosuppressant regimens in 1973, generalized WG was a fatal disease.

WG affects men and women equally. The mean age of presentation is 41 yrs, although the range is wide. WG affects mostly whites. The prevalence has been estimated to be 3 cases per 10,000 people, although that figure may underestimate the true prevalence, as milder and more limited forms have been recognized.

CAUSES

Pathophysiology

WG is associated with **c-ANCA.** The c-ANCA in WG has been identified as an antibody to PR3, a cytoplasmic glycoprotein present in active form in monocytes, endothelial cells, and in the azurophil granules of neutrophils. PR3 is involved in neutrophil migration and cytokine modulation. The role of c-ANCA in the pathogenesis of WG is controversial. Although animal studies show that serum anti-PR3 antibodies result in lesions similar to those found in WG, anti-PR3 antibodies are not present in all cases of WG. Immune complex deposition and complement activation are not features of WG.

Histopathologic findings depend on the organ sampled, the size of the specimen, and the manner in which it is prepared. Although open lung biopsies with adequate tissue may show the hallmark features of vasculitis, necrosis, and granulomatous inflammation, head and neck biopsies rarely display all three phenomena simultaneously. Hence, most specimens are compatible with, but not diagnostic of, WG. Renal biopsies show focal and segmental glomerulonephritis (FSGN) with occasional medium-vessel vasculitis and rare granulomatous changes. Immunofluorescent studies are negative for immune complex deposition or complement fixation.

Differential Diagnosis

The differential diagnosis of WG should be considered carefully. Inappropriate diagnosis of WG and subsequent treatment with potent immunosuppressants may prove fatal if the underlying disease is infectious. Causes include granulomatous disease (TB, histoplasmosis, cocciodiodomycosis, sarcoidosis), neoplastic disease (lymphoma, metastatic adenocarcinoma), CTDs (SLE, relapsing polychondritis, antiphospholipid syndrome, SS, MCTD, Still's disease), other small-vessel vasculitides, and Goodpasture's disease.

PRESENTATION

History and Physical Exam

WG can be divided into two phases: the *initial phase* and the *generalized phase*. The initial phase is characterized by granulomatous inflammation, usually in the upper airways. **Sinusitis** develops as the initial symptom in >50% of patients and develops in >85% of patients at some time during the course of illness. Other nasal symptoms include sinus obstruction, mucosal swelling, ulcers, septal perforations, epistaxis, serosanguinous discharge, and saddle nose deformity. Granulomatous inflammation can also occur in the oral cavity, retrobulbar space, and trachea. **Laryngotracheal disease** can be asymptomatic but can also present as hoarseness, stridor, or acute airway obstruction. Subglottic stenosis occurs in approximately 15% of adults and in approximately 50% of children affected with WG. Myalgias and arthralgias are also common presenting symptoms.

The generalized phase is characterized by systemic signs and symptoms of small-vessel vasculitis. Fever and weight loss are common. **Pulmonary disease** is one of the cardinal features of WG. Cough, hemoptysis, and pleuritis are common. Radiologic exams reveal fleeting infiltrates and multiple bilateral nodules with the tendency to cavitate. Diffuse pulmonary hemorrhage, pulmonary effusions, and mediastinal lymphadenopathy are less common. **Renal disease** develops in approximately 80% of patients, usually after other manifestations develop. The progression of disease can be rapid once glomerulonephritis develops; the mean survival time for untreated WG with FSGN is approximately 5 mos. WG may affect any segment of the urinary tract. Hematuria without RBC casts indicates nonrenal urinary tract involvement. Although most patients experience arthralgias, some patients exhibit arthritis. The patterns of **joint involvement** are variable and include monarticular, migratory oligoarticular, and polyarticular arthritides. The presence of symmetric polyarthritis can be mistaken for RA, especially when a positive value for RF is obtained. **Neurologic disease** develops in approximately 50% of patients but is rarely a presenting feature. Mononeuritis multiplex and symmetric polyneuropathy are the most common patterns. Cranial neuropathies also occur; cranial nerves II (optic neuritis), VI, and VII are the most common. The most common **GI manifestations** are abdominal pain, diarrhea, and bleeding from ulcerations in both the small and large intestines. The **cutaneous manifestations** are typical of the small-vessel vasculitides and include palpable purpura, ulcers, subcutaneous nodules, papules, and vesicles. They tend to parallel disease activity. WG can also have **ocular manifestations,** including keratoconjunctivitis, scleritis, episcleritis, pseudotumor of the orbit, conjunctivitis, and uveitis.

MANAGEMENT

Diagnostic Workup

The American College of Rheumatology 1990 classification criteria for WG requires the presence of at least *two* of the following four:

- Nasal or oral inflammation (painful or painless ulcers or purulent or bloody nasal discharge)
- Abnormal chest radiograph (nodules, fixed infiltrates, or cavities)
- Hematuria or RBC cast in urine sediment
- Pathologic evidence of granulomas, leukocytoclastic vasculitis, and necrosis

The yield of tissue diagnosis for WG depends on the biopsy site. *Head and neck biopsies tend to show nonspecific inflammation and are rarely diagnostic.* Transbronchial biopsies are also rarely diagnostic; however, when used in combination with bronchoalveolar lavage and cultures, they are useful for ruling out infections that mimic or complicate WG. The yield of open lung biopsy is high when larger samples are obtained and is frequently diagnostic, especially if lesions are radiographically evident. The presence of c-ANCA and, more specifically, anti-PR3 antibodies, supports the diagnosis, although c-ANCA may be negative in earlier and less fulminant forms of WG. Sinus CT scans are superior to plain sinus films and should be used to define the extent of sinus disease. Perform chest films on all patients, as asymptomatic patients may have significant radiologic abnormalities. Use chest CT scans in patients with hemoptysis with clear plain films, as early pulmonary hemorrhage may not be visible on plain films. Chest CT can be considered in patients with abnormal plain films to define extent of disease. Pulmonary function tests with flow volume loops may be useful to define irreversible extrathoracic or intrathoracic obstruction caused by airway granulomas. Then, if present, evaluate the airway by bronchoscopy. Monitor serum creatinine and evaluate hematuria by microscopy, looking for RBC casts that indicate glomerulonephritis. Renal biopsies show pauci-immune FSGN. Although biopsies are not pathognomonic for WG, perform them if there are diagnostic concerns. Elevated ESRs, leukocytosis, anemia of chronic inflammation or from hemorrhage, and thrombocytosis are common; leukopenia and thrombocytopenia are rare and should prompt a search for other diseases. Complement levels are normal or slightly elevated.

Treatment and Follow-Up

Base treatment on the objective presence of activity, the site of activity, and the severity of activity. Evaluate the presence and sites of activity by the diagnostic workup described above. Life-threatening disease or disease with high morbidity (e.g., lung, kidney, nervous system, and vision-threatening ocular disease) merit high-dose oral corticosteroids and immunosuppressants. **Oral prednisone,** 1 mg/kg qd, with **oral cyclophosphamide** (Cytoxan, Neosar), 2 mg/kg qd, are used for induction therapy. **Pulse IV methylprednisolone** (Medrol) (1000 mg qd) and higher doses of **oral cyclophosphamide** (3–5 mg/kg qd) may be used for the first 3 days in cases of immediately life-threatening fulminant disease (e.g., pulmonary hemorrhage or rapidly progressive glomerulonephritis). Because IV cyclophosphamide is ineffective, its use is inappropriate in induction therapy and is not recommended in maintenance therapy. **MESNA** may be given with oral cyclophosphamide to reduce bladder toxicities. Once remission has been achieved, switch cyclophosphamide to **oral methotrexate (Rheumatrex)** (20–25 mg/wk) for 2 yrs and then taper.

Prednisone and methotrexate (20–25 mg/wk) may be used for patients with significant cyclophosphamide-related side effects or who do not have immediately life-threatening disease. Taper prednisone doses with careful assessment of disease activity. Give **oral trimethoprim/sulfamethoxazole** (TMP/SMX) (Bactrim, Septra), 160 mg/ 800 mg three times a week, for *P. carinii* **pneumonia prophylaxis** while on immunosuppressants. The role of other immunosuppressants [e.g., azathioprine (Imuran)] for maintenance is being investigated. IV immune globulin and plasmapheresis are not effective. Anti-TNF therapy is under investigation.

For patients with WG limited to the upper airways, local therapy with nasal irrigation and nasal steroids may be given. Evidence suggests that **oral TMP/SMX** may be effective. Subglottic stenosis is treated with mechanical dilatation and intratracheal injection of a long-acting steroid.

Follow-up should include lab and radiographic studies of upper airway, lung, and kidney function. Anti-PR3 antibody levels correlate with disease activity in large groups of patients, but in individual patients, other direct studies of organ function are more useful. **Oral TMP/SMX,** 160 mg/800 mg bid, for 24 mos during remission has been shown to prevent relapses. Perform studies monitoring the toxicities of treatment.

KEY POINTS TO REMEMBER

- It is essential to monitor WG patients for opportunistic infections.
- WG is associated with c-ANCA, which is confirmed by anti-PR3 antibodies.
- Limited WG is a disease that is limited to the upper airways.
- Biopsies of upper airways usually provide limited help in establishing a pathologic diagnosis as these often consist of non-specific inflammation.

SUGGESTED READING

De Groot K, Gross WL. Wegener's granulomatosis: disease course, assessment of activity and extent, and treatment. *Lupus* 1998;7:285–291.

Duna GF, Galperin C, Hoffman GS. Wegener's granulomatosis. *Rheum Dis Clin North Am* 1995;21:949–986.

Hoffman GS, Specks U. Antineutrophil cytoplasmic antibodies. *Arthritis Rheum* 1998; 9:1521–1537.

Jennette JC, Falk RJ, Andrassy, et al. Nomenclature of systemic vasculitides: proposal of an international consensus conference. *Arthritis Rheum* 1994;2:187–192.

Langford CA, Hoffman GS. Wegener's granulomatosis. *Thorax* 1999;54:629–637.

Langford CA, Sneller MC. Update on the diagnosis and treatment of Wegener's granulomatosis. *Adv Intern Med* 2001;46:177–206.

Leavitt RY, Fauci AS, Bloch DA, et al. The American College of Rheumatology 1990 criteria for the classification of Wegener's granulomatosis. *Arthritis Rheum* 1990;33:1101–1107.

Mayet WJ, Helmreich-Becker I, Meyer zum Büschenfelde KH. The pathophysiology of anti-neutrophil cytoplasmic antibodies (ANCA) and their clinical relevance. *Crit Rev Oncol Hematol* 1996;23:151–165.

Stegeman CA, Cohen Tervaert JW, de Jong PE, et al. Trimethoprim-sulfamethaxazole (co-trimoxazole) for the prevention of relapses of Wegener's granulomatosis. *N Engl J Med* 1996;335:16–20.

25

Churg-Strauss Syndrome

Ernesto Gutierrez

INTRODUCTION

The Chapel Hill Consensus Conference defines *CSS*, also known as *allergic granulomatosis and angiitis*, as an **eosinophil-rich** and **granulomatous inflammation involving the respiratory tract** and necrotizing vasculitis affecting small- to medium-sized vessels associated with **asthma** and peripheral **eosinophilia.** It is a rare disease with an annual incidence of approximately 2.4 cases per million inhabitants. CSS tends to affect men slightly more often than women. The asthma associated with CSS usually begins in the fourth or fifth decade, although the age can vary.

CAUSES

Pathophysiology

The two diagnostic lesions are arterial and venous vasculitis and extravascular necrotizing granulomas, usually with eosinophilic infiltration of tissue. These findings coexist temporally only in a minority of patients. The signs and symptoms of CSS are caused by the effects these lesions have on the involved organ system at a given time and by the systemic effects of inflammation. The most commonly affected organ systems (in decreasing order) are pulmonary, neurologic, cutaneous, otorhinolaryngeal, musculoskeletal, GI, cardiac, and renal. p-ANCA—in particular, the anti-myeloperoxidase variant—has been associated with CSS in 70% of patients, but its role in pathogenesis is not well understood.

An association with leukotriene modifiers [zafirlukast (Accolate) and montelukast (Singulair)] has been recognized recently in patients with steroid-dependent asthma who were tapered from corticosteroids after initiation of the leukotriene modifier. Most of these patients had milder airway obstruction and a greater incidence of acute dilated cardiomyopathy than other patients with CSS. It is unclear whether the leukotriene modifiers induced the disease or the steroid tapering led to expression of patients with preexisting CSS.

Differential Diagnosis

The differential diagnosis includes PAN, MPA, WG, chronic eosinophilic pneumonia, and idiopathic hypereosinophilic syndrome (IHS). PAN usually spares the glomeruli and lungs, demonstrates arterial microaneurysms and stenoses, and tends to be negative for ANCA. MPA causes a necrotizing vasculitis of arterioles, venules, and capillaries without granulomas. It often involves the glomeruli and lungs. The key clinical, lab, and histologic findings should make the distinction between WG and CSS easy. Chronic eosinophilic pneumonia usually has no extrapulmonary findings, affects women, and has no granulomatous or vasculitic component. IHS typically has endomyocardial fibrosis and no vasculitic, granulomatous, asthmatic, or allergic component. IHS does not respond to systemic steroids.

PRESENTATION

History and Physical Exam

Three phases of CSS have been described. The first is a prodrome beginning in childhood and lasting up to 30 yrs characterized by **allergic rhinitis, sinusitis,** and **nasal polyposis. Asthma** develops later in life at an average age of 35 yrs. The asthma is usually severe and requires systemic corticosteroids.

The second phase is characterized by **peripheral blood and tissue eosinophilia.** Löffler's syndrome (transient, pulmonary, and acute eosinophilic infiltrates), chronic eosinophilic pneumonia, and eosinophilic gastroenteritis are common. The pulmonary infiltrates tend to be peripheral, patchy, parenchymal, migratory, and transient and are associated with eosinophilic pulmonary effusions, although these are neither sensitive nor specific pulmonary patterns.

The third phase is characterized by **small-vessel vasculitis,** with a mean time of onset of 3 yrs after the development of asthma. The symptoms are usually nonspecific **constitutional manifestations of systemic inflammation** (e.g., myalgias, arthralgias, fatigue, and weight loss). **Cutaneous signs** are similar to those of other vasculitides and include palpable purpura of the lower extremities, subcutaneous nodules of the scalp and lower extremities, livedo reticularis, and infarction. The asthma usually worsens during this phase. **Neurologic manifestations** are similar to those of PAN, with mononeuritis multiplex present in approximately 60–70% of cases. Distal symmetric peripheral neuropathies are also common, although occasional asymmetric peripheral neuropathies can occur. Cranial nerve palsies are less common, with ischemic optic neuritis being the most common. Cerebral infarctions can also occur.

Cardiac disease is the most common cause of mortality. Eosinophilic myocarditis and coronary vasculitis are the most common cardiac lesions and can lead to severe heart failure or MI. Pericardial effusions are also common but only occasionally lead to hemodynamic compromise. Endomyocardial fibrosis is rare. **GI tract manifestations** account for a substantial number of deaths and include tissue eosinophilic infiltration and/or mesenteric vasculitis with resultant ischemia, infarction, or perforation. **Renal involvement** tends to be mild. The most common renal manifestations are hematuria, albuminuria, and focal segmental necrotizing glomerulonephritis, although severe necrotizing glomerulonephritis has been described.

Systemic corticosteroid treatment for worsening asthma in patients with undiagnosed CSS in the earlier phases may blunt many of these signs and symptoms. There is no way to predict which patients with asthma will develop CSS.

MANAGEMENT

Diagnostic Workup

The American College of Rheumatology 1990 criteria for the classification of CSS require at least *four* of the following six:

- Asthma
- Eosinophilia >10%
- Mononeuropathy or polyneuropathy attributable to a systemic vasculitis
- Migratory or transient infiltrates on chest radiography
- Paranasal sinus abnormality (acute or chronic paranasal pain or radiographic opacification of paranasal sinuses)
- Extravascular eosinophils on biopsy

A patient with late-onset and worsening asthma, peripheral eosinophilia, and transient migratory lung infiltrates should raise suspicion for CSS. No test is specific for CSS. Biopsies of skin, nerve, or lung lesions may be diagnostic but may also be nonspecific, in which case they may be helpful in sorting through the differential diagnoses. Lab data supporting CSS include peripheral eosinophilia, elevated ESR, thrombocytosis, and elevated IgE levels. The presence of p-ANCA, specifically antimyeloperoxidase antibodies, may help support the diagnosis, but their absence does not rule out CSS. Measurement of urine protein and plasma creatinine and assessment of cardiac function provide prognostic information.

Treatment and Follow-Up

Treatment regimens include corticosteroids with or without additional immunosuppressants. The response to **oral prednisone**, 1 mg/kg qd, is dramatic. Within 1 mo, most patients are clinically improved and have a decreasing eosinophil count and ESR. Taper the steroid dose once the ESR is normal. **Pulse IV methylprednisolone (Medrol)**, 1000 mg qd for 3–5 days, is used for life-threatening disease. Recent studies suggest that combination therapy with **cyclophosphamide (Cytoxan, Neosar)** (usually 0.6 g/m^2 monthly IV doses with adjustments based on lab response or 2 mg/kg qd PO doses) has increased efficacy in those patients who have signs and symptoms of severe or life-threatening disease. **IV cyclophosphamide** is preferred for initial therapy, with oral forms reserved for severe disease or relapses. **High-dose IV immunoglobulins** may also be helpful. Most patients need long-term steroids because of residual asthma. There is little evidence to support plasma exchange. Patients receiving cyclophosphamide should receive **prophylaxis for _Pneumocystis carinii_ pneumonia with oral trimethoprim 160 mg/sulfamethaxazole 800 mg 3×/wk (Bactrim, Septra).**

Since the introduction of steroids and immunosuppressants, remission rates have been >75%. Follow-up involves clinical and lab assessment of disease status and monitoring of medication side effects and toxicities. Perform frequent eosinophil counts, as increases in counts tend to precede episodes of vasculitis. Factors associated with lower 5-yr survival rates include proteinuria >1 g/day, creatinine >1.58 mg/dL, cardiomyopathy, and GI tract or CNS involvement.

KEY POINTS TO REMEMBER

- Churg-Strauss vasculitis has a predilection for peripheral nerves and myocardium.
- Eosinophilia in the range of 5–20,000 eosinophils/μL commonly occurs with CSS.
- CSS is associated with asthma.

SUGGESTED READING

Choi YH, Im J, Han BK, et al. Thoracic manifestations of Churg-Strauss syndrome: radiological and clinical findings. _Chest_ 2000;117:117–124.

Cottin V, Cordier JF. Churg-Strauss syndrome. _Allergy_ 1999;54:535–551.

Eustace JA, Nadasdy T, Choi M. The Churg-Strauss syndrome. _J Am Soc Nephrol_ 1999;10:2048–2055.

Gayraud M, Guillevin L, le Toumelin P, et al. Long-term follow up of polyarteritis nodosa, microscopic polyangiitis, and Churg-Strauss syndrome. _Arthritis Rheum_ 2001;44:666–675.

Jennette JC, Falk RJ, Andrassy, et al. Nomenclature of systemic vasculitides: proposal of an international consensus conference. _Arthritis Rheum_ 1994;2:187–192.

Lhote FC, Guillevin L. Polyarteritis nodosa, microscopic polyangiitis, and Churg-Strauss syndrome: clinical aspects and treatment. _Rheum Dis Clin North Am_ 1995;21:911–947.

Manu S, Swanson, JW, Deremee RA, et al. Neurological manifestations of Churg-Strauss syndrome. _Mayo Clinic Proc_ 1995;70:337–341.

Masi AT, Hunder GC, Lie JT. The American College of Rheumatology 1990 criteria for the classification of Churg-Strauss syndrome (allergic granulomatosis and angiitis). _Arthritis Rheum_ 1990;33:1094–1100.

Weller PF, Plaut M, Taggart V, Trontell A. The relationship of asthma therapy and Churg-Strauss syndrome: NIH workshop summary report. _J Allergy Clin Immunol_ 2001;108:175–183.

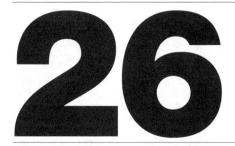

Microscopic Polyangiitis

Ernesto Gutierrez

INTRODUCTION

MPA is defined by the Chapel Hill Consensus Conference as a **necrotizing vasculitis affecting small vessels** (i.e., capillaries, venules, or arterioles) with few or no immune deposits. Necrotizing arteritis involving small- and medium-sized arteries may be present, necrotizing **glomerulonephritis** is very common, and pulmonary capillaritis often occurs. It was originally described as a microscopic variant of PAN in patients who had clinical manifestations of PAN and renal disease characterized by focal segmental necrotizing glomerulonephritis without granulomas. Hence, much of the literature groups MPA and PAN together. Unlike PAN, MPA is not associated with hepatitis B virus infection.

MPA affects men more often than women; the average age of onset is approximately 50 yrs. The prevalence and incidence of MPA are unknown but are thought to be less than that of PAN (see Chap. 23, Polyarteritis Nodosa).

CAUSES

Pathophysiology

The pathophysiology of MPA is poorly understood. Approximately 45% of cases are positive for antimyeloperoxidase (anti-MPO) antibodies, a specific type of **p-ANCA.** The role of anti-MPO antibodies in the pathogenesis is not well understood.

The characteristic pathologic lesion in MPA is focal segmental necrotizing vasculitis of arterioles, capillaries, and venules without granulomas. The vasculitic lesions may coexist with healed or normal vessels in different tissues or in different parts of the same tissue. Aneurysms like those in PAN are rare. Renal biopsies demonstrate segmental thrombosis, necrotizing glomerulonephritis, and proliferative crescents. Tubular damage and interstitial infiltration by mixed inflammatory cells are also common. The pulmonary capillaries and bronchial arteries are also commonly affected.

Differential Diagnosis

The differential diagnosis includes other causes of primary small-vessel vasculitis (e.g., cryoglobulinemia, WG, CSS, cutaneous vasculitis, and HSP), as well as vasculitides associated with CTD (e.g., SLE and RA).

As renal involvement is almost universal in MPA, consider causes of glomerulonephritis, both primary and secondary. The differential diagnosis of fulminant MPA with frank pulmonary hemorrhage and rapidly deteriorating renal failure includes fulminant WG and Goodpasture's syndrome.

Distinguishing PAN from MPA may be difficult, as the clinical manifestations of both are similar. Table 26-1 compares the two. Studies have suggested that, in patients with signs and symptoms of either MPA or PAN, the presence of ANCA in the correct clinical setting is diagnostic for MPA and, in most cases, rules out PAN. Abnormal angiograms effectively rule out MPA. Distinguishing between the two is important in determining the expected sequelae of each disease and in developing a therapeutic strategy.

TABLE 26-1. DISTINGUISHING FEATURES OF PAN AND MPA

Manifestation	PAN	MPA
Vasculitis	Necrotizing, medium- and small-sized arteries, may sometimes involve arterioles, and rarely granulomatous	Necrotizing small vessels, may sometimes involve small- and medium-sized arteries, no granulomas
Renal	Renal vasculitis with renovascular hypertension, infarcts, and microaneurysms; no RPGN	RPGN very common
Pulmonary	No hemorrhage	Hemorrhage common
Peripheral neuropathy	Present in 50–80%	Present in 10–50%
Relapses	Rare	Frequent
Lab data	ANCA positive in <20%, HBV may be present but uncommon, angiography commonly illustrates microaneurysms and stenoses	ANCA positive in 50–80%, HBV not present, normal angiography

HBV, hepatitis B virus; RPGN, rapidly progressive glomerulonephritis.
Adapted from Guillevin L, Lhote F. Distinguishing polyarteritis nodosa from microscopic polyangiitis and implications for treatment. *Curr Opin Rheumatol* 1995;7:20–24.

PRESENTATION

History and Physical Exam

The most common manifestations of MPA are constitutional, renal, pulmonary, GI, cutaneous, musculoskeletal, and neurologic. **Constitutional symptoms** (e.g., weakness, malaise, and arthralgias) are common in >60% of patients and are usually present for months or years before the onset of frank vasculitis. Hematuria and renal failure herald the onset of vasculitis. The characteristic **renal manifestation** in MPA is rapidly progressive glomerulonephritis, which is eventually present in all patients. Without treatment, renal function deteriorates rapidly. Nephrotic range proteinuria is common. **Pulmonary manifestations** range from scant hemoptysis during the early phase to frank pulmonary hemorrhage with fulminant disease. Pulmonary hemorrhage occurs in approximately 25% of patients and may be due to either capillaritis or bronchial arteritis. Patients may also present with clinical, radiologic, and pulmonary function findings suggesting interstitial fibrosis, a consequence of small-vessel vasculitis. The **GI, cutaneous, musculoskeletal,** and **neurologic manifestations** are similar to those of PAN, with a greater incidence of GI bleeding and a lower incidence of neuropathies in MPA (see Chap. 23, Polyarteritis Nodosa).

MANAGEMENT

Diagnostic Workup

The diagnostic workup of MPA includes assessment of renal, pulmonary, and nerve function (e.g., serum creatinine, urinalysis, spirometry, chest radiography, and nerve conduction studies). Almost all patients need renal biopsies to demonstrate the characteristic focal segmental glomerulonephritis. Cutaneous biopsies demonstrate leukocytoclastic vasculitis. Bronchoscopy with transbronchial biopsy and bronchoalveolar lavage is useful in demonstrating capillaritis and ruling out infectious causes of pulmonary hemorrhage. Lab findings include elevated ESRs, thrombocytosis, normochromic normocytic anemia of chronic inflammation, and, occasionally, eosinophilia. C3 and C4 levels are normal or elevated. p-ANCA is present in 50–80% of patients;

confirm this with anti-MPO antibodies. RF and ANAs may also be present in one-half and one-third of patients, respectively.

Treatment and Follow-Up

The initial therapy for MPA is the same as the treatment for PAN without hepatitis B virus infection. **Pulse IV methylprednisolone (Solu-Medrol)**, 1000 mg qd for 3 days, is followed by **prednisone PO**, 1 mg/kg qd. **Pulse IV cyclophosphamide (Cytoxan, Neosar)**, 0.5–1.0 g/m^2, is given with steroids every month depending on the patient's condition, response to previous therapy, renal function, and hematologic data (see Chap. 23, Polyarteritis Nodosa). Fulminant MPA with pulmonary hemorrhage and rapidly progressive renal failure is treated with the same regimen as that for immediately life-threatening fulminant WG, with **pulse IV methylprednisolone** and **daily oral cyclophosphamide** (see Chap. 24, Wegener's Granulomatosis). **Plasma exchange** may also be considered in refractory cases.

Maintenance therapy involves the substitution of cyclophosphamide with **azathioprine (Imuran)** after 4–6 mos. Prednisone is often continued. Relapses of MPA are common and usually occur during tapering of prednisone doses. Relapses are usually milder than the initial presentation and can often be treated with increased doses of prednisone. Occasionally, relapses may be severe enough that repeat induction therapy with cyclophosphamide is necessary.

Follow-up involves the clinical and lab assessment of disease activity as well as monitoring of medication toxicities.

KEY POINTS TO REMEMBER

- MPA often has anti-MPO.
- MPA is a small-vessel vasculitis with nongranulomatous pauci-immune glomerulonephritis.

SUGGESTED READING

Guillevin L, Lhote F. Distinguishing polyarteritis nodosa from microscopic polyangiitis and implications for treatment. *Curr Opin Rheumatol* 1995;7:20–24.

Guillevin L, Lhote F. Treatment of polyarteritis nodosa and microscopic polyangiitis. *Arthritis Rheum* 1998;12:2100–2105.

Guillevin L, Lhote F, Amouroux J, et al. Antineutrophil cytoplasmic antibodies, abnormal angiograms and pathological findings in polyarteritis nodosa and Churg-Strauss syndrome: indications for the classification of vasculitides of the polyarteritis nodosa group. *Br J Rheum* 1996;35:958–964.

Jennette JC, Falk RJ, Andrassy K, et al. Nomenclature of systemic vasculitides: proposal of an international consensus conference. *Arthritis Rheum* 1994;2:187–192.

Lhote F, Cohen P, Guillevin L. Polyarteritis nodosa, microscopic polyangiitis, and Churg-Strauss syndrome. *Lupus* 1998;7:238–258.

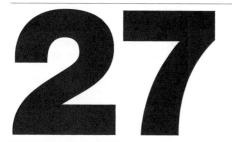

Henoch-Schönlein Purpura

Milan J. Anadkat and
Ernesto Gutierrez

INTRODUCTION

HSP is defined by the Chapel Hill Consensus Conference as **vasculitis with IgA-dominant immune deposits** affecting small vessels, including capillaries, venules, and arterioles. HSP affects the skin, kidneys, and GI tract and is associated with arthritis or arthralgias. Although HSP can be seen at any age, the majority of patients are children <10 yrs of age; the mean age is 6 yrs. HSP is slightly more common in men and boys and has an annual incidence of 14 cases per 100,000 people. It presents most commonly in the fall and winter months, often after a respiratory infection. Children generally have milder disease and are less likely to have nephritis. HSP is more severe and prolonged in adults; nephritis is generally more severe and renal failure more common.

CAUSES

Pathophysiology

HSP is characterized by deposition of IgA-dominant immune complexes in the walls of arterioles, capillaries, and post-capillary venules with resultant complement activation and leukocytoclastic vasculitis. Skin and GI manifestations are a direct result of inflammation and extravasation of blood cells. Renal biopsies demonstrate mesangial immune complex deposition, resulting in glomerulonephritis.

Although many cases follow respiratory infections and some are associated with administration of drugs and vaccines, no single dominant etiologic agent has been identified. Recent studies suggest that aberrant glycosylation within the hinge region of the IgA1 subtype may play a role in pathogenesis.

PRESENTATION

History and Physical Exam

The typical presentation of HSP is a child with colicky abdominal pain or lower extremity arthritis, usually preceded by signs and symptoms of an **upper respiratory tract infection** (e.g., fever, rhinorrhea, and cough). This is followed by bloody diarrhea and palpable purpura affecting the lower extremities and buttocks.

Palpable purpura is present in all patients with HSP. In children, it may be preceded by transient urticarial or maculopapular lesions. The purpura tends to occur in crops in regions such as the legs and buttocks. Individual lesions are 2–10 mm in diameter. Lesions may also appear in other areas of the body and often present before other manifestations. They typically last several days and resolve more quickly with bed rest.

Arthritis is the second most common manifestation of disease, present in 75% of patients. The knees, ankles, and feet are typically involved. The joints are typically warm and painful; joint effusions are not consistently present. The arthritis is usually self-limiting and nondeforming. It tends to be transient and rarely requires more than pain control.

GI involvement is another dominant feature of HSP, occurring in 50–75% of patients. Colicky abdominal pain and bleeding are the result of intestinal inflammation and edema. Potentially serious complications of HSP include intussusception, infarction, massive hemorrhage, and perforation. Unlike the typical ileocecal site of most intussusceptions, the intussusception seen in HSP is typically ileoileal.

Renal disease occurs in nearly 40% of patients. The most common renal manifestation is microscopic hematuria, but up to one-third of patients with nephritis have gross hematuria. HSP nephritis is typically not chronic and rarely leads to renal failure. Nephritis rarely precedes other manifestations; it usually arises 1–3 mos after the onset of other symptoms.

Occasionally, HSP affects the pulmonary vasculature, resulting in pulmonary capillaritis and alveolar hemorrhage. Coronary vessel vasculitis is rare.

Differential Diagnosis

The differential diagnosis of HSP includes other causes of small-vessel vasculitis [e.g., WG, MPA, cryoglobulinemic vasculitis (CV), and leukocytoclastic angiitis], PAN (in cases of unusually chronic or severe HSP), SLE, thrombotic thrombocytopenic purpura/hemolytic uremic syndrome, exanthematous drug eruption, purpura fulminans, and septic vasculitis.

Diagnostic Workup

The American College of Rheumatology 1990 criteria for the classification of HSP require the presence of *two* of the following four:

- Palpable purpura not related to thrombocytopenia
- Age ≤ 20 yrs at onset of symptoms
- Bowel angina, defined as either diffuse abdominal pain that is worsened by meals or the diagnosis of bowel ischemia, usually with bloody diarrhea
- Histologic changes showing granulocytes in the walls of arterioles or venules

In children with typical presentations, the diagnosis of HSP can be made once sepsis, thrombocytopenia, and clotting disorders are easily excluded. No invasive diagnostic studies are necessary. Basic lab data should include UA and serum creatinine levels. UA in patients with renal disease often demonstrates mild proteinuria and RBC casts. Renal biopsy is recommended in children with impaired renal function or marked proteinuria, as histologic lesions are indicators of prognosis. Other lab findings in patients with HSP include leukocytosis and elevated ESRs.

In adults, further studies are needed to rule out the other causes of small-vessel vasculitis. In addition, confirmatory biopsies of either skin or kidneys are often necessary. Skin biopsies demonstrate small-vessel leukocytoclastic vasculitis, most prominent in the post-capillary venules. Immunofluorescence studies show IgA-dominant immune complex vascular deposition. Findings on renal biopsies depend on degree of renal involvement. Biopsies in mild disease demonstrate focal mesangial proliferation with IgA-dominant immune complex deposition in the mesangial matrix. The renal biopsies in patients with more severe renal disease or with nephrotic range proteinuria are more likely to reveal marked cellular proliferation and crescentic glomerulonephritis.

MANAGEMENT

Treatment and Follow-Up

Most patients completely recover without specific therapy. **NSAIDs** are generally sufficient in relieving arthralgias and arthritis. **Corticosteroids** may be used for severe joint pain. Corticosteroids may also be used in severe abdominal pain, especially when intussusception is suspected. Do not use steroids for treatment of purpura; they play no role in decreasing the duration of disease or frequency of recurrences.

Long-term prognosis of HSP depends on the severity of renal impairment. Only 1% of patients develop end-stage renal disease. Patients with gross hematuria, nephrotic syndrome, or HTN are more likely to progress to end-stage renal disease. In those patients, renal biopsies provide prognostic information. Those with crescents involving >50% of the glomeruli have increased rates of chronic renal failure and end-stage renal disease. Therapeutic recommendations in patients with renal disease are therefore based on the pathologic findings. **Pulse IV methylprednisolone (Medrol)**, 30 mg/kg qd for 3 days, followed by **oral corticosteroids** is recommended for those with crescentic nephritis. Additional immunosuppressants (e.g., **azathioprine** or **cyclophosphamide**) are also recommended, but their additional benefits are not clear. **Plasmapheresis** and **IV immunoglobulins** may have a role in treating patients at risk for end-stage renal disease. Do not treat less severe nephritis.

HSP resolves within 2–4 wks. Recurrence of symptoms occurs in one-third of patients; resolution in these patients occurs within 4 mos. Repeat BP, serum creatinine, and UA at least every week in patients with mild renal disease while the disease is clinically active and once a month for 3 mos when the disease remits. Approximately 30–50% of patients with nephritis have persistent urinary abnormalities after long-term follow-up.

KEY POINTS TO REMEMBER

- HSP is more common in children but can occur in adults.
- Like IgA nephropathy, IgA deposits play a central role in the mechanism of disease in HSP.

SUGGESTED READING

Blanco R, Martinez-Taboada VM, Rodriguez-Valverde V, et al. Henoch-Schönlein purpura in adulthood and childhood: two expressions of the same syndrome. *Arthritis Rheum* 1997;40:859–864.

Flynn JT, Smoyer WE, Bunchman TE, et al. Treatment of Henoch-Schönlein purpura glomerulonephritis in children with high-dose corticosteroids plus oral cyclophosphamide. *Am J Nephrol* 2001;21:128–133.

Niaudet P, Habib R. Methylprednisolone pulse therapy in the treatment of Henoch-Schönlein purpura nephritis. *Pediatr Nephrol* 1998;12:238–243.

Saulsbury FT. Henoch-Schönlein purpura. *Curr Opin Rheumatol* 2001;13:35–40.

Saulsbury FT. Henoch-Schönlein purpura in children: report of 100 patients and review of the literature. *Medicine (Baltimore)* 1999;78:395–409.

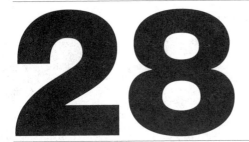

Cryoglobulinemia and Cryoglobulinemic Vasculitis

Ernesto Gutierrez

INTRODUCTION

Cryoglobulinemia refers to the presence of circulating cryoglobulins. Essential cryoglobulinemic vasculitis (CV) is defined by the Chapel Hill Consensus Conference as a vasculitis associated with cryoglobulinemia and with cryoglobulin immune deposits affecting small vessels such as capillaries, venules, or arterioles. Skin and glomeruli are often involved, but the musculoskeletal and nervous systems can also be affected. Cryoglobulinemia does not necessarily lead to CV, and cryoglobulinemia may cause disease in the absence of vasculitis.

CV affects patients in their 50s and 60s, with a female predominance of greater than 2:1. CV is commonly associated with lymphoproliferative diseases (e.g., multiple myeloma, leukemia, and lymphoma), chronic infections [e.g., hepatitis C virus (HCV)], and CTDs (e.g., SLE and RA). *Essential cryoglobulinemia* refers to the cryoglobulinemia with no known primary cause. Since the association between HCV and cryoglobulinemia was first recognized in 1990, it is recognized that many of the earlier reported cases of CV due to essential cryoglobulinemia were probably actually caused by HCV. >50% of HCV patients have either type II or type III cryoglobulinemia, but only approximately 25% of HCV patients with cryoglobulinemia have CV, mostly associated with type II cryoglobulins.

CAUSES

Pathophysiology

Cryoglobulins are immunoglobulins that reversibly precipitate at temperatures below body temperature. Three types of cryoglobulins have been described: Type I cryoglobulins are self-aggregating monoclonal antibodies, type II are monoclonal antibodies to polyclonal immunoglobulins, and type III are polyclonal antibodies to polyclonal immunoglobulins (see Chap. 5, Lab Evaluation of Rheumatic Diseases).

Type I cryoglobulins are most commonly associated with lymphoproliferative diseases. They are produced by monoclonal expansions of B-cell lymphocytes. They are more likely to produce vasoocclusive symptoms and less likely to produce vasculitis.

Type II and type III cryoglobulins are more often essential cryoglobulins, but they may be associated with lymphoproliferative diseases, chronic liver disease, and CTD. The pathogenesis of both types II and III cryoglobulinemia and CV is not well understood. Current investigations suggest that cryoglobulins are produced by low-grade localized clonal expansions of B-lymphocytes stimulated by a number of factors. It is believed that cryoglobulins affect different tissues in different ways. For example, patients with glomerulonephritis caused by immune complex deposition in type III cryoglobulinemia associated with HCV and hepatitis B virus (HBV) infections tend to lack the typical manifestation of small-vessel vasculitis (e.g., purpura, arthralgias, and polyneuropathy). Immune complex deposition consisting of type II IgM cryoglobulins, HCV RNA, IgG, and complement can be found in cutaneous biopsies of vasculitic lesions in patients with CV caused by type II cryoglobulins, whereas nerve biopsies with active disease often lack immune complexes, HCV RNA, and HCV proteins. Furthermore, renal biopsies often lack any HCV-related proteins. Biopsies with membranoproliferative glomerulonephritis may show deposition of type II IgM cryoglobulins with particular affinity to mesangial matrix proteins.

Differential Diagnosis

On clinical presentation of CV, consider other causes of small-vessel vasculitis (e.g., HSP), cutaneous vasculitides, and the ANCA vasculitides (e.g., MPA, WG, and CSS). Only CV is characterized by the presence of cryoglobulins. CV can be distinguished from the ANCA vasculitides by the absence of ANCA and the presence of low C4 levels and fluctuating C3 levels that correlate with disease activity.

PRESENTATION

History and Physical Exam

Constitutional symptoms (e.g., fever, myalgias, arthralgias, and weight loss) as well as skin involvement, weakness, peripheral neuropathy, and renal and liver disease are common manifestations of CV.

Palpable purpura is the most common symptom of CV. Lesions tend to involve the lower extremities, gradually extending proximally to the lower abdomen and occasionally involving the upper extremities but sparing the trunk and face. The rash can last for 1–2 wks and occurs once or twice a month; exposure to cold precipitates the lesions only in a minority of patients. Raynaud's phenomenon is also common. Livedo reticularis, urticaria, and subcutaneous nodules are less common. Type I cryoglobulins may cause occlusive symptoms (e.g., acrocyanosis, digital infarction, and ulcers).

Arthralgias affect the small distal joints more commonly than the larger proximal joints and may be exacerbated by cold. Arthritis is rare.

Symmetric peripheral neuropathy is the most common neurologic presentation and seems to occur more frequently in patients with type III cryoglobulinemia. The presentation is acute or subacute. Mononeuritis multiplex with a chronic or chronic-relapsing course can also occur. The neuropathy is characterized by axonal degeneration resulting initially in sensory deficits and followed later by motor deficits.

Renal disease is most common in patients with type II cryoglobulinemia. It occurs in approximately 25% of patients and usually follows the onset of purpura by approximately 4 yrs, although the two can occur concomitantly. Most patients present with non–nephrotic-range proteinuria, hematuria, and HTN; acute nephritis and nephrotic syndromes may also occur. Type I membranoproliferative glomerulonephritis accounts for approximately 80% of type II cryoglobulinemic nephropathy and is likely to present with chronic renal insufficiency. Mild mesangial proliferative nephropathy, acute vasculitis of the small and medium renal vessels, and thrombotic microangiopathy occur less commonly. Renal vasculitis and thrombotic microangiopathy may cause oliguria and rapidly progressive renal failure.

Liver disease is usually related to HCV infection. Hepatomegaly and splenomegaly are common. Liver specimens are characterized by diffuse lymphoid infiltration of liver parenchyma, ranging from minimal periportal infiltration to extensive nodular formation. As the liver disease progresses to cirrhosis, the likelihood of having a monotypic component of cryoglobulinemia, as well as the level of cryoglobulins, decreases.

Lymphadenopathy, mesenteric vasculitis, subclinical pulmonary fibrosis, and pulmonary vasculitis are less common manifestations of CV. Monosymptomatic courses of CV also exist, with predominantly skin, renal, or neural manifestations.

MANAGEMENT

Diagnostic Workup

The American College of Rheumatology does not have a set of criteria for the classification of cryoglobulinemia or CV.

The Gruppo Italiano di Studio delle Crioglobulinemie has offered a system of defining and characterizing symptomatic cryoglobulinemia:

- Cryocrit >1% for at least 6 mos
- At least two of the following: purpura, weakness, arthralgias, or C4 level <8 mg/dL
- Positive RF, characterized as either monoclonal or polyclonal
- Secondary if associated with CTD, chronic liver disease, or lymphoproliferative diseases
- Essential if without any underlying conditions
- Assessment of the extent of vasculitis (e.g., hepatic and renal involvement and neuropathies)
- Identification of microlymphoma-like nodules in the bone marrow

Once the diagnosis of cryoglobulinemia is established, perform a clinical and lab search for secondary causes of cryoglobulinemia. Causes include lymphoproliferative diseases (e.g., multiple myeloma, non-Hodgkin's lymphoma, chronic leukemias, Waldenström's macroglobulinemia, and immunoblastic lymphadenopathy), HCV infection, and CTDs (e.g., SLE, RA, SS, polymyositis, and dermatomyositis). Other viral infections (e.g., HIV, HBV, Epstein-Barr virus, CMV, influenza, and varicella) as well as bacterial endocarditis, syphilis, and some parasitic diseases can cause transient cryoglobulinemia.

The search for lymphoproliferative diseases should include a bone marrow biopsy, as many patients initially diagnosed with essential cryoglobulinemia may have lymphoproliferative diseases on biopsy. Examine the biopsy with caution, as most patients have abnormal biopsies characterized by reactive lymphocytosis. Furthermore, microlymphoma-like nodules that are present in essential cryoglobulinemia may be difficult to identify. As may be expected, patients with type II cryoglobulinemia should have some component of a B-cell lymphocyte clonal expansion on flow cytometry, but whether this represents a low-grade lymphoma or a potentially premalignant condition is unknown.

Evaluation for HCV must include testing for both HCV antibody and HCV RNA serum levels, even if liver enzyme tests are normal. Patients with negative serum HCV assays may have serum HCV RNA or HCV antibodies concentrated in circulating cryoglobulin immune complexes. Repeat testing after the serum is treated with acid to dissociate the immune complexes. Further problems arise in patients with cryoglobulinemia due to HCV infection. HCV infection commonly induces multiple autoantibodies, and patients may have features of certain autoimmune diseases, further confounding the diagnosis.

Other lab findings are consistent with systemic inflammation (e.g., elevated ESRs, normochromic normocytic anemia of chronic inflammation, and thrombocytosis). Low complement levels are present in approximately 90% of patients, and RF is present in approximately 75% of patients. Assess renal function with serum creatinine levels and urinalysis. Perform liver function tests. Assess cutaneous and sural nerve biopsies with immunofluorescence assays to identify immune complex deposition.

In summary, the diagnosis of CV is made by the presence of typical symptoms of CV, lab evidence of cryoglobulinemia, and evaluation for any secondary causes of cryoglobulinemia. Perform lab and pathologic assessment of organ involvement.

Treatment and Follow-Up

The treatment of cryoglobulinemia associated with lymphoproliferative diseases, CTD, and bacterial or parasitic infections is treatment of the underlying condition. **Plasmapheresis** may be used in cases of severe vasculitis.

The treatment of severe, life-threatening, essential or HCV-associated CV is the same as the induction treatment regimen used in severe, life-threatening WG, with **daily oral cyclophosphamide (Cytoxan, Neosar)** and **pulse IV methylprednisolone (Solu-Medrol, Medrol)** for 3 days followed by **daily oral prednisone** (see Chap. 24, Wegener's Granulomatosis). **Plasmapheresis** may be used in addition to immunosuppressive therapy to facilitate removal of cryoglobulins.

Treat severe, non–life-threatening disease with the same regimen used in PAN without HBV, with **monthly pulse IV cyclophosphamide** and **pulse IV methylpred-.nisolone** followed by **daily oral prednisone** (see Chap. 23, Polyarteritis Nodosa).

Once remission of severe disease is achieved, or if the presenting disease is mild, treat essential CV with **daily oral prednisone** and **weekly oral methotrexate (Rheu-**

matrex) as used in remission therapy for WG (see Chap. 24, Wegener's Granulomatosis). Patients with only skin manifestations and arthralgias may be treated symptomatically with NSAIDs.

The maintenance therapy for HCV-associated CV and induction therapy for mild HCV-associated CV is treatment of the HCV infection. The current treatment regimen is interferon-alpha, 3×10^6 units 3 times/wk, with the possible addition of ribavirin (Virazole). Corticosteroids may block viral elimination but may be necessary to control certain symptoms. Consultation with a hepatologist is advised.

Follow-up involves clinical and lab assessment of disease activity and organ function with the appropriate changes in medication regimens.

KEY POINTS TO REMEMBER

- Cryoglobulins can lead to a false positive RF.
- CV is often associated with decreased complement levels.

SUGGESTED READING

Della Rossa A, Trevisani G, Bombardieri S. Cryoglobulins and cryoglobulinemia: diagnostic and therapeutic considerations. *Clin Rev Allergy Immunol* 1998;16:249–264.

Dispenzieri A, Gorevic PD. Cryoglobulinemia. *Hematol Oncol Clin North Am* 1999;13:1315–1349.

Ferri C, La Civita L, Longombardo G, et al. Mixed cryoglobulinaemia: a cross-road between autoimmune and lymphoproliferative disorders. *Lupus* 1998;7:275–279.

Invernizzi F, Pietrogrande M, Sagramoso B. Classification of the cryoglobulinemic syndrome. *Clin Exp Rheumatol* 1995;13(S13):S123–S128.

Jennette JC, Falk RJ, Andrassy K, et al. Nomenclature of systemic vasculitides: proposal of an international consensus conference. *Arthritis Rheum* 1994;2:187–192.

Lambrecht P, Gause A, Gross WL. Cryoglobulinemic vasculitis. *Arthritis Rheum* 1999;42:2507–2516.

Vassilopoulos D, Calabrese LH. Hepatitis C virus infection and vasculitis. *Arthritis Rheum* 2002;46:585–597.

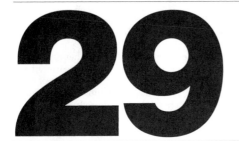

Cutaneous Vasculitis

Celso R. Velázquez

INTRODUCTION AND PATHOPHYSIOLOGY

Cutaneous vasculitis is a **small-vessel vasculitis affecting the skin.** It may occur as a result of a drug reaction or may be associated with systemic vasculitis (e.g., Henoch-Schönlein purpura), CTDs (e.g., SLE), malignancies, or infections (Table 29-1). As many as 15% of cases of cutaneous vasculitis are idiopathic.

Most cases of drug-induced cutaneous vasculitis do not involve other organs and resolve spontaneously. Some cases have a chronic course with remissions and recurrences. The **pathophysiology** of cutaneous vasculitis depends on the etiology. Certain infections cause direct invasion of blood vessels (e.g., *Neisseria, Rickettsia*) or may induce immune complex deposition (e.g., hepatitis B virus infection). Other vasculitides may also be immune-complex mediated (drug-induced or rheumatoid vasculitis) or due to immunoglobulin deposition (e.g., HSP). ANCA-associated vasculitis may involve the skin in addition to other organs, but the role of ANCA in these cases is unclear.

Leukocytoclastic vasculitis (LCV) is a pathologic term. *Leukocytoclasis* refers to the nuclear "dust" due to degranulation of neutrophils seen under light microscopy. Leukocytoclasia is nonspecific, and LCV may be seen with different causes of cutaneous vasculitis. **Necrotizing vasculitis** is synonymous with LCV. **Cutaneous leukocytoclastic angiitis** refers to isolated cutaneous vasculitis without systemic vasculitis or glomerulonephritis. **Hypersensitivity vasculitis** is a cutaneous vasculitis of the small vessels (arterioles and venules) secondary to an immune response to an exogenous substance. However, there is often no clear evidence of an immune response or an inciting agent. **Cutaneous leukocytoclastic angiitis,** or more simply, **cutaneous vasculitis,** may be the preferred term over **hypersensitivity vasculitis.**

Despite the confusing terminology, the **approach to vasculitis of the skin** is clear; aim the evaluation to answer the following questions: (a) Are the skin findings due to vasculitis? (b) What is the etiology? and (c) Are other organ systems involved?

PRESENTATION

History and Physical Exam

Cutaneous vasculitis usually appears suddenly, and the lesions are often painless. Myalgias or arthralgias may accompany the skin lesions. A history of a CTD (e.g., RA, SLE) is important, as are symptoms of an underlying systemic disease (fever, weight loss, hematuria, abdominal pain, joint pain, focal or generalized weakness). Examine the medication list for possible etiologic agents. Drug-induced vasculitis usually develops 7–21 days after starting drug.

Palpable purpura is the classic lesion of cutaneous vasculitis. Purpuric lesions are nonblanching and result from the extravasation of erythrocytes; the surrounding cellular infiltrate (neutrophils, lymphocytes) causes a palpable induration. Central necrosis may develop. Nonpalpable purpura, nodules, urticaria, vesicles, and shallow or deep ulcerations are also seen, sometimes in combination. Lesions usually occur in the lower extremities or in dependent locations. The physical exam aims to identify

TABLE 29-1. CAUSES OF CUTANEOUS VASCULITIS

Drugs (most common cause)	Penicillins, sulfonamides, allopurinol, thiazides, quinolones, propylthiouracil, hydantoins
Infections	*Neisseria, rickettsia, Streptococcus*, hepatitis virus
Connective tissue diseases	RA, SLE, SS
Systemic vasculitis (not associated with ANCA)	HSP, PAN, CV, urticarial vasculitis, Behçet's disease
ANCA-associated vasculitis	WG, CSS, MPA
Malignancies	Leukemia, lymphoma
Idiopathic	—

other organ system involvement and should include a musculoskeletal exam looking for arthritis and a neurologic exam to identify focal or diffuse weakness.

MANAGEMENT

Diagnostic Workup

A **skin biopsy** is essential to confirm the diagnosis. If possible, perform biopsies within 24–48 hrs after the appearance of a lesion. Examine specimens under light microscopy and direct immunofluorescence. Affected blood vessels are characterized by fibrinoid necrosis of the vessel wall with an inflammatory infiltrate within and around the vessel wall. Hemorrhage and fragments of leukocytes (leukocytoclasia) are also seen. Direct immunofluorescence may reveal immunoglobulin and complement deposition on the vessel wall. In particular, IgA deposition is characteristic of Henoch-Schönlein purpura. Cutaneous vasculitis associated with CTDs often has lymphocytic infiltration.

Investigate renal involvement with chemistries and UA. Blood cultures (and cultures from other sites) are mandatory in cases with fever. The ESR is often elevated but is nonspecific. Testing for ANA and RF is not recommended unless the clinical suspicion of SLE or RA exists. ANCA testing may be useful, as are hepatitis serologies and cryoglobulin determination. Chest radiographs or CT scans may be needed to evaluate the lungs and the upper respiratory tract.

Treatment and Follow-Up

In the absence of other organ involvement and underlying diseases, treatment of cutaneous vasculitis is symptomatic. Antihistamines and NSAIDs may be helpful. Some severe cases may require corticosteroids. If drug-induced vasculitis is suspected, stop the offending drug. Most cases of drug-induced cutaneous vasculitis resolve within weeks to a few months. The treatment of cutaneous vasculitis as a manifestation of an underlying disorder varies according to the type of disorder and the other organ involvement.

URTICARIAL VASCULITIS

Patients with urticarial vasculitis have urticarial wheals that may become necrotic. Skin biopsy reveals small-vessel vasculitis. Urticarial vasculitis should be suspected in patients who have urticarial lesions that persist for more than 24–48 hours. It may involve other organ systems; up to one-third of patients have renal or pulmonary involvement. Patients with urticarial vasculitis may have normal or decreased complement levels. Hypocomplementemic urticarial vasculitis is usually more severe and prolonged and may be associated with SLE. Urticarial vasculitis may require treatment with corticosteroids.

KEY POINTS TO REMEMBER

- Evaluate patients with vasculitis of the skin for other end-organ damage.
- Biopsy of any ulcer margin may show leukocytoclastic vasculitis, regardless of the ulcer etiology.

SUGGESTED READING

Gibson LE, Su WPD. Cutaneous vasculitis. *Rheum Dis Clin North Am* 1995;21:1097–1113.

Stone JH, Nousari HC. "Essential" cutaneous vasculitis: what every rheumatologist should know about vasculitis of the skin. *Curr Opin Rheumatol* 2001;13:23–34.

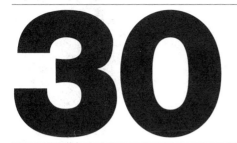

Thromboangiitis Obliterans

Ernesto Gutierrez

INTRODUCTION

Thromboangiitis obliterans (TAO), or *Buerger's disease*, is an **inflammatory disease of medium- and small-sized vessels** in the arms and legs characterized by segmental nonatherosclerotic thrombotic vessel stenosis and occlusion with subsequent limb ischemia and necrosis or thrombophlebitis.

TAO tends to affect male **smokers** <40 yrs. The incidence of TAO has decreased in the United States since its description in the first half of the twentieth century, despite the increasing numbers of tobacco smokers. The prevalence rate in the United States in 1986 was approximately 12.6 cases per 100,000. It is more common in the Middle and Far East and in Ashkenazi Jews in Israel. TAO accounts for 45–63% of the patients with peripheral vascular disease in India.

CAUSES

Pathophysiology

The cause of TAO is unknown. Tobacco use, either past or present, is strongly associated with TAO and is believed to be important in the pathogenesis, but its exact role remains to be elucidated. It has been suggested that arsenic poisoning can cause many of the same symptoms of TAO, and contamination of tobacco with arsenic can explain the epidemiologic national and international trends. Studies have demonstrated impaired mechanisms of endothelium-dependent vasodilation in response to acetylcholine in patients with TAO. Some authors suggest that previously unrecognized or underappreciated hypercoagulable states may be responsible for TAO or may have been misdiagnosed as TAO.

Pathologic findings in biopsies of affected arteries and veins vary according to the stage of disease. In the acute stage, vascular occlusion caused by a highly cellular and inflammatory thrombus consisting of neutrophils, multinucleated giant cells, and microabscesses with relative sparing of the vessel wall is seen. Later stages show organized thrombosis and fibrosis. Vascular wall architecture is maintained in all stages, in contrast to atherosclerotic stenosis or other vasculitic lesions where wall structure is disrupted.

Differential Diagnosis

The differential diagnosis includes atherosclerotic disease, hypercoagulable states, embolic disease, CREST-variant scleroderma, and other small-vessel vasculitides.

PRESENTATION

History and Physical Exam

The typical presentation of TAO is a male smoker <40 with ischemic signs and symptoms in the extremities (e.g., claudication or ulcerations). **Ulceration** is more common than **claudication** as an initial symptom because of the tendency of TAO to affect smaller arteries first. Pain at rest and sensory deficits are very common, usually from **ischemic neuritis. Migratory superficial thrombophlebitis** and **Raynaud's phenomenon** are present in 40–50% of patients. Signs of peripheral vascular disease (e.g., extremity poikilothermia, pallor, pulselessness, and paresthesia) are present in the affected as well as the unaffected limbs. An abnormal Allen test in a young male smoker with lower extremity ischemia suggests diffuse limb disease and is suggestive of TAO. TAO rarely affects the cerebral, coronary, mesenteric, pulmonary, iliac, or renal arteries, or the aorta.

MANAGEMENT

Diagnostic Workup

The American College of Rheumatology does not have diagnostic or classification criteria for TAO. Several authors have suggested criteria for diagnosis. Most criteria propose a combination of clinical, angiographic, histopathologic, and exclusionary findings. A commonly used set of criteria requires an age of onset <45 yrs, current or recent tobacco use, presence of distal-extremity ischemia manifested as claudication, rest pain, ulceration, or gangrene, and angiogram findings consistent with TAO. Autoimmune diseases, hypercoagulable states, diabetes mellitus, and proximal sources of emboli by echocardiography and angiography must be excluded.

Unlike other vasculitides, TAO does not have lab signs of systemic inflammation (e.g., elevated ESR, thrombocytosis, normochromic normocytic anemia, presence of autoantibodies, or serologic evidence of immune disease). Perform angiography in all four limbs, even those without clinical evidence of occlusive disease. Angiography of TAO shows segmental occlusive disease of small- and medium-sized vessels (e.g., palmar, plantar, tibial, peroneal, radial, ulnar, and digital arteries) with severe distal disease, distal collateralization, and normal proximal arteries. "Corkscrew" collaterals, referring to the anatomic pattern of vessels, are a common finding. Histopathologic exam is only necessary in cases that are atypical or that have confounding factors.

Treatment and Follow-Up

Crucial to the treatment of TAO is **complete smoking cessation.** Even second-hand smoke may be enough for disease progression. With smoking cessation, the disease remits and amputation can be avoided, but patients may still have claudication or Raynaud's phenomenon. Aspirin or other antiplatelet agents may be helpful. Daily IV iloprost, a prostacyclin analogue, may reduce ischemic symptoms more effectively than aspirin.

Surgical therapy for TAO includes amputation, sympathectomy, revascularization, and omental transfer. Sympathectomy may be helpful in healing superficial ulcerations. Revascularization is often not possible, because patients typically do not have a suitable distal target vessel. Omental transfer is becoming popular in India in cases refractory to sympathectomy and not amenable to surgical revascularization.

Follow-up involves continued efforts for smoking cessation and appropriate surgical interventions as necessary.

KEY POINTS TO REMEMBER

- TAO, or Buerger's disease, is often associated with smoking.
- Smoking cessation is essential for successful treatment of TAO.

SUGGESTED READING

Noël B. Buerger disease or arsenic intoxication? *Arch Intern Med* 2001;161:1016.

Noël B. Thromboangiitis obliterans: a new look for an old disease. *Int J Cardiol* 2001;78:199.

Olin JW. Thromboangiitis obliterans. *N Engl J Med* 2000;343:864–869.

Talwar S. Buerger's disease. *Int J Cardiol* 1999;68:241–242.

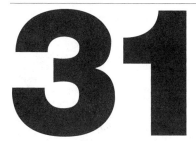

Behçet's Syndrome

Ernesto Gutierrez

INTRODUCTION

Behçet's syndrome (BS) is a **systemic vasculitis characterized by recurrent aphthous ulcers, genital ulcers, uveitis, and skin lesions.** BS is unique among the vasculitides in its ability to affect vessels of any size.

BS is most common along the ancient Silk Route extending from eastern Asia to the Mediterranean basin. Turkey has the highest prevalence of disease, estimated at 80–370 cases/100,000 population. Germans of Turkish origin have a prevalence of 21 cases/100,000, significantly higher than native Germans, who have approximately 0.5 cases/100,000. Prevalence rates in Japan, Korea, China, Iran, and Saudi Arabia are roughly 15 cases/100,000. BS is very rare in Western countries; the United Kingdom has 0.64 cases/100,000, and the United States has roughly 0.2 cases/100,000. BS is more common in females in the Far Eastern countries and more common in males in Middle Eastern countries. Age of onset is in the third or fourth decade.

CAUSES

Pathophysiology

BS is characterized by vascular injury, hyperfunctioning neutrophils, and immune dysfunction. Vascular injury consists of vasculitis of small vessels with subsequent vascular occlusion. Larger vessels demonstrate vasculitis of the vasa vasorum with aneurysm formation and superimposed hypercoagulability resulting in thrombosis. Active ulcerative lesions are infiltrated by hyperfunctioning neutrophils. Although neutrophils are found in active ulcers, they are not the primary abnormality in BS. It is believed that an unknown factor triggers local hypersecretion of cytokines that overstimulate the neutrophil. Immune dysfunction is characterized by lymphocytic infiltration of active lesions and clonal expansion of T cells. HLA-B51 has also been associated with disease in those countries with high prevalence rates. The main abnormality in BS has yet to be elucidated, but it is believed that the clinical manifestations are due to vasculitis of various-sized vessels in affected organs.

Differential Diagnosis

The differential diagnosis of BS depends on the clinical manifestations. If oral and genital ulcers are present, consider ReA. If ocular manifestations and acneiform nodules are present, seronegative arthropathies are in the differential. Ulcerative lesions in the colon have histologic similarity to ulcerative colitis. Erythema nodosum, ileocecal involvement, and ulcerative mouth lesions may suggest Crohn's disease. Sarcoidosis may also produce erythema nodosum. CNS involvement may mimic MS.

PRESENTATION

History and Physical Exam

The most common symptoms at presentation of BS in most series are **oral ulcers,** eye disease, and skin lesions.

Oral ulcers are usually present for years before other manifestations of BS. They are seen in all patients during the course of disease. The ulcer begins as a raised area of redness that soon ulcerates. Ulcers are painful, 2–10 mm in size, and round and have a sharp erythematous border, a necrotic white-centered base, and a yellow pseudomembrane. They appear on the gingiva, tongue, and buccal and labial membranes and heal within approximately 10 days. They tend to recur frequently during the first few years.

Ocular symptoms of BS include changes in visual acuity, pain, photophobia, lacrimation, floaters, and periorbital erythema. Approximately 10% of patients have eye disease at presentation, but approximately 50% have manifestations during the course of disease. Ocular manifestations as the initial symptom are more common in females, but eye involvement tends to be more severe in males during the course of disease. Blindness occurs in approximately 25% of patients. Anterior uveitis tends to be recurrent and self-limited, with repeated attacks causing iris deformity and glaucoma. A **hypopyon**, a layer of pus in the anterior ocular chamber, may be visible. Retinal disease is characterized by vasculitis causing vasoocclusive disease. The attacks are recurrent and episodic and result in painless, bilateral, and gradual visual loss. Retinal hemorrhage, exudative lesions, and cellular infiltration of the vitreous humor are visible on exam.

The **cutaneous manifestations** of BS include erythema nodosum, pseudofolliculitis, and acneiform nodules. Erythema nodosum is observed in approximately 50% of patients throughout the course of disease and is more common in females. Recurrent and painful subcutaneous nodules occur in the front of the legs and last for a few weeks. The nodules often leave an area of hyperpigmentation after spontaneous resolution and can occasionally ulcerate. Pseudofolliculitis and acneiform nodules are more common in men. The lesions are found on the back, face, neck, and along the hairline. Shaving often causes pseudofolliculitis.

Genital ulcers are rarely presenting symptoms of BS, but they appear in approximately 75% of patients over the course of disease. They are similar in appearance to oral ulcers, but they are more painful, last longer, recur less frequently, and leave scars. In young women, the appearance of ulcers may be related temporally to the menstrual cycle and may be the only manifestation of disease during early years.

Articular manifestations are common. The arthritis of BS is nondeforming, occasionally recurrent, and rarely chronic. It tends to be monoarticular, commonly affecting the knee, wrist, ankle, or elbow joints, but it can also be oligoarticular or polyarticular.

Venous thrombosis is a characteristic manifestation of BS. Superficial thrombophlebitis and deep venous thrombosis are common after injury to vessels, including cannulation by angiocatheters. Occlusions and aneurysms of major vessels can cause organ dysfunction, hemorrhage, or infarction (e.g., Budd-Chiari syndrome or pulmonary hemorrhage). Embolic events are rare.

CNS involvement in BS occurs in approximately 10–20% of patients. It is more common and more severe in males, particularly if the disease begins at a young age. Manifestations include aseptic meningitis, meningoencephalitis, focal neurologic deficits, and personality changes. These manifestations tend to develop more than 5 yrs after the time of diagnosis. Focal signs include pyramidal tract disease (e.g., spastic paralysis, Babinski sign, clonus, speech disturbances), brain stem disease (e.g., dysphagia and fits of laughter and crying), cerebellar ataxia, and pseudobulbar palsy. Sensory deficits are uncommon. Intracranial venous thrombosis can lead to intracranial HTN, seizures, and hemorrhage. Disease tends to recur and becomes irreversible: 40% have a relapsing-remitting course, 30% a secondary progressive course, and 16% a primary progressive course. In the terminal stage, approximately 30% of affected patients have dementia. Aseptic meningitis or meningoencephalitis early in the disease treated with steroids carries a good prognosis.

Other less common manifestations of BS include sterile tricuspid valve vegetations, epididymitis, and ileocecal, colonic, and esophageal ulceration.

MANAGEMENT

Diagnostic Workup

The International Study Group for Behçet's Disease published diagnostic criteria for BS in 1990. The observation by either patient or physician of oral aphthous ulcers, recurring at least three times over a 12-month period, is necessary for diagnosis. At least two of the following four are also necessary: (a) recurrent genital aphthous ulceration or scarring observed by patient or physician; (b) anterior or posterior uveitis, cells in vitreous humor, or retinal vasculitis observed by an ophthalmologist; (c) erythema nodosum or pseudofolliculitis observed by patient or physician or acneiform nodules in postadolescents not receiving steroids; and (d) positive pathergy test observed by physician at 24–48 hrs. The pathergy test is performed by using two SC pricks with blunt 20-gauge sterile needles to one arm and two SC pricks with sharp 20-gauge sterile needles to the other arm. A test is considered positive if a sterile erythematous papule >2 mm forms at 48 hrs.

Lab findings can include an elevated ESR, mild leukocytosis, and elevated immunoglobulins. T_2-weighted MRI of the brain can show multiple high-intensity focal lesions in the brain stem, basal ganglia, and white matter. CSF analysis may show elevated protein and IgG levels and pleocytosis with high numbers of both lymphocytes and neutrophils.

Treatment and Follow-Up

Treatment of BS depends on the manifestations. Mucocutaneous ulcers are treated with **topical steroids** [e.g., triamcinolone (Aristocort Topical, Kenalog, Triacet) ointment tid for oral ulcers and betamethasone ointment tid for genital ulcers]. **Oral colchicine,** 0.5–1.5 mg qd, may be used for the oral and genital ulcers, pseudofolliculitis, or erythema nodosum. Severe recurrent ulcerations can be treated with **azathioprine (Imuran),** 2.5 mg/kg qd; **thalidomide (Thalomid),** 100–400 mg qd, or **dapsone (Dapsone USP, DDS),** 100 mg qd. Thalidomide is the most effective agent, but its teratogenicity and peripheral neuropathy limit its use. **Prophylactic treatment** with both **benzathine penicillin and colchicine** may increase the rate of healing and decrease the frequency of recurrence.

Anterior uveitis is treated with **topical steroid drops** (e.g., betamethasone, 1–2 drops tid) and **mydriatic agents** [e.g., tropicamide (Mydral, Mydriacyl, Opticyl, Tropicacyl), 1–2 drops qd–bid]. Posterior uveitis is treated with **topical injection of steroids** (e.g., dexamethasone, 1.0–1.5 mg) and **oral prednisone,** 5–20 mg qd. **Pulse IV methylprednisolone (Medrol),** 1000 mg qd for 3 days, **and oral cyclosporin (Neoral, Sandimmune),** 5–10 mg/kg qd, is the recommended regimen for severe cases. Other immunosuppressants (e.g., **daily oral cyclophosphamide (Cytoxan, Neosar),** 2 mg/kg qd, **monthly IV cyclophosphamide,** 0.6 g/m², **oral azathioprine,** 2.5 mg/kg qd, **oral chlorambucil (Leukeran),** 5 mg qd, or **oral tacrolimus (Prograf),** 0.05–0.15 mg/kg qd) can be used. Colchicine may be used to prevent both anterior and posterior uveitis; prophylactic immunosuppression for those at risk for blindness is controversial.

CNS BS, including meningitis and meningoencephalitis early in the course of BS, is treated with **oral prednisone,** 1 mg/kg qd. Severe CNS disease may be treated with **pulse IV methylprednisolone,** 1000 mg qd for 3 days, followed by **oral prednisone,** 1 mg/kg qd, and an additional immunosuppressant (e.g., **oral cyclophosphamide,** 2–2.5 mg/kg qd, **monthly IV cyclophosphamide, daily oral chlorambucil,** or **oral methotrexate (Folex, Rheumatrex, Trexall),** 7.5–15 mg/wk).

Vasculitis is treated with **oral prednisone,** 1 mg/kg qd, and **monthly IV cyclophosphamide,** 0.6 g/m². Severe disease is treated **with pulse IV methylprednisolone,** 1000 mg qd for 3 days, and **oral cyclophosphamide,** 2–2.5 mg/kg qd, followed by **oral prednisone,** 1 mg/kg qd. Treat aneurysms surgically; however, they tend to recur. Anticoagulation with heparin or warfarin may be dangerous, as aneurysm formation underneath a thrombus is likely. Antiplatelet agents (e.g., daily aspirin) may be used.

Arthritis may be treated with **NSAIDs, colchicine,** or **sulfasalazine (Azulfidine).** Low-dose steroids (e.g., **oral prednisone,** 5–20 mg qd) and **azathioprine** may be used for refractory cases. **Prophylaxis** with **both benzathine penicillin and colchicine** may decrease the number of episodes of arthritis, although the severity, duration, and patterns of arthritis are usually not affected. GI manifestations are treated with **low-dose prednisone** and **sulfasalazine.** Surgery is necessary for patients with bowel perforation or recurrent bleeding. Surgical procedures can result in excessive infiltration of inflammatory cells into treated tissues. Consider intermediate doses of steroids perioperatively to prevent poor wound healing and avoid complications. The efficacy of infliximab has been documented in several case reports.

Follow-up involves assessment of disease activity by clinical history and assessment of drug toxicity.

KEY POINTS TO REMEMBER

- Recurrent oral and genital ulcers are a hallmark of BS.
- BS is more common in patients along the ancient Silk Route, especially in patients of Turkish, Mediterranean, Middle Eastern, and Japanese descent.

SUGGESTED READING

Barnes CG, Yazici H. Behçet's syndrome. *Rheumatology* 1999;38:1171–1176.
The International Study Group for Behçet's Disease. Criteria for diagnosis of Behçet's disease. *Lancet* 1990;335:1078–1080.
Kaklamani VG, Kaklamanis PG. Treatment of Behçet's disease—an update. *Semin Arthritis Rheum* 2001;30:299–312.
Kaklamani VG, Vaiopoulos G, Kaklamanis PG. Behçet's disease. *Semin Arthritis Rheum* 1998;27:197–217.
Sakane T, Takeno M, Suzuki N, et al. Behçet's disease. *N Engl J Med* 1999;341:1284–1290.

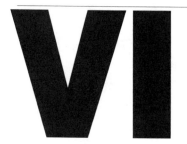

VI

**Infectious Causes
of Arthritis**

Infectious Arthritis

Kevin M. Latinis

32

INTRODUCTION

The acute onset of mono- or oligoarticular arthritis, especially in the setting of a fever and constitutional symptoms, should raise the suspicion of infectious arthritis. Delay in diagnosis can lead to rapid and severe joint destruction, causing significant morbidity and increased mortality. Early diagnosis with synovial fluid analysis and treatment with appropriate antibiotics help limit serious sequelae. **Bacterial arthritis is classically divided into GC and non-GC types.** Other etiologies include viral, mycobacterial, and fungal. The estimated incidence of infectious arthritis in the United States is approximately 20,000 cases annually. Lyme disease and rheumatic fever are discussed in Chap. 33, Lyme Disease, and Chap. 34, Acute Rheumatic Fever.

CAUSES

Pathophysiology

The majority of cases of bacterial arthritis in adults are caused by *Staphylococcus aureus*, accounting for up to 80% of confirmed cases. The second leading pathogen is *Streptococcus pneumonia,* followed by gram-negative bacteria, although any microbial pathogen is capable of causing infectious arthritis. The leading cause of bacterial arthritis in young, sexually active adults is *Neisseria gonorrhea*, with a male to female ratio of 1:4.

IV drug users, immunocompromised patients, patients with prosthetic joints, and patients with chronic debilitating diseases (e.g., cancer) are at higher risk of becoming infected, especially with gram-negative organisms. Immunocompromised patients are also at increased risk of developing opportunistic organisms (e.g., mycobacteria and fungi). Viral infections commonly associated with arthritis include hepatitis, rubella, mumps, Epstein-Barr virus, parvovirus, enterovirus, adenovirus, and HIV.

Several factors, including advanced age and comorbid conditions, predispose joints to develop bacterial infections. Patients with underlying arthritis, especially RA, are more prone to bacterial arthritis. Hematogenous spread is the most common route of inoculation; therefore, patients with sepsis or transient bacteremia are at increased risk. Additionally, suspect bacterial endocarditis, especially in patients with abnormal heart valves or IV drug abusers. Direct inoculation after joint manipulation via arthrocentesis or arthroscopy can occur, but risks are estimated to be <0.01% and 0.04–4%, respectively.

Bacterial colonization usually occurs within the synovial lining, followed by synovial fluid inoculation. The presence of bacteria induces an inflammatory response, recruiting leukocytes that propagate the inflammatory reaction through release of cytokines. Bacterial products, release of lysosomal enzymes, immune complex deposition, complement activation, metalloproteases, and chondrocyte inhibition all contribute to articular damage. Non-GC bacterial arthritis is typically more damaging.

Differential Diagnosis

In addition to infectious arthritis, the differential diagnosis of acute onset of monoarticular joint pain includes trauma, crystalline arthritis (gout and pseudogout), early stages of polyarticular diseases (e.g., RA and seronegative spondyloarthropathies), rheumatic fever, infectious bursitis, and Lyme disease.

PRESENTATION

History

Infectious arthritis usually occurs with the acute onset of pain, warmth, erythema, and swelling in a single joint. Fevers occur in most patients, although up to 20% of patients may be afebrile. Chills and rigors are unusual. 50% of cases involve the knees, followed by hips, shoulders, wrists, ankles, elbows, and small joints of the hands and feet. Up to 20% of cases may present with polyarticular symptoms. IV drug abusers tend to develop infectious arthritis in joints of the axial skeleton, including sternoclavicular and costochondral joints.

The history should elicit the presence of other rheumatologic diagnoses and comorbid conditions. Additionally, note any trauma, procedures such as arthrocentesis or surgeries, prosthetic joints, local infections such as cellulitis, urinary tract or respiratory infections, and high-risk sexual behavior or drug use.

Always consider GC arthritis in sexually active young patients, especially if there is a history of a new sexual partner, multiple partners, or high-risk sexual behavior. Other risk factors for GC infections include recent menses, pregnancy, or complement deficiencies. Tenosynovitis, dermatitis, and migratory polyarthritis is the classic triad for disseminated GC infections. Urethritis in men is more likely to be symptomatic than cervicitis in women.

Physical Exam

A careful joint exam should include the ability to bear weight, range of motion, and signs of soft tissue swelling, warmth, erythema, and synovitis within and around the suspected joints. In addition, the physical exam should include evaluation for fever and specific sites of infection. The respiratory exam should focus on evaluation for pneumonia, pharyngitis, and sinusitis. The cardiac exam should include evaluation for new murmurs or friction rubs. The genitourinary exam should include evaluation of flank pain (pyelonephritis), urethritis, and cervicitis. Perform a careful skin exam for signs of cellulitis or petechiae, papules, pustules, hemorrhagic bullae, or necrotic lesions, especially when entertaining the diagnosis of GC arthritis.

MANAGEMENT

Diagnostic Workup

An **initial joint fluid exam is critical in the diagnosis of infectious arthritis** and identification of the offending pathogen. Perform arthrocentesis in any patient presenting with monoarticular joint pain with an effusion. Note that patients with suspected infections involving prosthetic joints warrant prompt orthopedic consultation.

Evaluate synovial fluid for signs of xanthochromia, synovial fluid characteristics (cloudy versus clear), cell count with WBC differential, gram stain, culture, and polarizing microscopy for crystals. Chemistries such as LDH, glucose, and protein have limited value, although elevated LDH and low glucose are consistent with bacterial infections. The synovial fluid cell count in infectious arthritis indicates an inflammatory arthritis (>2000 WBCs); however, septic joints can produce WBC counts >50,000–100,000, with a predominance of polymorphonuclear neutrophils.

For difficult-to-access joints, radiographic assistance with ultrasound, fluoroscopy, or CT guidance may be necessary. Additionally, surgical or arthroscopic drainage is often necessary in cases of septic hip joints, septic arthritis with coexistent osteomyelitis, septic arthritis in a prosthetic joint, persistent infections, complex anatomy, or loculated effusions.

Routine gram stain provides the most rapid and helpful initial information to guide treatment. Perform routine cultures to isolate specific organisms. For non-GC infections, these are positive in 50–75% of infected joints not previously treated with antibiotics. Use of blood culture bottles may enhance recovery of pathogens.

For suspected GC infections in which gram stain and routine culture are much less sensitive (<50%), cultures of synovial fluid on chocolate agar or Thayer-Martin media may enhance recovery. PCR of synovial fluid to detect GC DNA may also increase diagnostic yield. In addition to synovial fluid cultures, culture samples from blood, cervix, urethra, rectum, pharynx, and skin lesions and analyze them for GC DNA.

Order cultures for unusual organisms in cases of TB exposure, penetrating trauma or animal bites, travel to areas endemic with particular fungal organisms, immunosuppressed patients, or monoarthritis refractory to conventional antibiotic therapy. For Lyme disease, serologies may improve diagnostic yield (see Chap. 33, Lyme Disease).

Perform radiographic analysis on all affected joints to help exclude fractures, tumors, and osteomyelitis. Additionally, x-rays may help confirm the presence of an effusion or other rheumatologic findings including erosions, joint space narrowing, or chondrocalcinosis.

Additional lab tests that may support the diagnosis of infectious arthritis include a CBC and indicators of inflammation, including ESR or CRP. The peripheral WBC count is elevated in approximately one-half of affected patients. Blood cultures may help identify causative organisms when synovial fluid tests are nondiagnostic. ESR and CRP are usually elevated and may be helpful in patients with an equivocal joint exam or concomitant osteomyelitis.

Treatment

The mainstay of **treatment of bacterial arthritis includes IV antibiotics and joint drainage.** For non-GC arthritis, base initial antimicrobial therapy on the results of the gram stain and the clinical setting. If no microorganisms are seen on gram stain, initiate empiric therapy for gram-positive and gram-negative organisms. Initial therapy with IV oxacillin (Bactocill, Prostaphlin) or nafcillin (Nafcil, Nallpen, Unipen), 2 g q4h, or cefazolin (Ancef, Kefzol), 1 g q8h, is appropriate for gram positives. If rates of methicillin/oxacillin-resistant *S. aureus* are high or if infections are acquired in hospital or nursing home settings or in patients with indwelling IV catheters, empiric therapy with vancomycin (Vancocin), 1 g q12h, is indicated. Follow vancomycin levels to ensure proper dosing. When available, culture results and antimicrobial sensitivities should guide further treatment. Most rheumatologists treat with IV therapy for 2–4 wks, and in most cases, this can occur on an outpatient basis.

For suspected GC arthritis, initiate empiric therapy for disseminated GC infection, as the gram stain will likely be negative. Therapy with IV ceftriaxone (Rocephin), 1 g q24h for 24–48 hrs after clinical improvement, followed by either oral cefixime (Suprax), 400 mg q12h; ciprofloxacin (Cipro, Cipro XR), 500 mg q12h; or ofloxacin (Floxin), 400 mg q12h for 1 wk.

As with most closed-space infections, drainage facilitates recovery. Most joints can be drained via arthrocentesis techniques. Daily aspiration is generally necessary, as certain joints (e.g., the knee) may continue to accumulate fluid for up to 10 days. Surgical consultation may be necessary for difficult-to-access joints (e.g., the hip) or for prosthetic joints or persistent infection despite repeated arthrocentesis that may require arthroscopy or open drainage.

Follow-Up

Follow clinical progression closely within the first few weeks of treatment with antibiotics. Repeat arthrocentesis should confirm sterilization of synovial fluid and decreasing WBC count. Failure to improve may warrant alteration in antibiotic regimen or surgical consultation for arthroscopic or open drainage. Early rehabilitation should include physical therapy with joint mobilization to prevent loss of joint range of motion.

Special Topics

Nonbacterial Arthritis

Arthralgias and nonbacterial septic arthritis are common with many viral infections. **Viral arthritis** tends to present with a symmetric polyarthralgia or polyarthritis and may be accompanied by a typical viral exanthem. The exact pathophysiology is unknown but may involve direct viral invasion of the joint or immune complex deposition. Supportive treatment with rest and NSAIDs is usually effective. The course is usually self-limited and resolves within 4–6 wks. Viral infections commonly associated with arthritis include hepatitis, rubella, mumps, Epstein-Barr virus, parvovirus, enterovirus, adenovirus, and HIV. If suspected, specific viral serologies may help support this diagnosis. Of note, in adults, parvovirus B19 arthritis can cause symmetric polyarthritis with morning stiffness similar to that of RA.

Septic Bursitis

Septic bursitis is overlooked easily, as the degree of synovial fluid inflammation is usually less than that with infectious arthritis. The olecranon and prepatellar bursa are the most commonly involved sites, and most patients provide a history of recent trauma or recurrent trauma due to an occupational predisposition. Cellulitis around the affected area can accompany the infected bursa. Gram-positive bacteria account for the majority of infections. Patients with infectious bursitis can often be treated as outpatients with oral antibiotics and daily percutaneous drainage as needed. Treat patients who fail to improve with at least 2 wks of IV antibiotics. Surgical resection of the bursa is occasionally necessary for patients who do not respond to antibiotics.

KEY POINTS TO REMEMBER

- Send synovial fluid for cell count with differential, crystal analysis, gram stain, and cultures.
- Gram stains rarely are positive with GC arthritis.
- Septic arthritis may be polyarticular in patients with underlying joint disease.
- The presence of crystals does not exclude the diagnosis of septic arthritis.

SUGGESTED READING

Baker DG, Schumacher RH. Current concepts: acute monoarthritis. *N Engl J Med* 1993;329:1013–1020.

Goldenberg DL. Septic arthritis. *Lancet* 1998;351:197–202.

Gupta MN, Sturrock RD, Field M. A prospective 2-year study of 75 patients with adult-onset septic arthritis. *Rheumatology* 2001;40:24–30.

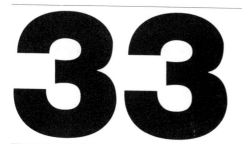

Lyme Disease

Kathryn H. Dao

INTRODUCTION

Lyme disease is a multisystem illness caused by the spirochete *Borrelia burgdorferi*, which is transmitted by the Ixodid tick. It was initially described in 1975 after an outbreak of juvenile arthritis in Old Lyme, Connecticut. In 1991, 9344 cases were reported, making it the most common vector-borne disease in the United States. It has been reported in 44 states, with a predominance of cases in the northeast, upper Midwest, and Pacific coastal regions. Late spring and summer are peak seasons.

CAUSES

Pathophysiology

Whether direct tissue damage by infection with *B. burgdorferi* or an immunologic reaction is responsible for the pathogenesis of the disease is unclear. The spirochetes have been isolated from all affected tissues except for peripheral nerve. Furthermore, spirochetes are potent inducers of inflammatory cytokines like IL-1. Patients with HLA-DR4 and HLA-DR2 are more susceptible to develop a chronic, erosive arthropathy similar to RA.

Differential Diagnoses

Other diseases to consider include syphilis, RA, adult-onset Still's disease, infectious endocarditis with embolic events, SLE, and other CTDs.

PRESENTATION

Clinical Presentation

Lyme disease has protean clinical manifestations and has been called "the great imitator." It can affect many organ systems and is thought to proceed in three stages.

Stage I is often heralded by a rash known as *erythema migrans*. The rash, occurring in 60–80% of patients, usually appears as an expanding annular red macule or papule 3 days to 1 mo after a tick bite. It generally resolves in 3–4 wks. Patients may also report malaise, headache, pharyngitis, fever, arthralgia, lymphadenopathy and fatigue.

Stage II occurs weeks to months after infection. 8% of patients progress and have cardiac and neurologic involvement, which may present as atrioventricular heart block, myocarditis, pericarditis, cardiomyopathy, Bell's palsy, meningoencephalitis, or radiculoneuritis. Mono- or oligoarthritis and acrodermatitis chronica atrophicans may also occur.

Stage III defines the period after 5 mo of infection. The most common late manifestation is episodic oligoarticular arthritis predominating in the lower extremities. Large effusions may be present. Chronic neurologic symptoms may persist, resembling organic brain disease. Demyelinating encephalopathy and chronic radiculoneuropathy are other manifestations.

Early studies have shown that, in patients who were not treated but were followed for several years, 18% developed arthralgias, 51% developed at least one episode of intermittent mono- or oligoarthritis lasting <1 yr, and 11% developed chronic synovitis in 1–3 large joints, of which >33% had evidence of radiographic disease.

MANAGEMENT

Diagnostic Workup

The Centers for Disease Control and Prevention developed a national surveillance case definition for Lyme disease that, for the purpose of case counting, requires the manifestation of erythema migrans or serologic confirmation of the disease and a late manifestation of the disease. **Serologic tests** may include detection of antibodies to *Borrelia* using ELISA, with positive tests confirmed by Western blot. IgM is generally seen within 2–4 wks after the onset of the rash. Sensitivity and specificity are low in early stages of infection. Other means of diagnosing infection are by direct visualization of the spirochete with a darkfield microscope, by skin biopsy specimens from erythema migrans (the yield is 57–86%), and through PCR of body fluids to detect *B. burgdorferi* DNA.

Treatment and Follow-Up

In the early stages of Lyme disease, **oral doxycycline** (Monodox, Periostat, Vibramycin), 100 mg PO bid for 20–30 days, is recommended; alternative antibiotics include beta-lactams, amoxicillin (Amoxil), and ceftriaxone (Rocephin). Oral antibiotics are used as initial therapy except in cases of neurologic or multisystem involvement, for which IV antibiotics are preferred. 15% of patients may still experience fatigue or arthralgias even after therapy; whether this is from continued infection or from an overactive immune response is unclear. Avoid intraarticular steroid injections for arthritis during periods of antibiotic therapy. Fibromyalgia and arthralgias as sequelae of infection may respond to exercise, antiinflammatory agents, and antidepressants (see Chap. 36, Fibromyalgia Syndrome). Patients with persistent Lyme arthritis may benefit from joint rest and aspiration of reaccumulated joint fluid. Arthroscopic synovectomy may be beneficial. Recent studies revealed no benefit of continued antibiotic therapy over placebo for persistent symptoms. Generally, antibiotic prophylaxis is not recommended after a tick bite, but a recent study evaluating the use of single-dose doxycycline prophylaxis after *Ixodes scapularis* tick exposure showed an efficacy of 87%. This study shows that prophylaxis may decrease incidence of disease in **endemic** areas when the tick is identified as the *I. scapularis* tick. Vaccination for Lyme disease remains controversial but is available for persons living in or visiting high-risk areas and who have frequent or prolonged exposure to Ixodid ticks.

KEY POINTS TO REMEMBER

- Lyme disease is endemic to the North Atlantic, Northern Midwest, and Pacific coastal regions.
- Suspect Lyme disease in patients with exposure to Ixodid ticks and with new rashes, arthritis, or neurologic symptoms.
- Interpret lab tests for Lyme disease with caution, as results may be variable between labs.

SUGGESTED READING

Klempner MS, Hu LT. Two controlled trials of antibiotic treatment in patients with persistent symptoms and a history of Lyme disease. *N Engl J Med* 2001;345:85–92.

Nadelman RB, Nowakowski J. Prophylaxis with a single-dose doxycycline for the prevention of Lyme disease after an *Ixodes scapularis* tick bite. *N Engl J Med* 2001;345:79–84.

Parola P, Raoult D. Ticks and tickborne bacterial diseases in humans: an emerging infectious threat. *Clin Infect Dis* 2001;32:897–928.

Rahn D, Malawista SE. Lyme disease: recommendations for diagnosis and treatment. *Ann Intern Med* 1991;114:472–481.

Shadick NA, Phillips CB, Logigian EL, et al. The long-term clinical outcomes of Lyme disease: a population-based retrospective cohort study. *Ann Intern Med* 1994;121:560–567.

Steere AC. Lyme disease. *N Engl J Med* 2001;345:115–124.

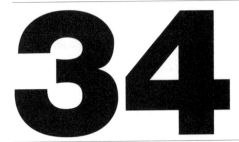

Acute Rheumatic Fever

Rebecca M. Shepherd

INTRODUCTION

Acute rheumatic fever (ARF) is a delayed sequela of a **group A streptococcal** pharyngeal infection occurring 2–3 wks after the initial infection. Various signs and symptoms, including arthritis, carditis, chorea, rash, and SC nodules, characterize ARF. ARF was associated with significant morbidity and mortality until the mid-1800s. At that time, there was a dramatic decline in cases, which has been attributed to changes in living conditions and the virulence of the organism. Additionally, the introduction of antibiotics in the 20th century significantly reduced the incidence of ARF. By 1962, the incidence had declined to 100 patients/100,000 in many European countries. ARF presently continues unabated in developing countries, however, with an estimated 10–20 million new cases a year. The incidence of disease in the United States is less than 1/100,000 children. Some areas of the United States have experienced an unexplained recent increase in disease incidence.

CAUSES

Pathophysiology

The pathogenesis of ARF is not clearly understood. A streptococcal pharyngeal infection, either clinical or subclinical, is necessary for the development of ARF. Cellulitis and glomerulonephritis, also caused by group A streptococcus, do not cause and are not features of ARF. Genetic susceptibility and molecular mimicry, involving the cross-reaction between group A streptococcal antigens and host antigens, likely play a role in the pathogenesis of ARF.

Differential Diagnosis

The differential diagnosis of ARF includes bacterial infections (e.g., septic arthritis, osteomyelitis, and bacterial endocarditis), viral infections (e.g., infectious mononucleosis and Coxsackie virus), RA, SLE, and malignancies (e.g., lymphoma and leukemia).

PRESENTATION

History and Physical Exam

ARF is characterized by a constellation of symptoms that arises 2–4 wks after pharyngeal infection. The classic manifestations include arthritis, carditis, neurologic involvement, and rash. **Arthritis** is usually the first symptom of ARF. It is a migratory polyarthritis of the larger joints, (e.g., knees, elbows, ankles, and wrists) and usually starts on the lower extremity. The involved joints become tender without evidence of inflammation. Joints may only be involved for a week before another joint becomes affected and the initial joint involvement subsides. Typically, 6–16 joints are affected. The synovial fluid is generally inflammatory but sterile. Salicylates and NSAIDs are effective, with quick resolution of joint symptoms and blunting of the migratory nature of disease. **Carditis** is an important manifestation of ARF, as it often results in long-term damage to the heart. ARF can involve any area of the heart, including pericardium, epicardium, myocardium, endocardium, and valvular structures. There may be no symptoms despite cardiac involvement, or patients may experience chest discomfort and dyspnea. Physical exam may elicit a new murmur. Mitral valvulitis can be distinguished by a high-pitched blowing murmur throughout systole, heard best at the apex. Associated with mitral valvulitis is the Carey Coombs murmur, a low-pitched diastolic murmur at the apex. Aortic valvulitis is a high-pitched decrescendo murmur along the left sternal border, heard best with the patient leaning forward. On exam, one may also find evidence of pericarditis, heart failure, or cardiomyopathy. The **neurologic** manifestation of ARF is best known as *Sydenham's chorea*, also called *chorea minor* and *the St. Vitus dance*. Chorea is characterized by nonrhythmic involuntary abrupt movements and muscle weakness. Usually the movements are more distinct on one side. Muscle weakness is rhythmic, with the strength increasing and decreasing on exertion. Frequently, emotional instability (e.g., crying, agitation, and inappropriate behavior) accompanies the chorea. **Skin manifestations** of ARF include erythema marginatum and SC nodules. Erythema marginatum is a faint, pink, nonpruritic rash that erupts across the trunk, upper arms, and legs; facial involvement does not occur. The lesion begins with a central area of normal skin and extends outward to a distinct border. It is transient, coming and going within hours and worsened by hot conditions (e.g., baths and showers). The rash usually occurs at the onset of disease, but it may recur at any time, including convalescence. SC nodules are firm, nontender nodules under noninflamed skin that occur on bony prominences and near tendons. They may be solitary or occur in groups; they are symmetric and usually resolve within 4 wks. The SC nodules of ARF differ from those of RA in that they are smaller and more transient, with a location nearer to the olecranon. Both erythema marginatum and SC nodules usually only occur in the presence of carditis.

MANAGEMENT

Diagnostic Workup

The diagnosis of ARF is clinical and based on the revised **Jones criteria** (Table 34-1). A diagnosis can be made if *two* major or *one* major and *two* minor criteria are present in the setting of a recent streptococcal pharyngeal infection.

Evidence of recent streptococcal infection includes increased streptococcal antibodies, (e.g., antistreptolysin O), positive throat culture for Group A beta-hemolytic

TABLE 34-1. REVISED JONES CRITERA FOR DIAGNOSIS OF ACUTE RHEUMATIC FEVER

Major manifestations	Minor manifestations
Carditis	Clinical findings
Polyarthritis	Arthralgia
Chorea	Fever
Erythema marginatum	Lab findings
Subcutaneous nodules	Elevated acute-phase reactants (ESR, CRP)
	Prolonged PR interval on ECG

Other manifestations include supporting evidence of preceding group A strep infection, positive throat culture or rapid streptococcal antigen test, and elevated or rising streptococcal antibody titer.

streptococci, and scarlet fever. Lab tests are nondiagnostic. CRP and Westergren sedimentation rate (ESR) may be elevated, and normochromic, normocytic anemia may be present.

Treatment and Follow-Up

Treatment of ARF should include **antibiotic treatment,** symptom relief, and prophylaxis. Antiinflammatory medications, especially aspirin, are useful in symptomatic relief. Arthritis and fever rapidly resolve once treatment is initiated; aspirin dosing is 4–8 g/day for adults. Continue antiinflammatory drugs until all symptoms are gone and the ESR and CRP are within normal range. Treatment of chorea includes the use of phenobarbital and diazepam.

Penicillin is the treatment of choice for ARF [Benzathine penicillin G (1.2 million units IM single dose or penicillin V, 250 mg tid PO × 10 days)]. Start antibiotics as soon as the diagnosis of ARF is suspected and continue them for a 10-day course. Either PO or IM penicillin can be given. If a penicillin allergy is present, erythromycin, 40 mg/kg/day in divided doses (maximum, 1 g/day), can be used. Family members should have throat culture and treatment if the culture is positive for beta-hemolytic streptococci.

Prophylaxis for ARF is important as symptoms can recur, most commonly within 2 yrs. Treatment with penicillin or erythromycin begins immediately after the initial 10-day antibiotic treatment course; duration of prophylaxis is controversial, but a 5- to 10-yr course is usually recommended (penicillin G, 1.2 million units IM every 4 wks; penicillin V, 250 mg bid; or erythromycin, 250 mg bid).

KEY POINTS TO REMEMBER

- ARF is classically characterized by symptoms of arthritis, carditis, chorea, erythema marginatum, and SC nodules occurring in temporal relationship to a beta-hemolytic streptococcal infection.
- Cardiac involvement with valvular damage is the most common long-term sequelae of ARF.
- Early treatment with antibiotics and long-term prophylaxis with antibiotics are important measures to prevent long-term sequelae.

SUGGESTED READING

Dajani AS, Ayoub E, Bierman FZ, et al. Guidelines for the diagnosis of rheumatic fever: Jones criteria, updated 1992. *Circulation* 1993;32:664.
Stollerman GH. Rheumatic fever. *Lancet* 1997;349:935.

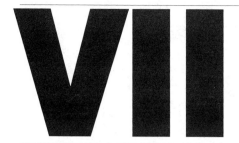

**Miscellaneous
Rheumatology
Consultations**

35

Inflammatory Myopathies

Celso R. Velázquez

INTRODUCTION

The inflammatory myopathies are a heterogenous group of disorders characterized by muscle weakness and inflammation of skeletal muscles (myositis). The three major distinct inflammatory myopathies are **PM, DM, and inclusion-body myositis (IBM).** Other inflammatory myopathies include juvenile dermatomyositis, malignancy-associated myositis, and myositis in overlap with other CTDs. Myositis is rare, with an incidence of 1/100,000. Women are affected twice as often as men. DM affects adults and children. PM is usually seen after the second decade of life. Unlike PM and DM, IBM affects men twice as often as women and is more common after age 50. The inflammatory myopathies are idiopathic but are believed to be immune mediated. Muscle biopsy specimens showing B- and CD4$^+$ T lymphocytes suggest cellular immune abnormalities. Multiple autoantibodies are found in patients, but it is unclear if they are pathogenic. Myositis-specific autoantibodies are found in up to 50% of patients and define groups of patients with uniform clinical features and prognosis (Table 35-1).

PRESENTATION

History and Physical Exam

All forms of inflammatory myopathy have in common **proximal, symmetric muscle weakness that progresses over weeks to months.** Shoulder and pelvic girdle muscles are most affected. Weakness of neck flexors and dysphagia occurs, but involvement of ocular and facial muscles is very rare and, if present, should suggest another diagnosis. Patients typically have difficulty getting up from a chair, lifting objects, or combing their hair. Systemic symptoms (e.g., fatigue, morning stiffness, anorexia) can accompany weakness. Muscle pain is rare. Tendon reflexes are normal except with severe atrophy. Sensation remains intact. IBM may present with weakness lasting years and some distal and asymmetric involvement. **Extramuscular manifestations** can occur at any time. Up to 40% of patients may have cardiac involvement that ranges from asymptomatic conduction defects to cardiomyopathy and heart failure. Pulmonary involvement is seen in 50% of patients. Dyspnea may be due to respiratory muscle weakness, but respiratory failure occurs rarely. Aspiration pneumonia is possible in patients with pharyngeal involvement. Alveolitis or slowly progressive interstitial lung disease may precede muscle involvement. DM has characteristic **cutaneous manifestations** that distinguish it from the other myopathies. Rashes often precede muscle weakness. Lilac papules (Gottron's papules) found on the dorsal aspect of MCP and interphalangeal joints, elbows, or knees are pathognomonic. Heliotrope rash is a purplish discoloration of the upper eyelids often associated with periorbital edema. An erythematous rash may be seen on the upper chest (in the shape of a V) and back and shoulders ("shawl sign") and may worsen with sun exposure. Periungual telangiectasias, irregular and thickened cuticles, and "mechanic's hands" (darkened horizontal lines across lateral and palmar aspects of fingers and hands) are also seen. Patients with classic cutaneous findings of DM but no clinical evidence of muscle disease have **amyopathic dermatomyositis.** Features of the inflammatory myopathies may also be seen in some patients with scleroderma, SLE, and MCTD.

TABLE 35-1. MYOSITIS-SPECIFIC AUTOANTIBODIES

Autoantibody	Clinical features	Treatment response
Antisynthetase (anti-Jo-1 is the most common)	Relatively acute onset of polymyositis or dermatomyositis	Moderate
	Interstitial lung disease	
	Fever	
	Arthritis	
	Mechanic's hands	
Anti-SRP	Polymyositis with very acute onset	Poor
	Severe weakness	
	Palpitations	
Anti-Mi2	Dermatomyositis with typical cutaneous findings	Good

SRP, signal recognition particle.

MANAGEMENT

Diagnostic Workup

The diagnosis of the inflammatory myopathies is based on history, physical exam, and selected tests. Table 35-2 lists the most frequently used diagnostic criteria. Exclude other causes of muscle weakness (Table 35-3). **Electromyography** (EMG) allows differentiation between neuropathic and myopathic conditions and should always be done. EMG is abnormal in 90% of patients. Needle insertion can damage muscle fibers for biopsy, so do EMG and biopsy on opposite sides. Myopathic changes seen on **muscle biopsy** include variation in fiber size, atrophy, regeneration, phagocytosis, inflammatory cells, and fibrosis. Inflammatory infiltrates are predominantly perivascular in

TABLE 35-2. BOHAN AND PETER'S CRITERIA FOR THE DIAGNOSIS OF POLYMYOSITIS AND DERMATOMYOSITIS

Symmetric proximal weakness.

Elevation of muscle enzymes.

Electromyographic findings of short, small, polyphasic motor unit potentials; fibrillations, positive sharp waves, and insertional irritability; and bizarre high-frequency repetitive discharges.

Muscle biopsy showing degeneration, regeneration, necrosis, atrophy, inflammatory infiltrate.

Typical skin findings of dermatomyositis.

Definite polymyositis requires four criteria (without rash).

Definite dermatomyositis requires three criteria (any three plus rash).

Multiple diseases must be excluded for these criteria to be applied, including neurologic disease, muscular dystrophies, infections, drugs and toxins, rhabdomyolysis, metabolic myopathies, and endocrinopathies.

Adapted from Bohan A, Peter JB. Polymyositis and dermatomyositis. *N Engl J Med* 1975;292:344–347,403–407.

DM. Intracellular lined vacuoles are characteristic of IBM. Similar vacuoles may also be seen in muscular dystrophies and toxic (alcohol, colchicine) myopathies. Special stains may reveal enzyme deficiencies characteristic of primary metabolic myopathies. **Skeletal muscle enzymes** [i.e., creatine phosphokinase (CK), aldolase, transaminases, lactate dehydrogenase] are almost always elevated. The most sensitive enzyme is CK; CK levels may reach 50× normal. Trauma, strenuous exercise, and IM injections can increase CK. Healthy black males have higher levels than whites. Routine blood counts and chemistries are usually normal. **Myositis-specific autoantibodies** are specific for inflammatory myopathies but are not very sensitive (Table 35-1). MRI detects muscle inflammation and may be useful to determine the best site for biopsy but is not used routinely. Evaluation of extramuscular features may require pulmonary function tests or swallowing studies.

Differential Diagnosis

Toxic Myopathies
See Table 35-3. Procainamide and penicillamine cause an immune-mediated myopathy. Statins and other lipid-lowering agents may cause mitochondrial dysfunction. Ethanol may cause a severe myopathy with rhabdomyolysis and a very high CK with acute intoxication. Chronic ethanol use is associated with a painless proximal muscle weakness and atrophy with normal CK. Corticosteroid myopathy is common and usually occurs after months of use. Patients with drug-induced myopathies improve after stopping the drug and do not require treatment with corticosteroids.

Myopathies and Cancer
Muscle weakness may precede or follow the diagnosis of cancer. The association is primarily with DM. Evaluation for occult malignancies in patients with myopathies should focus on common malignancies and be based on abnormalities on physical exam and lab tests.

Primary Metabolic Myopathies
Primary metabolic myopathies are rare diseases of muscle energy metabolism that may present with muscle weakness, elevated CK, and myopathic EMG. Patients with glycogen metabolism abnormalities or with myoadenylate deaminase deficiency (the most common metabolic myopathy) have exercise intolerance and may be asymptomatic at rest. The forearm ischemic exercise test is a standardized test that involves checking ammonia and lactate levels before and after vigorous forearm exercise with a BP cuff inflated above systolic pressure; it is a useful screening test. Suspect metabolic myopathies in patients who are young, have a family history of myopathy, or fail to respond to therapy.

Treatment

Physical therapy is essential to preserve muscle function and prevent joint contractures. **Prednisone** is the initial drug of choice. High doses of **1–2 mg/kg PO qd** are used. Some physicians use **bolus IV methylprednisolone (Medrol), 1 g IV qd for 3–5 days** in patients with severe disease and respiratory compromise. Maintain high doses of prednisone until strength and CK have normalized. Then, taper prednisone slowly by approximately 20% each month until the minimum dose that controls disease is reached. Multiple tapering regimens, including converting to alternate-day therapy, exist. Muscle strength almost always improves by the third month of therapy. Improvement in CK levels may precede or lag behind muscle strength improvement. Patients with inflammatory myopathies usually require prolonged courses of corticosteroids, so prevent side effects (e.g., osteoporosis) (see Chap. 50, Osteoporosis). Persistent disease activity beyond 3 mos despite prednisone therapy should lead to the consideration of another immunosuppressive agent and a reexamination of the diagnosis. Methotrexate (Folex, Rheumatrex, Trexall) and azathioprine (Imuran) are other commonly used immunosuppressive agents. Up to 90% of patients have a partial

TABLE 35-3. CAUSES OF MUSCLE WEAKNESS

Neuromuscular diseases
    Idiopathic inflammatory myopathies (polymyositis, dermatomyositis, and inclusion-body myositis)
    Muscular dystrophies (Duchenne's and others)
    Guillain-Barré and other neuropathies (diabetes, porphyria)
    Myasthenia gravis, Eaton-Lambert syndrome
    Myotonic diseases
    Metabolic myopathies
    Disorders of carbohydrate (McArdle's disease), lipid, and purine (myoadenylate deaminase deficiency) metabolism
    Mitochondrial myopathies
    Toxic myopathies
    Alcohol
    Amiodarone
    Clofibrate
    Cocaine
    Colchicine
    Corticosteroids
    Cyclosporine
    Gemfibrozil
    Heroin
    Hydroxychloroquine
    Ipecac
    Penicillamine
    Procainamide
    Statins
    Zidovudine
    Infections
    Viral (adenovirus, Epstein-Barr, HIV, influenza, rubella)
    Bacterial (streptococcus, staphylococcus, clostridia)
    Parasitic (toxoplasma, trichinosis, schistosomiasis, cysticercosis)
    Endocrine and electrolyte abnormalities
    Hypo- and hyperthyroidism
    Cushing's disease
    Addison's disease
    Hypokalemia, hypomagnesemia, hypo- or hypercalcemia
Rheumatic diseases
    PMR
    RA
    Systemic vasculitis
    Sarcoidosis
    SLE
Miscellaneous
    Paraneoplastic myopathies
    Fibromyalgia
    Psychosomatic

response. A delay in initiating treatment decreases the response rate. IBM responds less predictably to therapy. Cancer-associated myopathies may improve with successful treatment of the underlying malignancy.

KEY POINTS TO REMEMBER

- Patients with DM have a life-long increased risk of malignancies; therefore, maintain routine cancer surveillance.
- Proximal muscle weakness is the hallmark of the inflammatory myopathies.
- EMG and muscle biopsies are useful in the diagnostic workup of inflammatory myopathies.

SUGGESTED READING

Bohan A, Peter JB. Polymyositis and dermatomyositis. *N Engl J Med* 1975;292:344–347,403–407.

Buchbinder R, Forbes A, Hall S, et al. Incidence of malignant disease in biopsy-proven inflammatory myopathy. *Ann Intern Med* 2001;134:1087–1095.

Dalakas M. Polymyositis, dermatomyositis, and inclusion-body myositis. *N Engl J Med* 1991;325:1487–1498.

Miller FW. Myositis-specific autoantibodies: touchstones for understanding the inflammatory myopathies. *JAMA* 1993;270:1846–1849.

Plotz PH. Not myositis. *JAMA* 1992;268:2074–2077.

Wortmann RL, ed. *Diseases of skeletal muscle*. Philadelphia: Lippincott Williams & Wilkins, 2000.

Fibromyalgia Syndrome

Kathryn H. Dao

INTRODUCTION

Fibromyalgia syndrome (FMS) is a chronic musculoskeletal pain syndrome of unknown etiology that is characterized by **diffuse pain, tender points, fatigue, and sleep disturbance.** Studies in the 1980s estimated a prevalence of 2–5%, with a female to male ratio of 8:1. The mean age of patients is 30–60 yrs, but FMS may be present in children and the elderly. Many patients may have other rheumatologic disorders (e.g., RA, SLE, SS).

CAUSES

Pathophysiology

The pathophysiology of fibromyalgia is poorly understood. FMS represents a disorder of heightened pain response that may be a result of neuroendocrine axis alterations with subsequent disturbances in mood, sleep, and pain perception. Studies show that patients often have low serum serotonin, growth hormone, and cortisol levels and an elevated CSF substance P concentration. Substance P, regulated by serotonin, can cause exaggerated perception of normal sensory stimuli. Other objective abnormalities found in patients with FMS include sleep disturbances; patients infrequently progress to stages 3, 4, and REM sleep. Whether this has a direct effect on patients' symptoms or is an epiphenomenon is unclear.

Differential Diagnosis

Other diagnoses to consider include hypothyroidism, drug-induced myopathies (e.g., HMG-CoA inhibitors), PMR, myofascial pain, Lyme disease, sciatica, MS, metabolic myopathy, depression, temporomandibular joint syndrome, and other rheumatologic disorders (e.g., RA, SLE, SS, AS).

PRESENTATION

History and Physical Exam

The cardinal feature of FMS is diffuse soft tissue pain. Often described as burning, tingling, or gnawing, the pain may be located in the neck, back, chest, arms, or legs. In addition, patients may complain of morning stiffness, fatigue, sleep disturbances, or headaches. Commonly associated disorders include irritable bowel syndrome, chronic fatigue syndrome, depression, chronic muscle contraction headache, multiple drug allergies, premenstrual syndrome, and anxiety disorders. The physical exam is normal except for the presence of tender points, which are symmetric points of muscle and tendon insertions located throughout the body (Fig. 36-1).

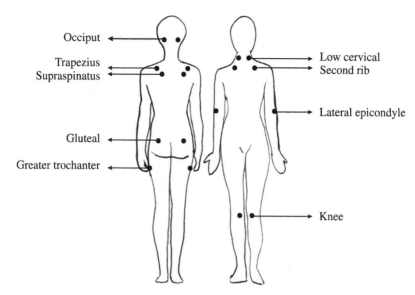

FIG. 36-1. Fibromyalgia tender points.

MANAGEMENT

Diagnostic Workup

The diagnosis of FMS is made clinically. The American College of Rheumatology 1990 criteria for the classification of FMS define fibromyalgia as a syndrome of widespread pain and tenderness at *11 or more* of **18 specific tender point sites** (Table 36-1). Lab tests and radiologic studies often are unrevealing but are helpful in excluding other diseases. Initial tests should include a CBC, an ESR, standard chemistries, and thyroid function studies. Due to the number of false positives, reserve testing for RF, ANAs, and Lyme antibodies for patients for whom clinical suspicion is high. Radiologic studies may be ordered for patients with evidence of arthritis or radiculopathy. Perform a careful sleep history and possible sleep study on obese patients and in males with fibromyalgia. Screen patients for coexistent depression, which commonly occurs in any patient with chronic pain.

Treatment and Follow-Up

Pharmacologic and nonpharmacologic therapies have been investigated for the management of FMS. Pharmacologic therapies with proven effectiveness target pain and abnormal sleep patterns. **Analgesics** that are helpful include muscle relaxants [e.g., carisoprodol (Soma) and cyclobenzaprine (Flexeril)], tramadol (Ultram), and acetaminophen. NSAIDs may also be used, but given the absence of tissue inflammation, they may not be better than placebo in treating patients with FMS. Topical agents (e.g., capsaicin cream and topical lidocaine) may be used as adjunctive therapies. Opioids generally are not recommended due to risk for habituation, but they can be used sparingly for severe pain with significant functional impairment. **Medications that target sleep patterns** by promoting stage 4 sleep and providing analgesic effects include amitriptyline (Elavil) and cyclobenzaprine. Amitriptyline is usually dosed 10–50 mg PO once at bedtime; cyclobenzaprine at 10–40 mg is given in divided doses. Trazodone (Desyrel) (25–100 mg at bedtime) may also be used. The role for SSRIs is emerging.

TABLE 36-1. THE AMERICAN COLLEGE OF RHEUMATOLOGY 1990 CRITERIA FOR THE CLASSIFICATION OF FIBROMYALGIA[a]

History of widespread pain

Definition: Pain is considered widespread when all of the following are present: pain in the left side of the body, pain in the right side of the body, pain above the waist, and pain below the waist. In addition, axial skeletal pain (cervical spine, anterior chest, thoracic spine, or low back) must be present. In this definition, shoulder and buttock pain is considered as pain for each involved side. "Low back" pain is considered lower segment pain.

Pain in 11 of 18 tender points sited on digital palpation

Definition: Pain on digital palpation must be present in at least 11 of the following 18 tender point sites:

Occiput: bilateral, at the suboccipital muscle insertions

Low cervical: bilateral, at the anterior aspects of the intertransverse spaces at C5-C7

Trapezius: bilateral, at the midpoint of the upper border

Supraspinatus: bilateral, at origins, above the scapula spine near the medial border

Second rib: bilateral, at the second costochondral junctions, just lateral to the junctions on upper surfaces

Lateral epicondyle: bilateral, 2 cm distal to the epicondyles

Gluteal: bilateral, in upper out quadrants of buttocks in anterior folds of muscle

Greater trochanter: bilateral, posterior to the trochanteric prominence

Knee: bilateral, at the medial fat pad proximal to the joint line

Perform digital palpation with an approximate force of 4 kg.

For a tender point to be considered "positive," the subject must state that the palpation was painful; "tender" is not to be considered "painful."

[a]For classification purposes, patients are said to have fibromyalgia if both criteria are satisfied. Widespread pain must have been present for at least 3 mos. The presence of a second clinical disorder does not exclude the diagnosis of fibromyalgia.

A nonpharmacologic therapy for FMS is exercise. Physical activity helps maintain function in patients. The goal is 20 mins of aerobic exercise daily. Behavioral therapy, cognitive behavior training, and biofeedback combined with relaxation and movement therapy have been proven effective. Other treatments include acupuncture. Support groups are also available for these patients. Finally, establishing a close patient-physician relationship with frequent visits often helps patients cope with their disease. A 1997 outcome study involving 538 patients over 7 yrs from six rheumatologic centers assessed status and disease severity over time. Functional disability worsened slightly, but health satisfaction improved slightly. Measures of pain, fatigue, sleep disturbance, anxiety, depression, and health status were essentially unchanged ($r = 0.82$).

KEY POINTS TO REMEMBER

- Depression, like fibromyalgia, can present with diffuse musculoskeletal complaints, sleep disorders, and weight changes.
- FMS often coexists with other rheumatic diseases.

SUGGESTED READING

Bennett RM, Gatter RA, Campbell SM, et al. A comparison of cyclobenzaprine and placebo in the management of fibrositis. *Arthritis Rheum* 1988;31:1535–1542.

Berman B, Ezzo J, Hadhazy V, et al. Is acupuncture effective in the treatment of fibro-myalgia? *J Fam Pract* 1999;48:213–218.

Goldenberg D, Mayskiy M, Mossey C, et al. A randomized, double blind crossover trial of fluoxetine and amitriptyline in the treatment of fibromyalgia. *Arthritis Rheum* 1996;39:1852–1859.

Goldenberg DL. Treatment of fibromyalgia syndrome. *Rheum Dis Clin North Am* 1989;15:61–71.

Millea P, Holloway R. Treating fibromyalgia. *Am Fam Physician* 2000;62:1575–1582.

Russell IJ. Fibromyalgia syndrome: formulating a strategy for relief. *J Musculoskeletal Med* November 1998:4–20.

Wolfe F, Anderson J, Harkness D, et al. Health status and disease severity in fibromyalgia. *Arthritis Rheum* 1997;40:1571–1579.

Wolfe F, Smythe HA, Yunus MB. The American College of Rheumatology 1990 criteria for the classification of fibromyalgia. Report of the Multicenter Criteria Committee. *Arthritis Rheum* 1990;33:160–72.

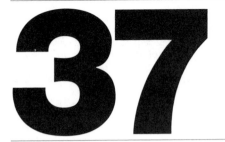

Sjögren's Syndrome

Ami N. Mody and
Kevin M. Latinis

INTRODUCTION

SS is a chronic inflammatory disorder characterized by **lymphocytic infiltration and autoimmune destruction of exocrine glands.** The salivary and lacrimal glands are commonly affected, leading to symptoms of **dry mouth** (xerostomia) and **dry eyes** (keratoconjunctivitis sicca). SS commonly occurs in patients with other systemic autoimmune diseases (e.g., RA, SLE, scleroderma, MCTD, and inflammatory myopathies). SS may also occur as a primary disease. The incidence of SS in the general population is estimated to range between 1/1000 and 1/100 new cases per year, depending on the diagnostic criteria used. The prevalence of SS is estimated to be 1 in 1250 in the general population. SS most often occurs in women (women:men ratio, 9:1) in their fourth and fifth decades of life and demonstrates a familial tendency.

CAUSES

Pathophysiology

The primary pathologic mechanism of SS consists of focal infiltration of lymphocytes, primarily CD4 T cells, into glandular tissue. The glandular endothelial cells acquire the ability to express HLA-DR class II molecules, allowing them to serve as antigen-presenting cells to the CD4 T cells. Further, capillaries within affected tissues develop characteristics of high endothelial venules, facilitating lymphocyte migration into the tissue. The CD4 T cells in SS patients produce increased IL-2 and interferon-gamma relative to normal controls, likely contributing to the inflammatory process. The autoimmune inflammatory process eventually leads to decreased exocrine secretions through a cellular-mediated glandular destruction. SS most commonly affects salivary and lacrimal glands but may occur in any exocrine glandular tissue.

Additional factors implicated in the pathogenesis of SS include autoantibody production, viral infections, and decreased glandular response to cholinergic stimuli. Antibodies against nuclear antigens SSA/Ro and SSB/La are commonly associated with SS; however, little evidence exists to support a causal role in the destruction of glandular tissue. Viral infections, including Epstein-Barr virus, retroviruses, and hepatitis C, are commonly associated with SS. These viral infections are not directly implicated in the glandular destruction of SS but may indirectly alter immune responses to favor autoimmune destruction.

The end effect of ocular discomfort in SS is mediated by inadequate tearing, causing increased friction between mucosal surfaces. This results in distortion of epithelial cells during the blinking process, leading to corneal irritation and abrasions. A localized inflammatory response is precipitated. Additionally, the loss of the nutritive effects of tears delays healing.

Similar pathologic processes affect the oral cavity. Inflammatory destruction of salivary glands leads to quantitative and qualitative changes in saliva production. The normal bacterial flora is altered by changes in salivation, leading to an increased frequency of dental caries, oral candidiasis, and periodontal diseases.

Differential Diagnosis

The differential diagnosis of SS includes any disease process that leads to symptoms of dry eyes and dry mouth. These include infiltrative diseases (e.g., sarcoidosis, amyloidosis, hemochromatosis, and lymphoma); infectious diseases [e.g., viral infections (HIV, hepatitis B and C, mumps, influenza, coxsackie A, CMV), syphilis, trachoma, TB, and bacterial infection]; fat deposition from diabetes, alcoholism, pancreatitis, cirrhosis, and hypertriglyceridemia; anticholinergic side effects from medicines (e.g., antidepressants, neuroleptics, antihypertensives, antihistamines, and decongestants); endocrine dysfunction including acromegaly, and gonadal hypofunction.

PRESENTATION

History and Physical Exam

Symptoms of SS develop insidiously, commonly over several years. Mucosal dehydration, manifested as **dry eyes and dry mouth,** is the most common complaint associated with SS. Symptoms of dry eyes include a foreign body sensation, itching, light sensitivity worse in the evening, and thick, crusting film present on awakening. Symptoms are commonly aggravated by airline travel, dry windy conditions, and use of contact lenses. Dry mouth often manifests as increased thirst and difficulty swallowing dry foods. Rapidly progressive dental caries, recurrent oral and gingival infections, and discomfort wearing dentures may all be associated with SS. Additional features of exocrine gland dysfunction include symptoms of dry skin (xerosis), vaginal dryness, and upper airway dryness creating a dry cough.

Salivary gland enlargement occurs in up to half of affected patients. The glands are usually firm, diffuse, and nontender, commonly with episodic swelling. A hard, nodular gland may suggest a neoplasm. This distinction is clinically significant, as there is an increased incidence of B-cell lymphomas in salivary glands affected with SS.

Extraglandular involvement of SS may also occur. Fatigue and arthralgias (sometimes arthritis) are common complaints with SS. Skin lesions include palpable purpura, urticaria, annular lesions, xerosis, and Raynaud's phenomenon. Respiratory involvement includes increased frequency of sinusitis, bronchitis, pneumonia, and pleural effusions. More severe complications include development of interstitial pneumonitis and pulmonary fibrosis. Cardiac involvement may include pericardial effusions or autonomic dysfunction. Neurologic complications may include cognitive dysfunction, demyelinating disease similar to MS, myasthenia gravis, and peripheral neuropathies. Renal involvement may manifest as renal insufficiency or chronic interstitial nephritis. GI manifestations include dysphagia, esophageal dysmotility, nausea, dyspepsia, atrophic gastritis, and hepatic abnormalities.

MANAGEMENT

Diagnostic Workup

A general diagnostic workup for SS should include the following lab tests: CBC, ESR or CRP, RF, ANA test, and serum protein electrophoresis. If the ANA is positive, obtain autoantibodies **SSA (Ro) and SS-B (La).** Most patients have a mild anemia, increased ESR or CRP, and positive RF and ANA, with the presence of SS-A and SS-B.

Functional studies may include Schirmer's test for tear secretion, rose bengal or fluorescein staining with slit-lamp exam to detect damaged corneal epithelium, and sialometry, sialography, or scintigraphy to measure salivary gland function.

Confirmation of SS can be obtained by performing a **minor salivary gland biopsy,** most often obtained from minor salivary glands in the lower lip. Findings of focal lymphocyte aggregates, plasma cells, and macrophages support the diagnosis.

Many criteria exist to aid in the diagnosis of SS. These criteria exist primarily to provide diagnostic criteria for entry into clinical studies and vary widely in their sensitivities and specificities for diagnosis. In general clinical practice, diagnosis of SS is supported by symptoms of dry mouth and/or dry eyes in the absence of other known causes and the presence of abnormal minor salivary gland biopsy or SS-associated autoantibodies.

Treatment and Follow-Up

Most patients with SS can be managed with education and simple **symptomatic relief** measures designed to keep mucous membranes moist. Encourage patients to avoid dry environments, wind, cigarette smoke, and medications with anticholinergic side effects. Humidifiers can counter low-humidity indoor environments, especially in winter months when centralized heating leads to dry air.

For dry eyes, patients should use **artificial tears** on a regular basis. Numerous brands are available, and patients are encouraged to try various formulas to find the most suitable one. In general, preservative-free solutions are better tolerated. Some patients may benefit from punctual occlusion to prolong the efficacy of artificial tears.

For dry mouth, patients are encouraged to **drink water frequently.** Stimulation of salivary glands with sugar-free gum or candy may also be useful. Patients should avoid dry foods. Some patients may benefit from treatment with the muscarinic agonist pilocarpine (Salagen), 5–10 mg PO qid, or Cevimeline (Evoxac), 30 mg PO tid; however, many patients experience side effects of increased urination and defecation, sweating, abdominal cramping, and flushing. Patients with xerostomia are at increased risk of dental caries and should be followed closely by a dentist. Topical fluoride treatments may help prevent tooth decay.

Dry skin can be managed with moisturizing lotions. Vaginal dryness is improved with lubricants. Arthralgias and other musculoskeletal complaints are often remedied with NSAIDs. For more severe joint and muscle pain, hydroxychloroquine (Plaquenil) at 400 mg PO qd may provide symptomatic relief. SS with severe disease manifestations of vasculitis, nephritis, interstitial lung involvement, or neuropathy may require the use of corticosteroids, azathioprine (Imuran), methotrexate (Folex, Rheumatrex, Trexall), or CYC (Cytoxan, Neosar).

KEY POINTS TO REMEMBER

- Patients with SS have a high risk of dental caries.
- Pilocarpine may benefit some patients with persistent symptoms of dry eyes and mouth.

SUGGESTED READING

Fox RI, Stern M, Michelson P. Update in Sjögren syndrome. *Curr Opin Rheum* 2000;2:391–398.

Vivino FB, Al-Hashimi I, Khan Z, et al. Pilocarpine tablets for the treatment of dry mouth and dry eye symptoms in patients with Sjögren syndrome: a randomized, placebo-controlled, fixed-dose, multicenter trial. *Arch Intern Med* 1999;159:174–181.

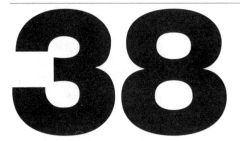

Scleroderma

Milan J. Anadkat and
Kevin M. Latinis

INTRODUCTION

Scleroderma is an autoimmune CTD characterized by progressive **skin thickening and tightening** and often associated with internal organ involvement. The estimated annual incidence of the disease in the United States is 1.9/100,000. Prevalence is estimated at 26/100,000. The disease occurs more often in women, with peak incidence in ages 40–60.

Scleroderma is subdivided according to different disease patterns: diffuse scleroderma, limited scleroderma, localized scleroderma, and scleroderma sine scleroderma. Scleroderma may also be part of overlap syndromes or MCTD.

Rapidly progressive diffuse scleroderma carries a poor prognosis and involves facial, truncal, extremity, and acral skin thickening along with extensive visceral organ involvement. Survival is approximately 50% at 10 yrs. The disease course is variable and often begins with the insidious onset of Raynaud's phenomenon and acral edema. Antitopoisomerase-I antibodies (anti-Scl-70) are present in 30% of patients.

Limited scleroderma is most often synonymous with the **CREST syndrome** (**c**alcinosis, **R**aynaud's phenomenon, **e**sophageal dysmotility, **s**clerodactyly, and **t**elangiectasias). It has a better prognosis, with 10-yr survival >70%. Skin involvement is generally limited to fingers, distal arms and legs, and the face, and it often begins with Raynaud's phenomenon. Anticentromere antibodies are present in up to 80% of cases. Visceral involvement may include interstitial lung disease, pulmonary HTN, or systemic HTN. This involvement tends to occur late in the disease course but can cause significant morbidity and increased mortality.

Scleroderma sine scleroderma is a rare manifestation of the disease in which visceral involvement precedes the typical skin changes of scleroderma. Localized scleroderma, including morphea and linear scleroderma, has only cutaneous disease activity and is not associated with underlying visceral involvement in most instances.

CAUSES

Pathophysiology

The pathogenesis of scleroderma involves three main disease processes. First, the presence of autoimmunity is nearly universal in scleroderma, with an estimated 75–95% of patients having ANAs present by the time of clinical presentation. This aspect of the disease is primarily T-cell mediated. Immune activation leads to the release of soluble mediators of inflammation (cytokines) that propagate the inflammatory reaction. The second feature displayed universally in scleroderma involves excessive fibrosis seen in the skin and other affected organs. This appears to be secondary to increased fibroblast activity with accelerated collagen deposition. Third, inflammation and fibrosis lead to a proliferative, obliterative vasculopathy affecting mostly small vessels (e.g., small arteries, arterioles, and capillaries). Large vessels may also be affected. Vasculopathy is the mechanism of most end-organ damage seen in scleroderma.

Differential Diagnosis

The differential diagnosis for scleroderma includes diseases that display similar skin findings, similar visceral involvement, and similar disease presentations. Skin thickening can be seen with diabetic digital sclerosis, chronic graft-versus-host disease, vinyl chloride exposure, vibration syndrome, bleomycin toxicity, complex regional pain syndromes/reflex sympathetic dystrophy, amyloidosis, porphyria cutanea tarda, acrodermatitis, scleredema, eosinophilic fasciitis, POEMS syndrome (**p**olyneuropathy, **o**rganomegaly, **e**ndocrinopathy, **m**onoclonal spikes, and **s**cleroderma-like skin changes), and carcinoid syndrome. Diseases with similar organ involvement include primary pulmonary HTN, interstitial pulmonary fibrosis, primary biliary cirrhosis, intestinal hypomotility, and collagenous colitis. Diseases that may present in a similar manner to scleroderma include SLE, MCTD, RA, and inflammatory myopathies.

PRESENTATION

History

The initial symptoms of scleroderma tend to be nonspecific and may consist of fatigue, weakness, and musculoskeletal complaints. **Raynaud's phenomenon,** present in virtually all patients with scleroderma, is often an early symptom. Patients experience episodic, bilateral color changes (white to blue to red) in their fingers, toes, ears, and nose lasting 10–15 mins and often precipitated by cold or emotional stress. These symptoms may persist for weeks to years before more specific clinical signs become apparent.

The extent of skin involvement often correlates with overall clinical course. Any involvement proximal to the elbow or knee joints typically corresponds to diffuse disease. Skin changes occur in 3 phases: edematous, fibrotic, and atrophic. Often, the first complaint specific for scleroderma is "swelling" or "puffiness" in the fingers or hands corresponding to the edematous phase of disease. Patients may also complain of pruritus, dry skin, tightening and decreased flexibility, and, occasionally, skin ulcerations.

GI complaints are common with scleroderma. Involvement may occur anywhere along the alimentary tract. Patients may note dry mouth, dysphagia, dyspepsia, nausea, vomiting, and early satiety. Patients may also experience cramping abdominal pain, diarrhea, weight loss, or fecal incontinence. Intestinal pseudoobstruction may occur secondary to hypomobility.

Musculoskeletal complaints tend to be nonspecific. Patients often experience generalized arthralgias and myalgias. Patients may also develop symptoms of CTS or trigeminal neuralgia.

Additional symptoms include dyspnea on exertion or nonproductive cough secondary to pulmonary involvement. These generally correspond with later stages of disease. Chest pain may occur due to esophagitis, pleurisy, pericarditis, musculoskeletal involvement, and, occasionally, coronary vasospasms. Nearly 50% of patients with scleroderma experience symptoms of major depression.

Physical Exam

Skin changes are variable, depending on the severity and extent of disease activity. Fibrotic activity within fingers leading to loss of the digital pad (sclerodactyly) is a common sign in scleroderma and a hallmark of the limited form of disease. As the disease progresses, flexion contractures may be appreciated at joints with occasional coexistence of ulcerations (due to skin atrophy). In systemic forms, cutaneous signs of inflammation (e.g., nonpitting edema and erythema) are seen early in the disease course. Hyper- and hypopigmentary changes may lead to a "salt-and-pepper" appearance of the skin. Signs of localized scleroderma tend to be unique in appearance. Morphea may appear as a solitary plaque or as multiple lesions. The presentation is usually that of expanding nonspecific erythema with a white, fibrotic center surrounded by a margin of lilac hyperpigmentation. The distribution tends to be asymmetric. On resolution, softening and pigmentation generally occurs. In linear scleroderma, a fibrotic band appears in nondermatomal distribution, typically involving the lower extremities. Midline facial involvement may also occur, revealing a "coup de sabre" deformity, which occasionally coexists with hemiatrophy and hair loss.

The color changes of Raynaud's phenomenon are transient and therefore not always apparent. Study of a patient's nailfold capillary bed can be beneficial for early diagnosis. Using a hand-held ophthalmoscope with power <20 diopters, nailfold capillaries are visualized through a water-soluble gel. In cases of secondary Raynaud's (associated with scleroderma or inflammatory myopathies), the exam reveals enlarged capillary loops, loss of normal capillary beds, and occasional capillary hemorrhages. SC calcinosis may be apparent with signs of local inflammation, induration, or ulceration; it tends to occur more often in the limited form of the disease.

A tight "purse-lip" appearance associated with decreased oral aperture is attributed to increased fibrotic activity within the perioral skin. In addition, telangiectasias may be appreciated over the face or gingival or oropharyngeal mucosa. When associated with the sicca complex (see Chap. 37, Sjögren's Syndrome), dry conjunctival and/or mucosal membranes with or without ulceration may be seen.

Musculoskeletal exam may reveal coarse friction rubs with joint movement when inflammation and fibrosis of tendon sheaths is significant, such as occurs in diffuse scleroderma. Muscle atrophy with weakness may become apparent over time. Patients with carpal tunnel compression due to fibrosis from scleroderma may have positive Tinel's or Phalen's tests.

In patients with renal involvement, BP is usually abnormal (>150/90); however, 10% of patients with scleroderma renal crisis are normotensive. Pulmonary disease may be difficult to assess by physical exam. Bibasilar rales may be heard with pulmonary fibrosis. Signs of right heart failure (e.g., a pulmonary artery tap, peripheral edema, ascites, and elevated jugular venous pulse) may occur with pulmonary HTN. Signs of cardiac involvement in scleroderma may include a pericardial rub with pericarditis, arrhythmias secondary to conduction system fibrosis, or signs of diastolic or systolic failure secondary to infiltrative fibrosis.

MANAGEMENT

Diagnostic Workup

The diagnosis of scleroderma is made clinically by the presence of characteristic findings as described in the section on Presentation. Most patients have characteristic skin sclerosis and Raynaud's phenomenon. Capillary dilatation or capillary dropout may be seen by capillaroscopy. Skin biopsy is usually not necessary. Diagnosis of limited scleroderma is supported by findings of calcinosis, abnormal esophageal motility, and telangiectasias in the presence of sclerodactyly and Raynaud's phenomenon. Diagnosis of diffuse scleroderma is supported by the finding of acute renal insufficiency with or without HTN, dyspnea with pulmonary interstitial fibrosis, pulmonary HTN, diarrhea and malabsorption, or hepatic dysfunction in conjunction with skin thickening. Scleroderma sine scleroderma involves the presentation of pulmonary, renal, cardiac, or GI disease secondary to vasculopathy or visceral fibrosis in the absence of typical skin findings.

Lab studies should include ANA with staining patterns and anti-Scl-70 (antitopoisomerase-I). **Most patients with scleroderma have a positive ANA.** Anti-Scl-70 antibodies are specific (but not sensitive) for diffuse scleroderma. The anticentromere staining pattern of the ANA is specific (but not sensitive) for limited scleroderma with the CREST syndrome. Less commonly assayed antibodies associated with scleroderma include anti-RNA polymerase I, II, and III and U3-ribonucleoprotein (RNP). Anti-U1-RNP antibodies are found in MCTD, and anti-PM-Scl antibodies may be present in overlap syndromes.

Direct additional testing at specific complaints. Esophageal motility can be evaluated by barium swallow or esophageal manometry. Pulmonary fibrosis is confirmed by high-resolution chest CT and restrictive pattern on pulmonary function testing. Pulmonary HTN and pericardial disease can be seen with two-dimensional echocardiography. Histologic analysis may be useful for liver disease and pulmonary fibrosis.

Treatment

There is no definitive therapy for scleroderma. Various lifestyle modifications may be proposed to patients to ameliorate symptoms. Avoiding cold temperature exposure, smoking, and stressful situations have proven to help patients with Raynaud's phenomenon. Avoiding excess bathing and using proper moisturizing creams can aid in skin care. Eating small, frequent meals while upright along with elevating the head while sleeping helps patients suffering from reflux symptoms. Aggressive physical therapy may be helpful early in the course of disease to minimize contractures and weakness. Wrist splints, local steroid injections, or surgical intervention may be used for symptoms of CTS.

Certain forms of pharmacotherapy have shown some benefit for patients with scleroderma. Slow-release preparations of calcium channel blockers, especially nifedipine (Procardia) at 10–20 mg PO tid, can provide modest relief of Raynaud's phenomenon. D-Penicillamine (Cuprimine, Depen) is an agent that interferes with cross-linking of collagen and has traditionally been used to treat diffuse scleroderma. Many retrospective studies support the use of penicillamine in doses of 500–1500 mg PO daily; however, recent randomized controlled trials have shown limited to no effect. NSAIDs or disease-modifying antirheumatic drugs [e.g., methotrexate (Folex, Rheumatrex, Trexall)] may be administered for signs of inflammation, including arthralgias and musculoskeletal pain.

For digital ulcerations, finger soaks in antiseptic fluid, proper drying, and occlusive dressing with antibiotic ointment is helpful. Give oral antibiotics for infected ulcers. Reserve surgical debridement and the use of IV antibiotics for deep infections. Amputation may ultimately be necessary.

For GI involvement, therapy is targeted at specific symptoms. Proton pump inhibitors and prokinetic agents are useful for reflux and aperistaltic symptoms. In addition, broad-spectrum antibiotics and supplemental fat-soluble vitamins can be given in instances of bacterial overgrowth and malabsorption, respectively. Periodic dilatations are effective in the management of esophageal strictures.

In cases of scleroderma renal crisis, **ACE inhibitors** are the mainstay of therapy. These agents are effective in reversing hyperreninemia, proteinuria, and HTN seen in scleroderma renal crisis. Emphasis is placed on early detection with rapid normalization of the patient's BP. In many instances, additional antihypertensive agents are necessary. Some patients may require dialysis for severe renal failure.

Pulmonary involvement significantly increases morbidity and mortality in scleroderma. Treatment of inflammatory alveolitis with oral CYC (Cytoxan, Neosar) (1–2 mg/kg/day) or monthly IV CYC (800–1400 mg) has shown benefit in lung function and survival. Pulmonary HTN occurring as a primary process in scleroderma or secondary to interstitial fibrosis has a significant increased mortality (50% survival in 1 yr). Recent studies using continuous IV epoprostenol (Flolan) or oral endothelin receptor antagonists demonstrated improved exercise capacity and cardiopulmonary hemodynamics and may increase survival. Other cardiopulmonary complications of scleroderma (e.g., arrhythmia, hypoxia, and thromboembolism) are treated with conventional supportive measures.

Many other therapies to treat manifestations of scleroderma, including CYC, corticosteroids, cyclosporine (Neoral, Sandimmune), methotrexate, azathioprine (Imuran), antithymocyte globulin, CAMPATH (lympholytic monoclonal antibody), colchicine, interferons alpha and gamma, oral and parenteral prostacyclin analogs, photophoresis, and plasmapheresis, have been tested or reported anecdotally but ultimately have limited utility. Currently, new treatments are being investigated. More profound immunosuppression with immunoablative conditioning treatment (usually high-dose chemotherapy with or without total body irradiation) followed by stem cell transplantation has shown success in phase II trials. Unfortunately, there is a significant procedure-related mortality, making careful patient selection critical and often limiting. Phase III trials are currently in progress.

KEY POINTS TO REMEMBER

- Most patients with scleroderma have Raynaud's phenomenon.
- ACE inhibitors are important for the treatment of HTN in patients with scleroderma.

- ACE inhibitors should be initiated immediately in the setting of scleroderma renal crisis.
- Pulmonary involvement significantly increases morbidity and mortality associated with scleroderma.

SUGGESTED READING

Badesch DB, Tapson VF, McGoon MD, et al. Continuous intravenous epoprostenol for pulmonary hypertension due to the scleroderma spectrum of disease. A randomized, controlled trial. *Ann Intern Med* 2000;132:425–434.

Binks M, Passweg JR, Furst D, et al. Phase I/II trial of autologous stem cell transplantation in systemic sclerosis: procedure related mortality and impact on skin disease. *Ann Rheum Dis* 2001;60:577–584.

Furst DE. Rational therapy in the treatment of systemic sclerosis. *Curr Opin Rheum* 2000;12:540–544.

Geirsson AJ, Wollheim FA, Akesson A. Disease severity of 100 patients with systemic sclerosis over a period of 14 years: using a modified Medsger scale. *Ann Rheum Dis* 2001;60:1117–1122.

Grassi W, Del Medico P, Izzo F, et al. Microvascular involvement in systemic sclerosis: capillaroscopic findings. *Semin Arthritis Rheum* 2001;30:397–402.

Pope JE, Bellamy N, Seibold JR, et al. A randomized, controlled trial of methotrexate versus placebo in early diffuse scleroderma. *Arthritis Rheum* 2001;44:1351–1358.

Rubin LJ, Badesch DB, Barst RJ, et al. Bosentan therapy for pulmonary arterial hypertension. *N Engl J Med* 2002;346:896–903.

Thompson AE, Shea B, Welch V, et al. Calcium-channel blockers for Raynaud's phenomenon in systemic sclerosis. *Arthritis Rheum* 2001;44:1841–1847.

White B, Moore WC, Wigley FM, et al. Cyclophosphamide is associated with pulmonary function and survival benefit in patients with scleroderma and alveolitis. *Ann Intern Med* 2000;132:947–954.

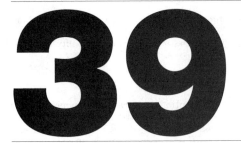

Antiphospholipid Syndrome

Kathryn H. Dao

INTRODUCTION

Antiphospholipid syndrome (APS) is a **hypercoagulable disorder** manifested by recurrent vasculopathic events associated with antibodies against phospholipids or plasma proteins bound to anionic phospholipids. The syndrome most commonly occurs in young females; however, both sexes and all ages may be affected. APS may be primary (with no concomitant disorder) or secondary when associated with another systemic disease (e.g., SLE). Thromboembolism occurs in 6–8% of patients with primary APS and in up to 50% of patients with secondary APS. Of note, APAs may be seen in other conditions (e.g., malignancy, viral infections, or lymphoproliferative disorders) but do not necessarily cause thrombosis.

CAUSES

Pathophysiology

The etiology of APS is poorly understood, although **APAs** are implicated in the disorder. Four types of APAs have been identified: the LAC, aCL antibodies, antibodies causing a false-positive serologic test for syphilis (STS), and anti-beta-2 glycoprotein-I antibodies (α-β-2gpI). APAs affect coagulation and thrombosis in different ways. These antibodies may bind to phospholipids or to epitopes exposed on plasma proteins that bind to phospholipids. For example, they can bind to platelet membrane phospholipids, leading to increased platelet adhesion and aggregation with resulting thrombosis and thrombocytopenia, or they can directly damage vascular endothelium, causing vasospasm and ischemia. Some studies propose that coagulation may result from disruption of the protein C pathway by APAs. Also, antibodies against β-2gpI (a naturally occurring anticoagulant bound by aCL and LAC) may induce a prothrombotic state. The importance of these antibodies in the pathogenesis of disease has been supported by animal studies that have shown that passive transfer of aCL antibodies may induce thrombocytopenia and fetal resorption.

Differential Diagnosis

Consider APS when a patient has unexplained or recurrent thromboses or thrombotic events at unusual sites (e.g., adrenal veins), when thrombosis occurs in a young patient, and when recurrent pregnancy losses occur in the second and third trimesters. Other diagnoses of prothrombotic events must be entertained: protein C or S deficiency, antithrombin III deficiency, factor V Leiden mutation, dysfibrinogenemias, hyperhomocystinuria, Behçet's syndrome, malignancies, thrombotic thrombocytopenic purpura, nephrotic syndrome, severe diabetes, paroxysmal nocturnal hemoglobinuria, pregnancy, smoking, estrogen therapy, and prolonged bedrest.

Although often associated with thromboses, APAs sometimes can be found in a healthy person or in those with lymphoproliferative disorders, viral infections (HIV), or malignancies. These individuals may not necessarily have APS. The prevalence of aCL antibodies in healthy populations is 2–5%.

TABLE 39-1. CLINICAL MANIFESTATIONS OF ANTIPHOSPHOLIPID SYNDROME

Cardiovascular: MI, angina, premature atherosclerotic valvular lesions, pseudoinfective endocarditis, intracardiac thrombosis

Dermatologic: livedo reticularis, splinter hemorrhages, skin infarcts, leg ulcers, superficial thrombophlebitis, blue toe syndrome, Raynaud's phenomenon, necrotizing purpura

Endocrine: adrenal insufficiency

GI: hepatic infarction, Budd-Chiari syndrome

Hematologic: thrombocytopenia, leukopenia, hemolytic anemia, positive Coomb's test

Musculoskeletal: deep venous thrombosis, AVN

Neurologic: cerebrovascular accidents, transient ischemic attacks, migraines, chorea, multiinfarct dementia, pseudotumor cerebri, peripheral neuropathy, myasthenia gravis, seizures, transverse myelopathy

Obstetric: eclampsia/preeclampsia; fetal wastage; intrauterine growth retardation; hemolysis, elevated liver enzymes, and low platelet count syndrome; oligohydramnios; chorea gravidarum; postpartum syndrome

Pulmonary: pulmonary embolus, nonthromboembolic pulmonary HTN

Renal: renal artery/vein thrombosis, HTN, glomerular thrombosis, renal insufficiency

PRESENTATION

History and Physical Exam

Obtaining a careful history to include or exclude the presence of other rheumatologic diagnoses and comorbid conditions is important. Because any blood vessel can be affected, clinical presentations may vary. Patients typically present in one of four ways: venous thrombosis, arterial thrombosis, pregnancy loss, or thrombocytopenia. Other manifestations can include livedo reticularis, Raynaud's phenomenon, dementia, premature atherosclerotic lesions, renal insufficiency, and pulmonary HTN (Table 39-1). When patients have multiorgan failure as a result of multiple-vessel occlusion occurring over a short time period, they are described as having "catastrophic antiphospholipid syndrome," which carries a mortality rate of 50% even with treatment.

MANAGEMENT

Diagnostic Workup

The International Consensus Statement on the preliminary classification criteria for *definite* APS was reported in 1998. The criteria stated that the diagnosis of APS should be considered when at least one clinical criterion and one lab criterion are met (Table 39-2). The clinical criteria include **vascular thrombosis and pregnancy morbidity,** and the lab criteria include the presence of **aCL antibody and the LAC.** Different assays are available to check for APAs (the LAC and aCL). The LAC is a misnomer; it was characterized by in vitro prolongation of clotting, but it confers a hypercoagulable state in vivo. It is not a specific analyte but a lab phenomenon and may be found in conditions other than SLE (see Chap. 5, Lab Evaluation of Rheumatic Diseases). Assays for the LAC include the dilute Russell viper venom time, aPTT, kaolin clotting time, and tissue thromboplastin inhibition; none has a >70% sensitivity to detect all LAC antibodies. The mixing of normal platelet-poor plasma to the patient's plasma will not correct a prolonged aPTT, but addition of excess phospholipids will.

aCL antibody tests are reported by different isotypes (IgG, IgA, IgM) and level of positivity. IgG and IgM aCL antibodies are clinically significant if they are associated with anti-β-2gpI antibody activity (currently, testing for activity is not widely avail-

TABLE 39-2. PRELIMINARY CRITERIA FOR THE DIAGNOSIS OF DEFINITE ANTIPHOSPHOLIPID SYNDROME

Clinical criteria

Vascular thrombosis: ≥ 1 clinical episodes of venous, arterial, or small-vessel thrombosis in any tissue or organ, which must be confirmed by imaging or Doppler studies or by histopathology, with the exception of superficial venous thrombosis. For histopathologic confirmation, thrombosis should be present without significant evidence of inflammation in the vessel wall.

Pregnancy morbidity: (a) ≥ 1 unexplained deaths of a morphologically normal fetus at or beyond the tenth week of gestation, with normal fetal morphology documented by ultrasound or by direct exam of the fetus, or (b) ≥ 1 premature births of a morphologically normal neonate at or before the 34th week of gestation because of severe preeclampsia or eclampsia or severe placental insufficiency, or (c) ≥ 3 unexplained consecutive spontaneous abortions before the 10th week of gestation, with maternal anatomic or hormonal abnormalities and paternal and maternal chromosomal causes excluded.

Lab criteria

Anticardiolipin antibody of IgG and/or IgM isotype in blood, present in medium or high titer, on ≥ 2 occasions, at least 6 wks apart, measured by a standardized ELISA for β-2-glycoprotein-I–dependent anticardiolipin antibodies.

Lupus anticoagulant present in plasma, on 2 or more occasions at least 6 wks apart, detected in the following steps: (a) prolonged phospholipid-dependent coagulation demonstrated on a screening test (e.g., aPTT, kaolin clotting time, dilute Russell's viper venom time, dilute prothrombin time), (b) failure to correct the prolonged coagulation time on the screening test by mixing with normal platelet-poor plasma, (c) shortening or correction of the prolonged coagulation time on the screening test by the addition of excess phospholipid, (d) exclusion of other coagulopathies (e.g., factor VIII inhibitor or heparin) as appropriate.

Definite antiphospholipid syndrome is considered to be present if at least one of the clinical criteria and one of the lab criteria are met.

Adapted from Wilson WA, Gharavi AE, Koike T, et al. International consensus statement on preliminary classification criteria for definite antiphospholipid syndrome. *Arthritis Rheum* 1999;42:1309–1311.

able). IgG is more specific than IgM. Level of positivity may be reported as low (<20 units), medium (20–80 units), or high (>80 units). Medium and high levels have high specificity for the diagnosis of APS.

Other lab tests to consider in the evaluation of the patient include CBC and blood chemistries (to evaluate for renal and liver dysfunction). Radiologic studies (CT/MRI) are helpful to assess damage and guide management.

Treatment and Follow-Up

Patients with high APA titers but no manifestation of thromboses are recommended to take **aspirin** (325 mg PO daily) as prophylaxis. Lifestyle modifications are recommended in this group, including smoking cessation, avoidance of supplemental estrogens, and controlling HTN and diabetes. In the Hopkins Lupus Cohort study, hydroxychloroquine (Plaquenil), 400 mg PO daily, has been found to be protective against future thrombosis by decreasing the titers of APAs; more studies are needed to make this recommendation for healthy patients with APAs.

For patients with documented thrombotic events, long-term intensive anticoagulation is recommended. Unfractionated IV heparin followed by **warfarin,** with a goal **INR of >2.5,** is the treatment of choice. The use of low-dose aspirin is optional. Significant bleeding may occur, but the risk of recurrent thrombosis outweighs the risk of major or even life-threatening bleeding. Cumulative life-threatening bleeding is estimated to be 9% at 8 yrs. Test proteins C and S before initiating warfarin therapy to guard against skin necrosis. If titers are low, initiation with warfarin should be <50% of the usual starting dose.

For patients with thrombocytopenia, high-dose corticosteroids are the treatment of choice. IV immune globulin, danazol (Danocrine), dapsone (Dapsone USP, DDS), and cyclosporin (Neoral, Sandimmune) have been tried with variable success. Splenectomy is often ineffective. Initiate anticoagulation after platelet counts reach 50,000 (if no contraindications are present) to prevent thrombotic complications.

In pregnant patients who have had prior events, prednisone (20–40 mg PO/day), heparin (5000–10,000 units SC injections bid), and aspirin (325 mg PO/day) increase the chance of a successful pregnancy. Hyperglycemia, preeclampsia, diabetes, infection, bleeding, osteoporosis, and AVN are potential maternal complications, and close monitoring is advised. In a large study of pregnant patients with APS, the live birth rates are 54% with aspirin and prednisone, 74% with heparin and aspirin, and 83% with heparin, prednisone, and aspirin. Women with thromboses should receive therapeutic doses of IV heparin during pregnancy, as warfarin is contraindicated due to teratogenic effects. The role of low-molecular-weight heparin is unclear. Counsel women who present with arterial thrombotic events not to become pregnant, as the greatest morbidity and mortality are seen in this group.

KEY POINTS TO REMEMBER

- Patients with aCL or APAs who have not had a thrombotic event do not need to be anticoagulated.
- Patients with APS should avoid smoking and exogenous estrogens.

SUGGESTED READING

Khamashta MA, Cuadrado MJ, Mujic F, et al. The management of thrombosis in the antiphospholipid-antibody syndrome. *N Engl J Med* 1995;332:993–997.

Levine JS, Branch W, Rauch J. The antiphospholipid syndrome. *N Engl J Med* 2002;346:752–763.

Myones BL, McCurdy D. The antiphospholipid syndrome: immunologic and clinical aspects. Clinical spectrum and treatment. *J Rheumatol* 2000;27[Suppl 58]:20–28.

Petri M. Hydroxychloroquine use in the Baltimore lupus cohort: effects on lipids, glucose, and thrombosis. *Lupus* 1996;5[Suppl 1]:S16–S22.

Petri M. Pathogenesis and treatment of the antiphospholipid antibody syndrome. *Med Clin North Am* 1997;81:151–176.

Triplett DA. Many faces of lupus anticoagulants. *Lupus* 1998;7[Suppl 2]:S18–S22.

Wilson WA, Gharavi AE, Koike T, et al. International consensus statement on preliminary classification criteria for definite antiphospholipid syndrome. *Arthritis Rheum* 1999;42:1309–1311.

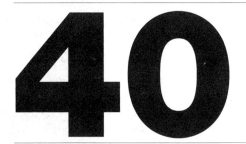

Mixed Connective Tissue Disease

Kathryn H. Dao

INTRODUCTION

MCTD is a specific overlap syndrome characterized by clinical features of SLE, scleroderma, and polymyositis in the presence of antibodies to U1-ribonucleoprotein (RNP). MCTD patients do not fulfill criteria for any one CTD but have "mixed" findings. In addition, it is distinguished from undifferentiated connective tissue disease (UCTD), which is a disorder characterized by incomplete features and nonspecific clinical and lab abnormalities (see Chap. 41, Undifferentiated Connective Tissue Diseases). The prevalence of MCTD is estimated to be 10/100,000, with a female to male ratio of 9:1. Several studies have described an association with DR4, especially in patients with erosive arthritis. A possible link with vinyl chloride exposure has been described in MCTD patients.

CAUSES

Pathophysiology

The pathophysiology of MCTD is poorly defined. MCTD is characterized by high titers of **anti-U1-RNP antibodies;** hence, an assumption is made that anti-U1-RNP and its antigen are involved in the pathogenesis of the disease. Whether this is a direct effect or an epiphenomenon is unclear. U1-RNP is a uridine-rich RNA particle found in the spliceosome complex that is required to splice pre-messenger RNA to mature RNA. The antigenic targets in U1-RNP are U1-RNA and U1-specific polypeptides (70 kD). The pathogenic stimulus to anti-U1-RNP production is unknown, but one study reported that microbial agents (e.g., recombinant CMV glycoprotein B) can initiate an immune response against U1-RNP.

PRESENTATION

History and Physical Exam

Patients display "mixed" features of different CTDs. Patients may initially present with features suggestive of one disorder (e.g., SLE), but they eventually develop other features and are diagnosed with MCTD. Of note, patients seldom develop psychosis, seizures, or diffuse proliferative glomerulonephritis, which may be present in SLE patients. Raynaud's phenomenon with associated hand edema is a very common feature; it can also occur in scleroderma, eosinophilic fasciitis, and other overlap syndromes. Arthralgias and arthritis lack a unique pattern. Myositis and fibrosing alveolitis are important features of MCTD. Pulmonary HTN is the principal cause of death in patients with MCTD. Other clinical features include photosensitivity, calcinosis, telangiectasia, dysphagia, trigeminal neuralgia, and sicca symptoms.

MANAGEMENT

Diagnostic Workup

In 1986, the International Symposium on Mixed Connective Tissue Disease and Antinuclear Antibodies proposed classification criteria for MCTD that included the

TABLE 40-1. PRELIMINARY DIAGNOSTIC CRITERIA FOR THE CLASSIFICATION OF MCTD

Common symptoms

   Raynaud's phenomenon

   Swollen fingers or hands

Anti-U1 snRNP positive

Mixed findings

   SLE-like findings: polyarthritis, lymphadenopathy, facial erythema, pericarditis or pleuritis, leukopenia, thrombocytopenia

   Systemic sclerosis–like findings: sclerodactyly, pulmonary fibrosis with restrictive lung changes (forced vital capacity <80% or diffusing capacity of lung for CO <70%), hypomotility or dilatation of the esophagus

   Polymyositis-like findings: muscle weakness, elevated creatine kinase, myogenic pattern on electromyography

Diagnosis of MCTD when all 3 conditions are fulfilled:

   Presence of one or both common symptoms

   Positive anti-U1 snRNP antibody

   Presence of ≥ 1 findings in at least 2 of the 3 disease categories under "mixed findings"

snRNP, small nuclear ribonucleoprotein.
From Kasukawa R, Tojo T. Preliminary diagnostic criteria for classification of mixed connective tissue disease. Conference in Amsterdam. Elsevier, 1987:33–40.

presence of serum RNP antibodies and core clinical features as seen in Table 40-1. The sine qua non for diagnosis is the presence of U1-RNP antibodies, also known as "anti-RNP;" this test can be ordered as part of the extractable nuclear antigen lab panel. Patients with MCTD often have a positive ANA; however, other antibodies may also be present, including RF, anti-Jo-1, anti-La, and aCL. The aCL in MCTD are β-2-glycoprotein-I independent, explaining the lack of association with thromboembolic events. A distinction of MCTD is the lack of anti-Sm and anti–double stranded DNA antibodies, the presence of which would suggest SLE. Blood counts may reveal a thrombocytopenia or leukopenia; ESR and serum immunoglobulins are often elevated.

Treatment and Follow-Up

There is no specific treatment for MCTD. Treatment is feature-specific and directed toward symptom relief. Antiinflammatory agents or analgesics are helpful for musculoskeletal complaints; steroids and/or cytotoxic agents are often used in patients with myositis, synovitis, or severe multiorgan involvement. Follow patients long term with physical exams, BP checks, and routine lab tests for CBC, muscle enzymes, and UA looking for protein. The disease may eventually evolve into a more distinct clinical entity.

KEY POINTS TO REMEMBER

- MCTD is a unique clinical entity characterized by features of SLE, polymyositis, scleroderma, and a positive anti-RNP antibody.
- MCTD is a distinct diagnostic entity not to be confused with overlap connective tissue disease.

SUGGESTED READING

Burdt MA, Hoffman RW. Long-term outcome in mixed connective tissue disease. *Arthritis Rheum* 1999;42:899–909.

Hoffman RW, Greidinger EL. Mixed connective tissue disease. *Curr Opin Rheumatol* 2000;12:386–390.

Kasukawa R, Tojo T, et al. Preliminary diagnostic criteria for classification of mixed connective tissue disease. Conference in Amsterdam. Elsevier, 1987;33–40.

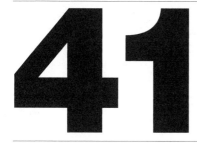

Undifferentiated Connective Tissue Diseases

Kathryn H. Dao

INTRODUCTION

Approximately 25% of patients with systemic rheumatic complaints do not meet the American College of Rheumatology criteria for one defined rheumatic disorder. They may present with early Raynaud's phenomenon, inflammatory polyarthritis, or non-specific clinical and lab abnormalities. These patients are categorized as having undifferentiated connective tissue disease (UCTD) if they have systemic features that overlap two or more disorders but cannot be definitely diagnosed as having one specific rheumatic disease. Many clinical features may be shared with RA, SS, SLE, systemic sclerosis, and inflammatory myopathies. Serologic abnormalities may include positive ANA, RF, anti-Ro/anti-La, anti-centromere, anti-Sm, and anti–double stranded DNA antibodies.

Evolution to a discrete disease may occur. In a North American study of 143 patients with UCTD, 29% of individuals met criteria for the diagnosis of SLE, 3% for RA, 15% for systemic sclerosis, and 3% for MCTD; 6% of patients underwent complete remission, whereas the remainder kept their original diagnosis. Analgesics, antiin-flammatory agents, and steroids are often used to treat symptoms. Methotrexate may be used for arthritis or chronic synovitis. Treatment is directed toward clinical manifestations (see Chap. 12, Systemic Lupus Erythematosus; Chap. 38, Scleroderma; and Chap. 10, Rheumatoid Arthritis). Follow patients with UCTD long term to assess progression to a specific disease or remission.

SUGGESTED READING

Cervera R, Khamashta MA, Hughes GR. "Overlap" syndromes. *Ann Rheum Dis* 1990;49:947–948.

Williams HJ, Alarcon GS, Joks R, et al. Early undifferentiated connective tissue disease. VI. An inception cohort after 10 years. *J Rheumatol* 1999; 26:816–825.

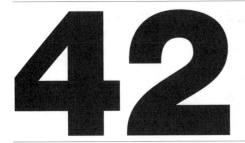

Adult-Onset Still's Disease

Kevin M. Latinis

INTRODUCTION

AOSD is a relatively rare inflammatory condition consisting of a constellation of clinical and lab findings similar to those of **systemic juvenile arthritis (Still's disease).** It is characterized by daily high, spiking fevers; arthritis; and an evanescent rash that typically occurs during febrile periods.

The incidence of AOSD is estimated to be 0.16 new cases/100,000 patients/year. It occurs in a bimodal distribution between ages 15–25 and 36–46, with no gender predilection.

CAUSES

Pathophysiology

The etiology of AOSD is poorly understood. However, immune-mediated mechanisms and a number of viral and bacterial infections have been speculated to play a role.

Differential Diagnosis

The diagnosis of AOSD is one of exclusion, as many other clinical conditions can mimic its onset. The differential diagnosis includes RA, viral or postviral arthritis, infectious arthritis, acute systemic viral or bacterial infections, malignancy, and SLE.

PRESENTATION

History and Physical Exam

Patients can present with myriad symptoms. Many of these are required for diagnosis (see Diagnostic Workup). Patients tend to present with a history of high, spiking **fevers,** often >39°C. The fevers classically follow a quotidian or double quotidian pattern of daily or twice daily peaks, often with afebrile periods between spikes. The fevers typically occur in late afternoon or evening and follow a regular cycle.

Coincident with fevers is the appearance of a characteristic salmon-colored macular or maculopapular **rash.** The rash of Still's disease usually is found on the trunk or extremities and may be precipitated by rubbing (the Koebner phenomenon). Its transient nature may make it difficult to identify on routine exam.

Arthritis and arthralgias involving the knees, wrists, ankles, elbows, PIPs, and shoulders are common manifestations of AOSD. Oligoarticular joint involvement is usually gradual in onset and mild in nature but may progress to a more clinically severe arthritis. Arthrocentesis reveals an inflammatory fluid.

Additional clinical findings may include pharyngitis, lymphadenopathy, splenomegaly, hepatomegaly, and cardiopulmonary involvement, including pericarditis, pleural effusions, or pulmonary infiltrates.

MANAGEMENT

Diagnostic Workup

The diagnosis of AOSD is a clinical diagnosis and involves diagnostic exclusion of other possible conditions. There are no confirmatory lab or radiographic tests; however, diagnostic criteria have been created to assist in the diagnostic workup.

Major Criteria

- Fever of $\geq 39°C$ lasting ≥ 1 wk
- Arthralgias or arthritis lasting ≥ 2 wks
- Characteristic rash (described in the section History and Physical Exam)
- Leukocytosis ($> 10,000$ cells/mm^3) with a predominance of neutrophils

Minor Criteria

- Pharyngitis
- Lymphadenopathy
- Hepatomegaly or splenomegaly
- Abnormal liver function tests
- Negative ANA and RF

Exclusions

- Current infections
- Malignancy, especially lymphoma
- Other active rheumatologic diseases

These diagnostic criteria carry an estimated sensitivity of 93% when *five* of the above features are present with at least *two* from the major criteria.

Lab and radiographic abnormalities may occur with AOSD and lend support to the diagnosis, but no test alone is specific for the disease. Order the following tests when entertaining the diagnosis of AOSD: CBC with differential, liver function tests, ESR, serum ferritin, ANA, RF, and radiographs of affected joints.

A CBC usually reveals a leukocytosis with a predominance of neutrophils; a normocytic, normochromic anemia; and thrombocytosis. The ESR is most often elevated, consistent with an inflammatory condition. Liver function tests may demonstrate elevated aminotransferases, alkaline phosphatase, and LDH. Serum ferritin levels can be markedly elevated. Elevated ferritin levels correlate with disease activity and have been proposed as markers of treatment response. ANA and RF are usually negative (see minor diagnostic criteria listed above) but may be present in low titers in some patients.

Radiographic findings in AOSD are relatively uncommon. When present, findings consistent with the diagnosis of AOSD include nonerosive narrowing of CMC and intercarpal spaces within the wrist (with sparing of MCP joints), sometimes leading to ankylosis of the wrist.

Treatment and Follow-Up

NSAIDs and aspirin are effective in most patients with AOSD for relief of mild to moderate inflammatory symptoms. Monitoring for liver and GI toxicity is recommended. For more severe manifestations, **corticosteroids** may be indicated. Oral prednisone dosed at 0.5–1.0 mg/kg daily or IV methylprednisolone (Medrol) followed by oral prednisone is usually effective to relieve more severe inflammatory manifestations of AOSD. Local joint injections with steroids may provide symptomatic relief. Few studies have evaluated the efficacy of other agents to treat AOSD. However, a few small studies suggest that oral methotrexate (Folex, Rheumatrex, Trexall) in doses up to 20 mg/wk is effective as a steroid-sparing agent. Anecdotal evidence also suggests that hydroxychloroquine, azathioprine, CYC, cyclosporine, sulfasalazine, IV immunoglobulin, etanercept, infliximab, or anakinra may be useful in the treatment of AOSD.

The course of AOSD is variable. Approximately one-third of patients experience complete resolution within a year of onset. One-third of patients experience a cyclic relapsing pattern of the disease. The remaining one-third of patients experience a chronic active disease often associated with destructive arthritis.

KEY POINTS TO REMEMBER

- Consider AOSD in a fever of unknown origin evaluation.
- Serum ferritin may be very elevated in active Still's disease.

SUGGESTED READING

Fautrel B, Borget C, Rozenberg S, et al. Corticosteroid sparing effect of low dose methotrexate treatment in adult Still's disease. *J Rheumatol* 1999;26:373–378.

Fautrel B, Le Moel G, Saint-Marcoux B, et al. Diagnostic value of ferritin and glycosylated ferritin in adult onset Still's disease. *J Rheumatol* 2001;28:322–329.

Fujii T, Akizuki M, Kameda H, et al. Methotrexate treatment in patients with adult onset Still's disease: retrospective study of 13 Japanese cases. *Ann Rheum Dis* 1997;56:144–148.

Masson C, Le Loet X, Liote F, et al. Comparative study of six types of criteria in adult Still's disease. *J Rheumatol* 1996;23:495–497.

Ohta A, Yamaguchi M, Tsunematsu T, et al. Adult Still's disease: a multicenter survey of Japanese patients. *J Rheumatol* 1990;17:1058–1063.

Schwarz-Eywill M, Heilig B, Bauer H, et al. Evaluation of serum ferritin as a marker for adult Still's disease activity. *Ann Rheum Dis* 1992;51:683–685.

Yamaguchi M, Ohta A, Tsunematsu T, et al. Preliminary criteria for classification of adult Still's disease. *J Rheumatol* 1992;19:424–430.

Relapsing Polychondritis

Ernesto Gutierrez

INTRODUCTION

Relapsing polychondritis (RP) is a rare disease characterized by **recurrent inflammation of cartilaginous structures,** most commonly the outer ear, nose, tracheobronchial tree, and peripheral and axial joints. RP can also affect other proteoglycan-rich structures (e.g., the eye, heart, vessels, and inner ear).

RP occurs mostly in white patients aged 40–60 yrs. It tends to occur with equal frequencies in both sexes, but some recent case series report a female predominance. >30% of cases are associated with either a myelodysplastic syndrome or an autoimmune disease, including primary systemic vasculitides and CTDs.

CAUSES

Pathophysiology

Strong evidence suggests that RP is caused by an immune-mediated attack on cartilaginous structures. Both humoral and cell-mediated mechanisms are thought to be involved. 20–50% of patients have serum antibodies to collagen II, which is normally found in large amounts in cartilage. HLA-DR4 has been associated with increased risk for RP.

Differential Diagnosis

The differential diagnosis depends on manifestations of RP. Saddle nose deformity and laryngotracheal chondritis can be mistaken for WG, although RP is confined strictly to cartilaginous portions of the airways. Arthritis can mimic RA. Ocular symptoms and arthritis can be mistaken for seronegative spondyloarthropathies.

RP is also associated with a number of vasculitides, CTDs, and hematologic and autoimmune diseases. These include most other rheumatic diseases and CTDs, myelodysplastic syndromes, lymphoma, pernicious anemia, acute leukemias, hypothyroidism, Hashimoto thyroiditis, Graves' disease, ulcerative colitis, myasthenia gravis, primary biliary cirrhosis, and diabetes mellitus.

PRESENTATION

History and Physical Exam

The main manifestations of RP are otorhinolaryngeal disease, respiratory compromise, arthritis, and ocular inflammation.

The most common symptom is **auricular chondritis,** characterized by the sudden onset of unilateral or bilateral auricular swelling, pain, warmth, and erythema or violaceous discoloration. The inflammation affects the cartilaginous structures of the ear with sparing of the lobulus. The episode usually resolves with or without treatment within days or weeks. Recurrent attacks result in soft, nodular, and deformed ears. RP can also cause both conductive and neurosensory hearing loss, which occurs in approximately 50% of patients. **Conductive hearing loss** is caused by collapse of auricular cartilage or by swelling of the external auditory canal or eustachian tubes. Serous or purulent otitis media can also occur. **Neurosensory hearing loss** is caused by vasculitis of the cochlear branch of the internal auditory artery. Vasculitis of the vestibular branch is also common, resulting in dizziness, vertigo, nausea, vomiting, and ataxia. If acute, these symptoms can mimic a posterior circulation stroke. Although the hearing loss is often permanent, vestibular symptoms usually improve. **Nasal chondritis** occurs in approximately 50% of patients. It is more common in women and in those <50 yrs. It presents as severe nasal pain, a sensation of nasal and adjacent tissue fullness, and, occasionally, epistaxis. Recurrent attacks result in saddle nose deformity.

Respiratory tract involvement is the main cause of death in some case series. Inflammation of the cartilage in the larynx, trachea, and bronchial tree causes hoarseness, throat pain, difficulty talking, aphonia, dyspnea, cough, stridor, wheezing, and choking. Obstruction can occur in varying degrees and at different levels. Total obstruction of the upper airways can occur from attempted bronchoscopy, intubation, or tracheostomy. Involvement of the lower airways is often asymptomatic until detected by radiographs, bronchoscopy, or spirometry. Respiratory infections are common and result from impaired drainage of secretions caused by airway collapse and impaired mucociliary function. Parenchymal pulmonary disease is not a feature of RP.

Arthritis is the second most common manifestation of RP. It is a presenting symptom in 30% of patients but occurs in up to 80% of patients during the course of disease. The arthritis is nondeforming and nonerosive. The most commonly affected joints are the MCP, PIP, knee, ankle, wrist, and MTP. Acute monoarthritis and tenosynovitis can also occur.

The eye is involved in approximately 50% of patients. **Eye inflammation** is more common in men and is frequently associated with systemic manifestations. Inflammation affects any part of the eye, most commonly as scleritis, episcleritis, keratoconjunctivitis sicca, and peri-orbital edema; uveitis, keratitis, corneal thinning, proptosis (from inflammation of posterior globe elements), and retinal vasculitis can also occur.

RP can also affect the kidney, skin, and cardiovascular and nervous systems. The **kidney** is affected in approximately 15% of patients, and the most common histopathologic findings are mild mesangial proliferation and focal segmental necrotizing glomerulonephritis caused by glomerular deposition of C3, IgG, or IgM. **Skin involvement** occurs in approximately 20% of cases. Palpable purpura, urticaria, and angioedema are the most common cutaneous manifestations; livedo reticularis, migratory superficial thrombophlebitis, erythema nodosum, erythema multiforme, and panniculitis are rare. **Cardiovascular involvement** includes aortic and mitral inflammation with subsequent aortic root dilatation, valvulitis, papillary muscle dysfunction, valvular regurgitation, and atrioventricular conduction blocks.

MANAGEMENT

Diagnostic Workup

The American College of Rheumatology does not have a set of classification criteria for RP. The most widely accepted criteria are that of McAdam et al. The presence of ≥ *3* of the following 7 defines RP:

- Bilateral auricular chondritis
- Nasal chondritis
- Nonerosive seronegative inflammatory polyarthritis
- Ocular inflammation defined as conjunctivitis, keratitis, scleritis, episcleritis, or uveitis
- Respiratory tract chondritis
- Cochlear and/or vestibular dysfunction (e.g., neurosensory hearing loss, tinnitus, and/or vertigo)
- Cartilage biopsy compatible with chondritis

Lab findings of RP are nonspecific markers of inflammation: elevated ESR, normochromic normocytic anemia of chronic inflammation, leukocytosis, thrombocytosis, and hypergammaglobulinemia. Perform CT of the neck and lungs to assess the laryngotracheobronchial tree. Perform spirometry with inspiratory and expiratory volume curves, which may show a variety of dynamic intrathoracic or extrathoracic obstructive patterns.

Treatment and Follow-Up

Corticosteroids are the main form of therapy for RP. **Oral prednisone,** 1 mg/kg qd, is often necessary to suppress inflammation. **Pulse IV methylprednisolone (Medrol),** 1000 mg qd for 3 days followed by **daily PO prednisone,** is used for acute airway closure. Other **immunosuppressants** have been tried as steroid-sparing drugs, with **methotrexate (Folex, Rheumatrex, Trexall)** being the most effective. Other treatments (e.g., dapsone, colchicine, azathioprine, cyclosporin, penicillamine, and plasma exchange) have been tried and are less effective. Focal segmental glomerulonephritis is treated with steroids and either **daily PO or monthly IV cyclophosphamide. Surgical management** of respiratory tract RP includes tracheostomy or bronchial stent placement, although iatrogenic trauma may cause complete obstruction.

Most patients experience intermittent episodes of inflammation and develop some degree of disability (e.g., bilateral deafness, impaired vision, phonation difficulties, or cardiorespiratory problems). Follow-up involves clinical assessment of disease activity and pulmonary status.

KEY POINTS TO REMEMBER

- RP may be present with other CTDs.
- Corticosteroids are the mainstay of treatment for RP.

SUGGESTED READING

McAdam LP, O'Hanlan MA, Bluestone R, et al. Relapsing polychondritis: prospective study of 23 patients and review of the literature. *Medicine (Baltimore)* 1976;55:193–215.

Molina JF, Espinoza LR. Relapsing polychondritis. *Ballière's Best Pract Res Clin Rheumatol* 2000;14:97–109.

Park J, Gowin KM, Schumacher HJ Jr. Steroid sparing effect of methotrexate in relapsing polychondritis. *J Rheumatol* 1996;23:937–938.

Sarodia BD, Dasgupta A, Mehta AC. Management of airway manifestations of relapsing polychondritis. *Chest* 1999;116:1669–1675.

Trentham DE, Le CH. Relapsing polychondritis. *Ann Intern Med* 1998;129:114–122.

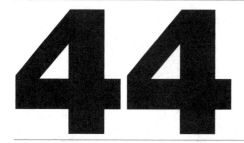

Deposition and Storage Disease Arthropathies

Giancarlo A. Pillot and
Kevin M. Latinis

INTRODUCTION

Arthropathies can result from the deposition of naturally occurring metal ions or accumulation of abnormally processed biochemical intermediates. Most of these diseases are relatively rare and are often mistaken for more common arthropathies. However, many of these diseases have unique characteristics with varying prognoses and treatments, and, hence, accurate diagnosis is important to guide appropriate therapy.

HEMOCHROMATOSIS

Hemochromatosis is a disease of **excess iron accumulation.** The classic familial form has an inheritance that follows an autosomal-recessive inheritance pattern with variable penetrance. Secondary etiologies usually involve iron overload from multiple transfusions. The disease mainly affects the liver, leading to cirrhosis. However, iron that exceeds the liver's storage capacity deposits in other organs, including the pancreas, heart, and pituitary gland, as well as in the joints, causing an arthropathy. Death typically occurs by liver failure, liver cancer, or complications of diabetes or cardiomyopathy.

Chronic, progressive arthritis is a frequent complaint (40–60% of patients) and often predates other symptoms of iron overload. Involvement may include multiple joints: hips, wrists, knees, ankles, shoulders, and the PIP joints. However, involvement of the MCP joints is most common. Classically, arthritis of hemochromatosis is similar to OA and is suspected in patients (particularly men) who present with involvement of MCP and wrist joints. Radiographically, arthritis of hemochromatosis resembles OA with cystic lesions and joint space narrowing. Osteopenia and chondrocalcinosis may also be present radiographically.

Elevated serum iron and ferritin and increased transferrin saturation support the diagnosis. Liver biopsy with staining for iron stores or genetic testing for specific gene defects provides a more definitive diagnosis. Treatment is aimed at reduction of excessive iron through phlebotomy or iron chelators. Symptomatic relief of arthritis can be managed with NSAIDs; use caution to avoid hepatically metabolized agents.

WILSON'S DISEASE

Wilson's disease is an **autosomal-recessive disease of excess copper accumulation** and storage. The disease primarily affects the liver (cirrhosis), kidneys (renal tubular damage), brain (movement disorders and lenticular degeneration), and cornea (Kayser-Fleischer rings) but may also lead to arthropathy (resembling OA) in up to 50% of affected patients.

Commonly affected joints include the knees, shoulders, ankles, and spine, but MCP joints, feet, wrists, hips, and neck can also be involved. Joint manifestations are similar to those of OA, with mechanical pain and crepitus without swelling or warmth. Radiologic findings include osteophyte formation and subchondral cysts. Osteoporosis is commonly present.

Diagnosis is made by the presence of decreased serum ceruloplasmin and either Kayser-Fleischer rings or increased liver copper concentration on biopsy. Other lab abnormalities include increased urinary copper excretion and elevated liver transaminases. Treatment consists of chelation therapy with penicillamine. This treatment often also improves the symptoms of arthritis. Additionally, arthritis can be treated symptomatically with NSAIDs. Liver transplantation is sometimes necessary for end-stage liver disease.

OCHRONOSIS (ALKAPTONURIA)

Ochronosis is a manifestation of the disease **alkaptonuria,** in which pigmented polymers of homogentisic acid accumulate in cartilage, skin, and sclera. Alkaptonuria is a rare **autosomal-recessive disease resulting from the deficiency of homogentisic acid oxidase, an enzyme in the metabolism of phenylalanine.** Alkalinization and oxidation of homogentisic acid causes the metabolite to turn black, causing black urine and pigment deposits in the joints, cartilage, skin, and sclera.

Joint manifestations usually include a progressive degenerative arthropathy initially involving the spine. The knees, hips, and shoulders may also be affected, with relative sparing of the small peripheral joints. Decreased mobility and joint stiffness are the most common complaints. Osteochondral bodies may form in or around joints and cause mechanical complications. Joint effusions and crepitus may also occur. Other manifestations of ochronosis include pigment deposition in the skin, cartilage of the ears and nose, and sclera.

Radiographically, ochronosis resembles OA. Spinal involvement leads to disc calcification, disc narrowing, spinal collapse, and eventual fusion. SI and apophyseal joints are generally spared. Diagnosis is supported by evidence of black urine and arthritis. Synovial fluid analysis may reveal small, pigmented particles resembling ground pepper. Therapy involves symptomatic treatment of the arthropathies with analgesics or NSAIDs. No treatment currently exists for the metabolic defect.

GLYCOLIPID STORAGE DISEASES

Multicentric reticulohistiocytosis is a rare disease primarily affecting middle-aged women and is characterized by inflammatory arthritis and cutaneous lesions. The arthritis is an erosive, symmetric, polyarticular process with synovitis and is often mistaken for RA. Joint involvement includes the interphalangeal joints, shoulders, knees, hips, feet, ankles, elbows, and spine. Joint manifestations often precede skin lesions and may progress to arthritis mutilans in severe cases. Skin lesions include papules and nodules that are typically firm and may be flesh colored, red, brown, or yellow. Skin involvement may appear anywhere but most commonly occurs on the dorsum of the hands and fingers, ears, elbows, face, and often the oral, nasal, or pharyngeal mucosa.

The pathophysiology of multicentric reticulohistiocytosis is poorly understood. It is often associated with other diseases [e.g., infections (in particular, tuberculosis), malignancies, and autoimmune diseases]. Diagnosis is made by biopsy of affected tissue demonstrating the presence of multinucleated giant cells and glycolipid-laden histiocytes, which stain positive with periodic acid–Schiff stain. When a diagnosis is established, evaluate the patient for TB and occult malignancies as well. Spontaneous remission may occur in some patients; however, most patients experience a chronic course. Treatment is based on anecdotal experience and includes the use of corticosteroids, CYC, chlorambucil, methotrexate, or cyclosporin A.

Gaucher's disease and **Fabry's disease** are rare glycolipid storage diseases that include arthritic manifestations. These diseases are caused by known biochemical defects in glycolipid metabolism leading to accumulation of metabolic intermediates in various tissues, including bones, cartilage, and joint tissue. Details of the biochemical defects and disease manifestations are beyond the scope of this manual and should be sought in more comprehensive sources.

KEY POINTS TO REMEMBER

- Arthropathies in association with other disease-specific findings should raise suspicion for deposition and storage disease arthropathies.
- Prognosis of both hemochromatosis and Wilson's disease depends on the extent of systemic organ involvement.
- Treatment of deposition and storage disease arthropathies mainly consists of NSAIDs and analgesics as tolerated.

SUGGESTED READING

Bulaj ZJ, Ajioka RS, Phillips JD, et al. Disease-related conditions in relatives of patients with hemochromatosis. *N Engl J Med* 2000;343:1529–1535.

Klippel JH, Weyand CM, Wortmann RL, eds. *Primer on the rheumatic diseases*, 11th ed. Atlanta: Arthritis Foundation, 1997.

McDonnell SM, Phatak PD, Felitti V, et al. Screening for hemochromatosis in primary care settings. *Ann Intern Med* 1998;129:962–970.

Menerey KA, Eider W, Brewer GJ, et al. The arthropathy of Wilson's disease: clinical and pathologic features. *J Rheumatol* 1988;15:331–337.

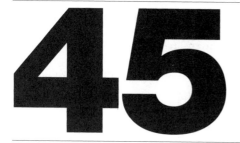

Complex Regional Pain Syndromes/ Reflex Sympathetic Dystrophy

Chakrapol Lattanand

INTRODUCTION

Complex regional pain syndrome type 1 (CRPS1), formerly known as *reflex sympathetic dystrophy* (RSD), describes a rare syndrome consisting of pain, altered skin color, altered skin temperature, edema, and reduced range of motion of an extremity. The pain follows an initiating noxious event to the affected limb but is not limited to the distribution of a single nerve. Much controversy continues surrounding the description and recognition of the disorder. CRPS1 is synonymous or closely related to the following disorders: RSD, Sudeck's atrophy, shoulder-hand syndrome, sympathalgia, algodystrophy, and posttraumatic vasomotor disorders. In 1993, the International Association for the Study of Pain provided a consensus statement on nomenclature: *RSD* was defined as complex regional pain syndrome type 1, and the disorder *causalgia* became complex regional pain syndrome type 2.

Limited data exist regarding the epidemiology of CRPS1. Some documentation has been provided in Sweden. In 1993, of 2458 cases described as pain in an extremity, 29 cases were causalgia and 80 cases were RSD, or CRPS1.

CAUSES

Pathophysiology

The etiology of CRPS1 is unknown. Postulated mechanisms include the following: aberrant healing response, an exaggerated inflammatory response, protection and disuse of an injured limb, a dysfunctional sympathetic nervous system, myofascial dysfunction, and CNS abnormalities. Psychological and behavioral factors (e.g., stress) surrounding the inciting event may also play a role.

PRESENTATION

History and Physical Exam

Onset of symptoms usually occurs within 1 mo of an inciting event. Clinical signs and symptoms are outlined in the diagnostic criteria (Table 45-1). Less common clinical findings include trophic changes (atrophy of the skin, nails, and soft tissues), motor dysfunction (weakness, tremor, and dystonia), and osteoporosis (Sudeck's atrophy of bone).

Classically, CRPS1 has been described as following three stages: Stage 1 involves constant pain of a burning quality, localized to area of injury. This stage may last from a few weeks to up to 6 mos. Stage 2 involves gradual decrease of pain, spread of edema, and increased atrophy. This stage typically lasts 3–6 mos. Finally, stage 3 involves marked trophic changes, with weakness and limited motion.

MANAGEMENT

Diagnostic Workup

Diagnosis is made by the presence of clinical criteria as described above. Supplemental tests may support the clinical diagnosis but are not routinely used. **Three-phase bone**

TABLE 45-1. SYMPTOMS OF COMPLEX REGIONAL PAIN SYNDROMES (CRPSs)

1. Presence of an initiating noxious event (e.g., surgery or trauma) or cause of immobilization.
2. Continuing pain, allodynia (distress from painful stimulus), or hyperalgesia with pain disproportionate to inciting event.
3. Edema, changes in skin blood flow, or abnormal sudomotor activity (change in skin color or increased/decreased sweating) in region of pain.
4. Exclusion of existing condition that would otherwise account for the degree of pain and dysfunction.

CRPS type 1 requires criteria 2–4 to be satisfied. CRPS type 2 requires criteria 2–4 but follows a nerve injury.

scintigraphy demonstrates a reduction in blood flow during the early phase and increased periarticular uptake during the third phase. Sensitivity is on the order of 44–67% and specificity of 86–92%. Thermography is a side-to-side temperature difference for which $>1.1°C$ is required for significance. Laser Doppler flowmetry, which demonstrates changes in peripheral blood flow, may be an early predictor of sympathetic dysfunction. Quantitative sweat testing [Quantitative Sudomotor Axon Reflex Test (QSART)] shows abnormalities of resting and evoked sweat production and may reflect pathologic changes of peripheral autonomic function. Muscle strength and joint testing may provide a baseline and serve as prognostic indicators. Finally, psychological screening and testing may be useful to identify confounding psychological issues.

Treatment and Follow-Up

Goals of therapy include restoration and normalization of function. An interdisciplinary approach and patient education are emphasized. Physical therapy is the primary modality to achieve measurable rehabilitation goals. Medications, regional anesthesia, and other treatment modalities are used to allow progress and achieve goals of physical therapy by relieving pain and increasing patient compliance with a rehabilitation program. Referral to a pain management service may also be helpful.

Pharmacologic management includes NSAIDs, opioids, anticonvulsants, local anesthetics, mexiletine, corticosteroids, calcitonin, capsaicin cream, alpha blockers (in those who respond to a trial of phentolamine infusion), and clonidine (transdermal, intraspinal, and epidural). Regional anesthetic techniques are indicated to provide analgesia to facilitate physical therapy, and sympatholysis is indicated in cases with unequivocal evidence of sympathetically maintained pain. Sympathetic blocks may be diagnostic and therapeutic for sympathetically maintained pain. Methods include stellate ganglion blocks, lumbar blocks, local IV guanethidine and bretylium blocks, and IV phentolamine infusion. Therapeutic neurolytic sympatholysis is achieved with injection of phenol prepared with radiocontrast media or by using radiofrequency techniques. Duration of effect is normally 3–6 mos. Epidural catheters can infuse long-acting local anesthetic (bupivacaine) and opioid and can be retained up to 6 mos. There are no clinical trials to support efficacy of any of these modalities.

Other treatment options exist but also have not been supported by large clinical trials. Neuromodulation by spinal cord stimulation or percutaneous nerve stimulation may provide some relief. Surgical sympathectomy may facilitate pain relief in patients with nonsustained relief from sympathetic blockade. Intrathecal baclofen has been reported to improve dystonia in some patients with CRPS.

KEY POINTS TO REMEMBER

- CRPS is a clinical diagnosis. However, three-phase bone scan may help support the diagnosis.
- Allodynia (distress from painful stimuli) is a common characteristic of CRPS.

SUGGESTED READING

Galer B, Schwartz L, Allen R. Complex regional pain syndromes—type I: reflex sympathetic dystrophy and type II: causalgia. In: Loeser J, ed. *Bonica's management of pain*, 3rd ed. Philadelphia: Lippincott Williams & Wilkins, 2001:388–411.

Manning D. Reflex sympathetic dystrophy, sympathetically maintained pain, and complex regional pain syndrome: diagnoses of inclusion, exclusion, or confusion? *J Hand Ther* 2000;13:260–268.

Merskey H, Bogduk N, eds. *Classification of chronic pain: descriptions of chronic pain syndromes and definitions of pain terms*, 2nd ed. Seattle: IASP Press, 1994:40–42.

Stanton-Hicks M, Baron R, Boas R, et al. Complex regional pain syndromes: guidelines for therapy. *Clin J Pain* 1998;14:155–166.

Stanton-Hicks M, Janig W, Hassenbusch S, et al. Reflex sympathetic dystrophy: changing concepts and taxonomy. *Pain* 1995;63:127–133.

Neuropathic Arthropathy

Shannon C. Lynn

INTRODUCTION

Neuropathic arthropathy (NA), also known as **Charcot joints,** describes an arthropathy associated with an underlying neurologic deficit. NA was first reported by Charcot in patients with tabes dorsalis (neurosyphilis involving the posterior columns of the spinal cord and dorsal roots) who had joint deformity and destruction. NA is also associated with diabetes mellitus, syringomyelia, leprosy, MS, polio, and sympathetic nerve injury. **Diabetes mellitus is the most common cause of NA in the United States.**

CAUSES

Pathophysiology

The pathogenesis of NA is not completely understood, but decreased neuronal stimulation, autonomic dysfunction, and increased vascularity of involved joints are thought to play a role. Charcot theorized that the degeneration of nerves leads to bone atrophy. Virchow and Volkman hypothesized that, without the protective warning sense of pain, joints are susceptible to repeated trauma that eventually leads to joint destruction. However, one-third of patients do not have a neurologic deficit before the onset of the arthropathy. The current understanding is that increased vascularity and autonomic dysfunction lead to arteriovenous shunting and dysregulation of the vasoconstrictive response, which results in bone atrophy and joint destruction.

Two phases of NA have been described. The first stage is the atrophic, resorptive, or hyperemic phase, characterized by replacement of bone by more vascular connective tissue. The second stage is the hypertrophic reparative sclerotic phase, characterized by excessive formation of bone.

Differential Diagnosis

The differential diagnosis includes OA, AVN, septic arthritis, cellulitis, osteomyelitis, crystalline arthropathies, hemophilia, and RA.

PRESENTATION

History and Physical Exam

The patient usually presents with an acutely inflamed joint, often after minor trauma. The joint may have the cardinal signs of inflammation (e.g., warmth, erythema, swelling, and loss of function); pain may or may not be present. Of those patients who have pain, one-third have decreased response to deep pain and proprioception on exam. NA can precede the detection of a neurologic abnormality. Diabetic patients with NA of a foot joint usually have absent patellar deep tendon reflexes. The presentation of acute NA may be complicated by ulceration on the plantar surface, forefoot, or midfoot if the toes, metatarsus, or lesser tarsi are involved. This clinical presentation can easily be confused with osteomyelitis. Later in the course of the disease, the joint may feel like "a loose bag of bones."

TABLE 46-1. JOINT INVOLVEMENT IN CONDITIONS ASSOCIATED WITH NEUROPATHIC ARTHROPATHY

Disease	Joints involved
Syringomyelia	Shoulder, elbow, spine
Neurosyphilis	Hip, knee
Diabetes mellitus	Ankle, foot (especially tarsometatarsal and MTP)

Table 46-1 lists the most commonly involved joints in those conditions associated with NA.

MANAGEMENT

Diagnostic Workup

WBC count and ESR are usually normal, even in the acute phase when the joint is hot, swollen, and erythematous. Synovial fluid has only been studied in the hypertrophic phase. The fluid is usually clear, straw colored, and viscous, with a normal WBC count. The fluid may also be bloody or xanthochromic and contain lipid crystals or droplets in patients with intraarticular fractures. Calcium pyrophosphate or hydroxyapatite crystals may complicate the picture.

Radiologic evaluation usually begins with plain films. Plain films often show joint "3D distention" (i.e., dislocation, destruction, and degeneration in a distended joint). The distention is a result of fluid accumulation, hypertrophic synovitis, osteophytes, and subluxation. A bone scan may be helpful to rule out infection. MRI may also be useful to identify ligament tears and intraarticular fragmentation.

Treatment and Follow-Up

Early diagnosis and treatment are imperative to improve long-term outcomes. After infection has been excluded, treatment involves **immobilization and NSAIDs** to control swelling.

Eichenholtz has defined treatment by stages in diabetic patients with NA of the foot and ankle. The first stage, known as the *dissolution* or *inflammatory phase*, is characterized by swelling, redness, warmth, and loss of foot function. The treatment is strict prohibition of weight-bearing activity for 6–12 wks or until skin temperature is normal to limit persistent inflammation. Stage two is the *healing phase*, characterized by a reduction in swelling and a return of joint function. Plain films show evidence of consolidation of bony fragments. The foot is still very vulnerable to further injury, and treatment consists of orthotic shoes and/or braces. In the third phase, known as the *resolution* or *remodeling phase*, the joint demonstrates increased stability, but function may still be abnormal. The joint demonstrates the classic "Charcot deformity." Radiographs show bony consolidation and reduced bony fragmentation. The patient still requires protective footwear.

Surgical interventions are indicated only when the patient has failed casting, bracing, or orthotic footwear or has a malaligned, unstable, or nonreducible fracture. Arthroplasty is generally contraindicated because of increased rates of loosening and breakage of the prosthesis in a neuropathic joint.

Small, nonrandomized studies suggest that pamidronate may be beneficial in patients with NA. One small study shows promise with the use of pamidronate infusion for the treatment of acute NA in diabetics. This study included six diabetic patients with severe peripheral sensory neuropathy. Each patient presented with a swollen, hot foot. The diagnosis of NA was confirmed by radiographs and bone scans. Each patient was treated with IV pamidronate (Aredia) infusion of 30 mg followed by 60 mg infusions q2wks for five cycles. Response was monitored by skin temperature of the affected joint and patients' symptoms. All patients showed a statistically significant decrease in skin temperature after the first pamidronate infusion, and each patient reported a subjective improvement. Pamidronate warrants further investigation with double-blind randomized controlled studies.

Complications of NA include nerve root impingement or entrapment secondary to bony overgrowth, cord compression when the axial skeleton is involved, stress fractures, and secondary infections.

Frequent monitoring of joint stability and encouraged use of protective devices are recommended to avoid progression of joint destruction.

KEY POINTS TO REMEMBER

- Diabetes mellitus is the most common cause of NA in the United States.
- X-rays of affected joints show dislocation, destruction, and degeneration of a distended joint.

SUGGESTED READING

Allman RM, Brower AC, Kotlyarov EB. Neuropathic bone and joint disease. *Radiol Clin North Am* 1988;26:1373–1381.

Eichenholtz SN. *Charcot joints*. Springfield IL: Charles C. Thomas, 1966.

Guis S, Pellissier JF, Arniaud D, et al. Healing of Charcot's joint by pamidronate infusion. *J Rheumatol* 1999;26:1843–1845.

Klenerman L. The Charcot joint in diabetes. *Diabet Med* 1996;13[Suppl 1]:S52–S54.

Selby PL, Young MJ, Boulton AJ. Bisphosphonates: a new treatment for diabetic Charcot neuroarthropathy? *Diabet Med* 1994;11:28–31.

Sequeira W. The neuropathic joint. *Clin Exp Rheumatol* 1994;12:325–337.

Sinacore DR, Withrington NC. Recognition and management of acute neuropathic (Charcot) arthropathies of the foot and ankle. *J Orthop Sports Phys Ther* 1999;29:736–746.

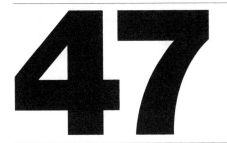

Sarcoid Arthropathy

Giancarlo A. Pillot and
Rebecca M. Shepherd

INTRODUCTION

Sarcoidosis is a granulomatous inflammatory disease of unknown etiology that can involve any organ, most commonly the **lung, skin, eye, and joints.** The prevalence of sarcoidosis is 10–20 cases/100,000 population. The incidence is higher among blacks than other races. The disease also varies by geographic region and may have a genetic component.

CAUSES

Pathophysiology

The etiology of sarcoidosis is unknown. Sarcoidosis is characterized by **noncaseating granulomas** occurring at any site in the body. The granuloma is a chronic inflammatory reaction comprised of macrophages, lymphocytes, monocytes, and epithelial cells. Multinucleated giant cells are frequently found in the center of the granuloma. Granuloma formation is thought to occur because of an exaggerated immune response to an unidentified antigenic stimulus. Theories concerning the possible antigen include infection (e.g., *Propionibacterium* species), genetic factors, environmental factors, and immunodeficient states.

Differential Diagnosis

The differential diagnosis of sarcoidosis includes HIV, TB, neoplastic processes (i.e., lymphoma or bronchogenic carcinoma), syphilis, and fungal infections. Acute joint manifestations can mimic infectious arthritis, gout, RA, ARF, hemochromatosis, hemarthrosis, and vasculitic syndromes.

PRESENTATION

History and Physical Exam

Sarcoidosis occurs most commonly in patients aged 20–40 yrs. The lung is the most commonly involved organ, occurring in 86% of patients. Patients usually present with fatigue and **pulmonary symptoms,** (e.g., cough, dyspnea, and chest pain). Extrapulmonary involvement frequently accompanies the pulmonary symptoms. **Lymph nodes, liver, and spleen** are frequently involved. Heart, kidney, and pancreas are less commonly involved. Sarcoidosis of the musculoskeletal system occurs in 15–25% of patients. **Acute sarcoid arthritis** occurs most commonly as a polyarthritis of the knees, ankles, elbows, and wrists. Erythema, warmth, swelling, and tenderness of joints occur. Involvement is usually symmetrical, and periarticular swelling, rather than joint effusions, is common. Acute arthritis commonly occurs in the presence of **erythema nodosum** and acute **uveitis.** The triad of acute arthritis, erythema nodosum, and bilateral hilar adenopathy is **Löfgren's syndrome** and has a good prognosis. Acute arthritis usually lasts several weeks to months and often does not recur. **Chronic sarcoid arthritis** is rare and typically nondestructive. It presents several months after the onset of disease. It is most common in the knee but also involves the ankles and PIP joints. The arthritis is not associated with erythema nodosum. Periosteal bone resorption appears as cysts. Joint destruction can occur rarely with shortening and deformity of the phalanges. Sarcoidosis affects the muscle in the form of myopathy, atrophy, myositis, or palpable nodules. Asymptomatic granulomatous involvement of the muscles is documented frequently at autopsy. Sarcoidosis causes lytic and sclerotic lesions in the bone, both of which can be painful. Typically, lesions occur in the hands and feet but can potentially involve any bone. Along with bone resorption, the lesions contribute to a high risk of fracture in sarcoid patients.

MANAGEMENT

Diagnostic Workup

Diagnosis of sarcoidosis is made by histologic evidence of noncaseating granulomas. Biopsy of the affected organ is the most effective way to demonstrate the granulomas. Biopsy of lymph nodes, skin, and lacrimal glands often yields diagnostic histology. Biopsy of lung tissue requires fiberoptic bronchoscopy with transbronchial lung biopsy. Biopsy is required for diagnosis if any other diagnoses (e.g., tuberculosis) are being considered, as treatment is vastly different. Often, however, a diagnosis can be tentatively made based on symptoms, signs, and supporting data. Chest radiograph findings in sarcoidosis include bilateral hilar lymphadenopathy, diffuse parenchymal changes, or a combination of both. Pulmonary function tests demonstrate a restrictive pattern with normal flow rates but may be normal. Serum ACE levels are high in three-fourths of untreated patients. 1,25-dihydroxyvitamin D levels may also be elevated. These serum levels, however, are nondiagnostic. Joint involvement is characterized by noninflammatory synovial fluid in both acute and chronic forms of arthritis. Synovial biopsy occasionally reveals granulomas but is not often performed. Acute onset of joint symptoms in a sarcoidosis patient should prompt the consideration of infectious arthritis. In patients with muscular complaints, a muscle biopsy can reveal granulomas.

Treatment and Follow-Up

Control mild symptoms with **NSAIDs. Corticosteroids** are used for patients with moderate to severe symptoms, including musculoskeletal symptoms. There is some controversy regarding whom to treat, because sarcoidosis clears spontaneously in approximately 50% of patients. The choice to use corticosteroids is typically guided by persistence of symptoms for >2–3 mos, unless there is significant respiratory impairment or worrisome symptoms (e.g., eye involvement, significant heart involvement, neurologic impairment, or severe fevers, fatigue, and weight loss). Although corticosteroid therapy clearly reduces inflammation and symptoms attributable to disease, there is a paucity of data regarding the optimal dose and duration of treatment. Initial doses of prednisone, 1 mg/kg/day PO for 4–6 wks followed by slow tapering over 2–12 mos, are used. Disease can often recur after withdrawal of steroids, requiring reinitiation of therapy. Relapse of spontaneous remission, however, is rare. Most (90%) of patients have remission with few sequelae. Other possible treatment modalities include chloroquine, colchicine, allopurinol, and cyclosporine. Low-dose methotrexate (7.5–20 mg PO weekly) may be helpful as a steroid-sparing agent.

KEY POINTS TO REMEMBER

- The triad of polyarthritis, erythema nodosum, and bilateral hilar adenopathy due to sarcoidosis is known as *Löfgren's syndrome* and carries a favorable prognosis.
- Diagnosis of sarcoidosis should include evaluation of pulmonary and other systemic organ involvement.

SUGGESTED READING

Barnard JS, Newman LS. Sarcoidosis: immunology, rheumatic involvement, and therapeutics. *Curr Opin Rheumatol* 2001;13(1):84–91.
Newman LS, Rose CS, Maier LA. Sarcoidosis. *N Engl J Med* 1997;336:1224.
Pettersson T. Sarcoid and erythema nodosum arthropathies. *Ballière's Best Pract Res Clin Rheumatol* 2000;14(3):471–476.
Wilcox A, Bharadwaj P, Sharma OP. Bone sarcoidosis. *Curr Opin Rheumatol* 2000;12(4):321–330.

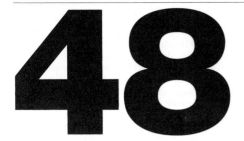

Amyloidosis and Amyloid Arthropathy

Rebecca M. Shepherd

INTRODUCTION

Amyloidosis is the term used to describe a group of diseases characterized by the deposition of fibrils in the extracellular tissue. The fibrils are 5- to 25-kD subunits of normal proteins formed into antiparallel beta-pleated sheets. There are >50 proteins now identified that form these amyloid sheets; the most common forms of amyloidosis are AL, AA, familial transthyretin, and dialysis-related amyloidosis (DRA). The number of total cases of the systemic amyloidoses is not known. The incidence of AL amyloidosis is approximately 5.8–12.8/million person years. The prevalence of DRA correlates with length of treatment with hemodialysis; at 12 yrs of dialysis, 50% of patients have DRA, and 100% have it at 20 yrs.

CAUSES

Pathophysiology

Amyloid deposits are rigid linear fibrils of indefinite length that form cross beta-pleated sheets. AL amyloidosis, also called *primary amyloidosis*, is a disorder in which fragments of immunoglobulin monoclonal light chains deposit in end organs. >50 monoclonal proteins have been identified. AL amyloidosis is most often associated with plasma cell dyscrasias (e.g., multiple myeloma) but can occur without evidence of blood dyscrasias. Most patients have an M protein in the serum and/or urine. Secondary amyloidosis is not caused by deposits of immunoglobulin light chains but from a deposition of a protein called *amyloid A* (AA). Secondary amyloidosis occurs in the setting of chronic inflammation, especially rheumatic diseases (e.g., RA, juvenile chronic polyarthritis, and AS) and IBD. Chronic infections (e.g., osteomyelitis, TB, leprosy, and bronchiectasis), chronic viral infections (e.g., HIV), and chronic IV drug use are also associated with AA. The familial amyloidoses are a group of autosomal-dominant diseases in which mutant proteins form and precipitate. The most common disease is transthyretin-derived amyloid, in which the normal transthyretin protein is unstable. DRA develops from the deposition of beta$_2$-microglobulin (B2M). B2M is normally secreted by cells in the body and is catabolized and secreted by the kidneys. In patients with renal failure, B2M is not easily cleared by hemodialysis and, thus, accumulates in the serum and tissue.

Differential Diagnosis

The differential diagnosis for amyloidosis includes light chain deposition disease, chronic infection, and malignancy. Differentiate amyloid arthropathy from RA, OA, hemarthrosis, and sarcoidosis.

PRESENTATION

History and Physical Exam

Clinical manifestations are determined by the end organs involved. Symptoms of fatigue, weight loss, and anorexia are common. Primary amyloidosis is characterized by widespread organ involvement, whereas secondary amyloidosis is more commonly localized to the liver and spleen. **Renal** involvement is the most common and serious manifestation of amyloidosis. Proteinuria is the initial manifestation, often leading to nephrotic syndrome and eventually the need for dialysis. Adrenal insufficiency can occur with renal involvement. **Cardiac** involvement occurs in 80–90% of patients with amyloidosis. Amyloid infiltrates the myocardium and coronary vessels, leading to heart failure, conduction disturbances, and ischemic symptoms from insufficient blood flow through the coronary arteries. **GI involvement** is seen in all types of amyloidosis. Macroglossia is common and can cause dysphagia and obstructive sleep apnea. Dysfunctional motility is common, as are obstruction, diarrhea, and malabsorption syndromes. The liver and spleen are heavily infiltrated with amyloid but without significant organ dysfunction. **Respiratory** symptoms are less common, but amyloid can deposit anywhere along the respiratory tract, and symptoms are related to the location of deposition. Amyloid can deposit in the **peripheral and autonomic nervous systems.** Sensory and motor disturbances occur in any distribution, and orthostasis and impotence can occur. Peripheral neuropathy occurs in 25–30% of patients with AL disease but less commonly in patients with AA disease. **Musculo-skeletal** involvement can occur with both primary and secondary amyloidoses. **Joint deposition** of amyloid often mimics the clinical picture of RA and can be found in all joints at postmortem. AL amyloidosis causes an arthropathy that is subacute, progressive, and symmetric in nature, with the shoulders, wrists, knees, and MCP and PIP joints most commonly involved. The joints are only mildly tender, with minimal morning stiffness. **CTS** is common in patients with B2M disease, and the incidence is directly related to the duration in years of hemodialysis. **Subcutaneous nodules** are present in 60% of cases. AL amyloidosis can be associated with soft tissue swelling and synovial deposition in up to 75% of cases. The **"shoulder pad"** sign refers to deposition of amyloid in the glenohumeral joint. **Palmar fascia** can become nodular and thickened with resultant pain, contractures, and weakness. Muscles can also be involved to produce pseudohypertrophy with weakness and pain. Periarthritis of the scapulohumeral joint occurs with synovial tissue and subacromial bursa involvement, imitating a rotator cuff tear or bursitis. Patients undergoing dialysis for 8 yrs often develop bilateral effusions, frequently of the knees and shoulder. Cystic lesions of the bone containing amyloid occur in DRA and usually involve the ends of long bones and predispose to fractures.

MANAGEMENT

Diagnostic Workup

Amyloidosis is diagnosed by demonstration of amyloid in a tissue biopsy. Biopsy of the affected organ has the highest yield. In AL or AA amyloidosis, biopsy yields a positive diagnosis in the following organs: kidney or liver, >90%; abdominal fat pad, 60–80%; rectal, 50–70%; bone marrow biopsy (in suspected AL), 50–55%; skin, 50%. Gingival biopsy has low yield. For B2M amyloidosis, carpal tunnel biopsy is preferred. Once biopsy is obtained, tissue is stained with alkaline Congo red, and immunohistochemical techniques are performed. In musculoskeletal amyloidosis, joint aspirate is noninflammatory in nature with a predominance of mononuclear cells. The amyloid in the aspirate stains with Congo red. If AL amyloidosis is suspected, send serum and urine protein electrophoresis to identify paraproteins and perform a bone marrow biopsy to search for populations of plasma cells. In the 10% of AL amyloidosis without paraprotein excretion, diagnosis can be difficult. AL and AA amyloidosis can usually be differentiated, however, by the clinical setting and medical history.

Treatment and Follow-Up

Systemic amyloidosis is a chronic, progressive disease that is difficult to treat. **The goal of therapy is to prevent further amyloid deposition and promote reabsorption of the fibrils.** AL amyloidosis has a poor prognosis with a median survival of 1–2 yrs. The end organ affected predicts prognosis; heart involvement is associated with 6-mo survival, and kidney involvement is associated with 21-mo survival. Chemotherapy with melphalan and melphalan plus prednisone has shown some survival benefit. Prognosis, even with treatment, remains poor. The prognosis for AA amyloidosis is affected by the course of the underlying chronic disease. For all patients with AA amyloidosis, the average 4-yr survival is 50–60%. The therapy for AA amyloidosis includes treatment of the underlying inflammatory disease and the use of oral colchicine (600 mg PO bid). The mechanism of action of colchicine is not clear, but it likely reduces the production of amyloid fibrils. Dimethyl sulfoxide, chlorambucil, and methotrexate have also been used successfully in small studies. Treatment of amyloid arthropathy is again based on treatment of the underlying disease process. NSAIDs may help with joint tenderness and stiffness.

KEY POINTS TO REMEMBER

- Amyloid arthropathy is managed by treatment of the underlying precipitating cause and the use of colchicine and NSAIDs.
- Diagnostic workup for amyloid arthropathy should include evaluation for other systemic organ involvement.

SUGGESTED READING

Buxbaum J. The amyloidoses. In: Klippel J, Dieppe PA, eds. *Rheumatology*, 2nd ed. St. Louis: Mosby–Year Book, 1998:1–10.

Falk RH, Comenzo RL, Skinner M. The systemic amyloidoses. *N Engl J Med* 1997;337:898–908.

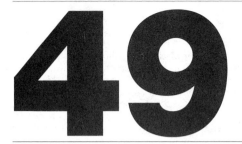

Miscellaneous Conditions Affecting the Skin

Celso R. Velázquez

ERYTHEMA NODOSUM

The lesions of erythema nodosum (EN) are cutaneous nodules that vary in size from 1 to 10 cm and usually appear acutely over the anterior aspect of the legs and, less commonly, on the thighs and forearms. The nodules are usually tender and may be surrounded by erythema and bruising. EN may be associated with infections (streptococcus, TB, histoplasmosis), medications (sulfonamides, penicillin, oral contraceptives), sarcoidosis, IBD, spondyloarthropathies, and malignancies. Löfgren's syndrome is the triad of hilar lymphadenopathy, EN, and polyarthritis seen in acute sarcoidosis. The lesions of EN may resolve spontaneously in weeks or become chronic. Histopathology reveals septal panniculitis without vasculitis. Treatment is symptomatic with NSAIDs. Severe and unresponsive cases may require oral corticosteroids. Oral potassium iodide may also be useful.

PYODERMA GANGRENOSUM

Pyoderma gangrenosum (PG) is characterized by painful ulcers that usually appear on the lower extremities. PG often begins as an inflammatory nodule or pustule that ulcerates and enlarges and can reach sizes of up to 20 cm in diameter. The ulcers appear necrotic, with violaceous, undermined borders. PG is associated with IBD, seronegative RA, and hematologic malignancies. An important characteristic of PG is pathergy: Normal skin of patients with PG that is subjected to trauma may develop the lesions. Débridement or biopsy may therefore worsen the lesions. Histopathology may show marked neutrophilic infiltration but may also be inconclusive. PG may improve with treatment of the associated disorder, but oral corticosteroids are the mainstay of treatment. Secondary infection must be treated if present.

SWEET'S SYNDROME

Sweet's syndrome is a rare condition that may be associated with many different diseases. It has been described in patients with malignancies (both hematologic and solid tumors), infections, IBD, certain medications (antibiotics, granulocyte colony-stimulating factor), RA, sarcoidosis, and Behçet's syndrome. It is characterized by tender red or purple papules or nodules with sharply demarcated borders that appear most commonly over the upper extremities, face, and neck. The lesions may mimic EN when they appear on the lower extremities. Cutaneous manifestations are usually accompanied by fever and leukocytosis. Arthralgias, arthritis, and CNS and renal involvement sometimes occur. Histopathology shows a dense neutrophilic infiltrate without evidence of leukocytoclastic vasculitis. Prednisone at doses of up to 60 mg PO qd provides prompt relief of cutaneous and systemic manifestations.

KEY POINT TO REMEMBER

Diagnosis of EN, PG, or Sweet's syndrome should prompt evaluation of associated diseases.

SUGGESTED READING

Callen JP. Pyoderma gangrenosum. *Lancet* 1998;351:581–585.

Cohen PR, Kurzrock R. Sweet's syndrome: a neutrophilic dermatosis classically associated with acute onset and fever. *Clin Dermatol* 2000;18:265–282.

Hannuksela M. Erythema nodosum. *Clin Dermatol* 1986;4:88–95.

50

Osteoporosis

Latha Sivaprasad,
Jason D. Wright, and
Rebecca M. Shepherd

INTRODUCTION

Osteoporosis is the **most common metabolic disease in the United States.** The NIH published a consensus statement in March 2000 describing osteoporosis as a "skeletal disorder characterized by compromised bone strength predisposing to an increased risk of fracture." The World Health Organization defines osteoporosis as a bone density of 2.5 SD below the mean for young adult white women. Osteoporosis affects an estimated 10 million people, and an additional 18 million people have low bone mass. White postmenopausal women are at most risk for osteoporosis and related fracture; this population suffers three-fourths of all hip fractures. Men and black women have lower hip fracture rates, as do Hispanic women and Native Americans. Osteoporosis is a common comorbidity in patients with rheumatologic disease because of the increased use of corticosteroids.

CAUSES

Pathophysiology

Osteoporosis is characterized by either **low bone density or poor bone quality.** Bone quality is determined by architecture, turnover, damage, and mineralization. Bone mineral density (BMD) is determined by peak bone mass and amount of bone lost. Loss of bone mass occurs when resorption, a result of osteoclast activity, occurs more quickly than bone formation, a consequence of osteoblast activity. After age 40, cortical bone is lost at a rate of 0.3–0.5%/yr. Trabecular bone loss may begin at an even younger age. This loss of cortical and trabecular bone accelerates after menopause. Histologically, the bone has decreased cortical thickening and decreased number and size of the trabeculae of cancellous bone.

Low BMD correlates with increased risk of primary osteoporosis. Predictors of low BMD include female gender, increased age, estrogen deficiency, white race, low weight and body mass index, family history of osteoporosis, smoking, history of fracture, late menarche, and early menopause. Secondary causes of osteoporosis are extensive. They include diseases of hormone disregulation, including Cushing's syndrome, hypogonadism, hyperthyroidism, diabetes mellitus, and hyperparathyroidism. Malnutrition, malabsorption syndromes, pernicious anemia, parenteral nutrition, and gastrectomy are predisposing factors. Certain drugs and toxins (e.g., corticosteroids, anticonvulsants, heparin, lithium, thyroxine, cytotoxic drugs, ethanol use, and tobacco) have been implicated. Severe liver and renal disease, chronic obstructive pulmonary disease, hemochromatosis, and mastocytosis also indicate higher risk of osteoporosis. Rheumatologic diseases that predispose to osteoporosis include amyloidosis, AS, multiple myeloma, RA, and sarcoidosis. **Glucocorticoid use is the most common form of drug-related osteoporosis and is often seen in patients with rheumatic diseases.** Patients who receive glucocorticoids (e.g., prednisone at >5 mg PO/day) for >2 mos are considered at high risk for excessive bone loss.

Differential Diagnosis

The differential diagnosis of osteoporosis includes osteomalacia, metastatic malignancy to bone, multiple myeloma, hyperthyroidism, hyperparathyroidism, renal osteodystrophy, malabsorption syndromes, vitamin deficiencies, and Paget's disease.

PRESENTATION

History and Physical Exam

Osteoporosis is commonly asymptomatic until back pain or fractures occur. Vertebral compression fractures most commonly occur in the T-11 to L-2 region and may present as loss of height rather than back pain. Other common fracture sites are the wrist (Colles' fracture), hip, and pelvis. Physical exam may reveal scoliosis, kyphosis, or tenderness along the spine. Signs and symptoms of secondary causes can be elicited during the history and physical exam (e.g., hypogonadism, evidence of thyroid disease, and cushingoid features).

MANAGEMENT

Diagnostic Workup

Consider the diagnosis of osteoporosis and fracture risk in all postmenopausal women and patients with high risk of secondary causes. Limited lab testing (e.g., thyroid hormone levels, protein electrophoresis, parathyroid hormones, vitamin D level, urine calcium, and cortisol) can be helpful in diagnosing secondary causes. Radiographs demonstrate osteopenia and compression fractures. Evaluation of BMD, however, is the most effective way to diagnose osteoporosis. Measuring BMD at any skeletal site has value in predicting fracture risk. Hip BMD, however, is the best predictor of hip fractures and is also good at predicting fractures at other sites. BMD is expressed as two values: the Z-score (the expected BMD for the patient's age and sex) and the T-score (the expected BMD for young adults). The T-score is more helpful in assessing fracture risk. The difference between the patient's score and the norm is expressed as SD above or below the mean. The World Health Organization definition for BMD in white women is as follows: normal is 1 SD of a normal adult (T-score, >−1), osteopenia is 1–2.5 SD below the normal adult (T-score, −1 to −2.5), and osteoporosis is 2.5 SD below the normal adult (T-score, <−2.5).

BMD testing techniques include dual-energy x-ray absorptiometry (DXA or DEXA), single-energy x-ray absorptiometry, peripheral DXA or DEXA (pDXA or pDEXA), radiographic absorptiometry, quantitative CT, and ultrasound densitometry. DEXA measures BMD in the spine, wrist, and hip. The test is quick and precise, with minimal radiation exposure.

Test BMD in all postmenopausal women <65 yrs who have one or more additional risk factors for fracture, all women >65 yrs, postmenopausal women who present with fracture, and women who have been on hormone replacement therapy (HRT) for long periods of time. To diagnose and prevent glucocorticoid-induced osteoporosis, obtain a baseline assessment of BMD of the hip or spine by DXA or quantitative CT before initiating any long-term (>6 mos) therapy.

Treatment and Follow-Up

Recommendations for all patients include adequate intake of **calcium and vitamin D,** regular weight-bearing exercise, and avoidance of tobacco and alcohol use. All adults should receive at least 1200 mg/day of elemental calcium and vitamin D of 400–800 IU/day. Initiate pharmacologic therapy to reduce fracture risk in women with BMD T-scores <−2 in the absence of risk factors, and in women with T-scores <−1.5 if risk factors are present. Women >70 yrs with multiple risk factors are at high enough risk to begin treatment without BMD testing. HRT has been shown in observational studies to decrease vertebral fractures by 50–80% and all fractures by 25% with 5 yrs of treatment. There are, however, no randomized controlled trials. Assess the risk–benefit ratio with each patient individually. Bisphosphonates have been demonstrated to reduce the incidence of fracture by 50% in all patients with osteoporosis. Use alendronate (Fosamax) or risedronate (Actonel) if a patient does not use HRT. Alendronate (5 mg PO qd or 35 mg PO qwk) or risedronate (5 mg PO qd or 35 mg PO qwk) is used for prevention, whereas alendronate (10 mg PO qd or 70 mg PO qwk) or risedronate (5 mg PO qd or 35 mg PO qwk) is used for treatment of osteoporosis. Other bisphosphonates (e.g., pamidronate, ibandronate, etidronate, and tiludronate) are not FDA approved but are undergoing clinical trials. Raloxifene (Evista), a selective estrogen receptor modulator, is an alternative treatment for osteoporosis that reduces the risk of vertebral fracture by 40–50%. Calcitonin, a hormone that inhibits bone resorption, is FDA approved for the treatment of osteoporosis but is far less effective than HRT or alendronate. The newest FDA-approved agent for the treatment of osteoporosis is recombinant human PTH (1–34) (teriparatide, Forteo), 20 µg SC daily. Sodium fluoride is also being studied as a treatment for osteoporosis. The role of monitoring the response to treatment is controversial. Commonly, however, caregivers restudy BMD annually or biannually.

For steroid-induced osteoporosis, randomized controlled studies demonstrate calcium carbonate, 1000 mg PO qd, and vitamin D, 500 IU PO qd, to be effective preventive therapy for some patients receiving prednisone. Studies also show that bisphosphonates are effective in both the prevention and treatment of corticosteroid osteoporosis. Postmenopausal women receiving HRT and men should receive alendronate, 5 mg PO qd or 35 mg PO qwk, or risedronate, 5 mg PO qd or 35 mg PO qwk. Women not on HRT should receive alendronate, 10 mg PO qd or 70 mg PO qwk, or risedronate, 5 mg PO qd or 35 mg PO qwk. The role of monitoring is the same as in other patients with osteoporosis.

For severe or bisphosphonate-refractory osteoporosis, Forteo (recombinant PTH) is used at 20 µg SC qd.

KEY POINTS TO REMEMBER

- Patients on steroids should have a bone density test performed and take prophylactic or therapeutic bisphosphonates, if tolerated.
- Osteoporosis is a common comorbidity in patients with rheumatic conditions.
- All patients with osteopenia or osteoporosis or who are taking steroids should receive supplemental calcium and vitamin D.

SUGGESTED READING

American College of Rheumatology Ad Hoc Committee on Glucocorticoid-Induced Osteoporosis. Recommendations for the prevention and treatment of glucocorticoid-induced osteoporosis. *Arthritis Rheum* 2001;44:1496–1503.

Buckley LM, Leib ES, Cartularo KS, et al. Calcium and vitamin D supplementation prevents bone loss in the spine secondary to low dose corticosteroids in patients with rheumatoid arthritis: a randomized, double-blind, placebo controlled trial. *Ann Intern Med* 1996;125:961–986.

Eastell R. Treatment of postmenopausal osteoporosis. *N Engl J Med* 1998;338:736.

Osteoporosis prevention, diagnosis, and therapy. NIH consensus development conference statement online 2000 March 27–29; [cited 2001, October 12];17(1):1–36.

Reid DM, Hughes RA, Laan RF, et al. Efficacy and safety of daily risedronate in the treatment of corticosteroid-induced osteoporosis in men and women: a randomized trial. *J Bone Miner Res* 2000;15:1006–1020.

Saag KG, Emkey R, Schnitzer T, et al. Alendronate for the treatment and prevention of glucocorticoid-induced osteoporosis. *N Engl J Med* 1998;339:292–299.

Sambrook PN, Birmingham J, Kelly P, et al. Prevention of corticosteroid osteoporosis: a comparison of calcium, calcitriol, and calcitonin. *N Engl J Med* 1993;328:1747–1752.

51

Avascular Necrosis

Shannon C. Lynn

INTRODUCTION

AVN, also known as *osteonecrosis* and *aseptic necrosis*, involves vascular compromise to bone with subsequent **bone death.** Incidence is estimated at 15,000 cases annually in the United States, with a male to female ratio of 8:1. It accounts for 10% of the 500,000 joint replacements performed annually. The majority of patients are <50 yrs, although AVN can affect persons of any age. Various bones can be affected, including the femur (femoral head and condyles), tibia (tibial plateau), humerus (humeral head), vertebrae, and small bones of the foot, ankle, and hand. Osteonecrosis of the hip causes the most severe and debilitating impairments.

CAUSES

Pathophysiology

The pathogenesis of AVN is poorly understood. The circulatory compromise to the bone is thought to occur by one of four mechanisms: (a) mechanical vascular interruption, (b) thrombosis and embolism, (c) injury to a vessel wall (vasculitis, radiation injury, or spasm), or (d) venous occlusion (blood flow is impeded as venous pressure is greater than arterial pressure). Any of these events may lead to medullary infarction in the fatty marrow, resulting in bone death with subsequent cell necrosis. This leads to acidification of the tissue and release of lysosomes, ultimately leading to tissue saponification.

Risks for developing AVN include oral corticosteroid use, alcohol abuse, SLE, RA, trauma, sepsis, renal failure, sickle cell disease, vasculitis, Gaucher's disease, dysbaric conditions (caisson disease), radiation injury, cancer, pregnancy, and trauma.

Differential Diagnosis

Other diagnoses to consider include infection, fractures, tumors, soft tissue injuries, and exacerbation of existing joint disease.

PRESENTATION

History and Physical Exam

Patients commonly present with vague and mild joint pain, but acute, severe pain presentations are also possible. Early in the course of the disease, pain is increased with activity, but over time it progresses to pain with rest. More severe pain can occur with larger infarcts (most often associated with Gaucher's disease, dysbarism, and hemoglobinopathies). The physical exam is usually nonspecific but may reveal local tenderness, swelling, and decreased range of motion of the affected joint. Large effusions are sometimes seen when the knee is involved.

MANAGEMENT

Diagnostic Workup

Lab tests are useful only for finding an underlying cause of AVN or excluding other diseases. **Radiologic evaluation plays a key role in helping make the diagnosis.**

TABLE 51-1. RADIOGRAPHIC STAGING OF AVN

Stage	Marcus (1–6)	Stage	Ficat (I–IV)
1	Increased density of the femoral head	I	No findings
2	Increased intensity of the zonal increase described in stage 1	II	Subchondral radiolucency but no femoral head deformity
3	Subchondral radiolucency (crescent sign)	III	Progression of stage II
4	More progressive deformity	IV	Early OA
5, 6	Further progression		—

Evaluation may begin with plain radiographs, but early in the disease these can be normal; other imaging studies that are useful include CT, MRI, and technetium 99m bone scans. The MRI is the most sensitive study available for evaluation of osteonecrosis. The earliest sign is marrow edema, later followed by marrow necrosis and cortical bone changes. Classically, the "double-line sign" is seen: high signal intensity within two parallel lines of decreased signal intensity on a T2-weighted MRI image. Bone scans that are obtained early in the disease demonstrate a dead central area surrounded by increased activity described as the "doughnut sign." With disease progression, the bone scan shows only a uniformly high level of activity.

Classically, staging of AVN is done by plain radiographs. Two techniques for staging exist. The first, by Marcus, describes six stages; the second technique, by Ficat, uses only four stages (Table 51-1). Both staging techniques are based on disease of the femoral head.

Treatment and Monitoring

Treatment varies according to site and whether an underlying cause is found; cessation of the offending agent may be beneficial. Involvement of the distal femur or proximal tibia often necessitates only temporary immobilization of the knee with weight-bearing limitations, along with antiinflammatory medications and physical therapy. Osteonecrosis of the hip usually requires more aggressive therapy. Early involvement of the hip can be treated with weight-bearing limitation and exercise. Regardless of site, prompt orthopedics consult is important, as some cases of early bone involvement may benefit from débridement of necrotic bone with subsequent bone grafting. Other surgical modalities include (a) "core decompression," which decreases the intramedullary pressure; (b) osteotomy of the proximal femur or rotation of the femoral head to redistribute pressure away from the affected bone, and (c) prosthetic replacement. Prosthetic replacement remains the most popular surgical option. Progression of disease remains unpredictable. Complications include incomplete fractures and superimposed degenerative arthritis.

KEY POINTS TO REMEMBER

- AVN can be an adverse complication caused by chronic steroid use.
- Limiting cumulative steroid dose is a key to preventing steroid-induced AVN.

SUGGESTED READING

Chang C, Greenspan A, Gershwin ME. Osteonecrosis: current perspectives on pathogenesis and treatment. *Semin Arthritis Rheum* 1993;23:47–69.

Mankin HK. Nontraumatic necrosis of bone (osteonecrosis). *N Engl J Med* 1992;326: 1473–1479.

Wolfe CJ, Taylor-Butler K. Avascular necrosis: a case history and literature review. *Arch Fam Med* 2000;9:291–294.

Index

Page numbers followed by *t* indicate tables; numbers followed by *f* indicate figures.